AAU-7915
VC-Grad-Re'

47.50

HANDBOOK OF ADOLESCENT INPATIENT PSYCHIATRIC TREATMENT

HANDBOOK OF ADOLESCENT INPATIENT PSYCHIATRIC TREATMENT

Edited by

Harinder S. Ghuman, M.D.

Associate Clinical Professor of Psychiatry and Behavioral Sciences,
George Washington University, Washington, D.C.;
Teaching Staff, The Sheppard and Enoch Pratt Hospital,
Towson, Maryland

and

Richard M. Sarles, M.D.

Clinical Professor of Psychiatry and Pediatrics, Director of Child and
Adolescent Psychiatry, University of Maryland School of Medicine,
Baltimore, Maryland

with a Foreword by

E. James Anthony, M.D.

Director of Child and Adolescent Psychotherapy,
Chestnut Lodge Hospital, Rockville, Maryland

BRUNNER/MAZEL *Publishers* • NEW YORK

Library of Congress Cataloging-in-Publication Data
Handbook of adolescent inpatient psychiatric treatment / edited by
  Harinder S. Ghuman and Richard M. Sarles: with a foreword by E.
James Anthony
      p.   cm.
Includes bibliographical references and index
ISBN 0-87630-731-4
  1. Adolescent psychotherapy—Residential treatment. I. Ghuman,
Harinder S. II. Sarles, Richard M. (Richard Milford)
  [DNLM: 1. Psychotherapy—in adolescence. 2. Adolescent, Institu-
tionalized. 3. Mental disorders—in adolescence. 4. Mental Disor-
ders—therapy. WS 463 H236 1994.]
RJ503.H267 1994
616.89'14'0835—dc20
DNLM/DLC
for Library of Congress   93-42921
                                                               CIP

Published by
BRUNNER/MAZEL, INC.
19 Union Square West
New York, New York 10003

Manufactured in the United States of America
    10 9 8 7 6 5 4 3 2 1

CONTENTS

PREFACE vii
ACKNOWLEDGMENTS xi
FOREWORD by E. James Anthony xiii
CONTRIBUTORS xvii

PART I   General Considerations
1. INDICATIONS FOR INPATIENT TREATMENT AND
   TYPES OF SETTINGS by Harinder S. Ghuman
   and Richard M. Sarles 3
2. EVALUATION AND TREATMENT PROCESS
   by Harinder S. Ghuman 18

PART II   Therapeutic Interventions
3. INDIVIDUAL PSYCHOTHERAPY by Donald H. Saidel 37
4. GROUP PSYCHOTHERAPY SETTING, STRUCTURE,
   AND PROCESS by Harinder S. Ghuman and
   Erika E. Wilmoth 52
5. NURSING SERVICES: COACHING THE PATIENT TO
   IMPROVED MENTAL HEALTH by D. Heidi Waltos 71
6. SOCIAL WORK SERVICES by Louise R. Hopkins 90
7. PHARMACOTHERAPY IN CHILDREN AND
   ADOLESCENTS by Paramjit T. Joshi, Joseph T.
   Coyle, and John T. Walkup 104
8. OCCUPATIONAL THERAPY, ART THERAPY,
   THERAPEUTIC RECREATION, AND VOCATIONAL
   SERVICES FOR INPATIENT ADOLESCENTS
   by Janice J. Jaskulski, Erika Grant, Gregory Kearney,
   and Vera Roth 132
9. SPECIAL EDUCATION IN AN INPATIENT SETTING
   by Burton Lohnes 149

PART III   Special Treatment Considerations

10. TREATMENT OF EATING DISORDERS by Elizabeth
    Williams, David Roth, and Fereidoon Taghizadeh 165
11. INTEGRATING ALCOHOL AND DRUG ABUSE
    TREATMENT INTO AN ADOLESCENT PSYCHIATRIC
    HOSPITAL PROGRAM by Steven L. Jaffe 181
12. SECLUSION, ECT, AND HYDROTHERAPY
    by Paramjit T. Joshi, Harinder S. Ghuman, and
    Erika E. Wilmoth 189
13. DEVELOPMENTAL CONSIDERATIONS IN THE
    INPATIENT TREATMENT OF ADOLESCENTS
    by Thomas R. Pentz 203
14. LIMIT SETTING WITH ACTING-OUT ADOLESCENTS
    by Harinder S. Ghuman and Richard M. Sarles 224

PART IV Special Issues

15. TEAMWORK WITHIN THE TREATMENT TEAM
    by Harinder S. Ghuman and Erika E. Wilmoth 241
16. ADMINISTRATION OF AN ADOLESCENT
    INPATIENT PSYCHIATRIC TREATMENT
    PROGRAM by Richard M. Sarles 254
17. LEGAL ISSUES IN ADOLESCENT
    INPATIENT PSYCHIATRY by Daniel J. Moore 261
18. RESEARCH ISSUES IN ADOLESCENT INPATIENT
    PSYCHIATRY by Wells Goodrich 277
19. FUNDING, THIRD-PARTY PAYERS, AND
    MANAGED CARE by Steven S. Sharfstein 293

NAME INDEX 303
SUBJECT INDEX 309

PREFACE

The Sheppard and Enoch Pratt Hospital has been treating severely emotionally disturbed adolescents for a number of years. During this time, we have had the opportunity to build upon the principles and techniques of acknowledged experts and leaders, and have gained a great deal of experience and wisdom ourselves. Our treatment teams had the time to deliver intensive, in-depth treatment, which included three weekly individual psychotherapy sessions, three weekly group therapy sessions, daily activity therapy, and intensive milieu program, daily ward meetings, weekly family therapy, and a daily therapeutic school program. This time- and energy-intensive program is for severely disturbed, treatment-resistant patients.

It seemed desirable that the lessons learned by our staff and the wisdom gained should be recorded and disseminated to other professionals engaged in the arduous and draining, but overall rewarding, inpatient work. It was ironic that as we all worked on this book, from inception to completion, our ability to continue our intensive treatment programs was almost completely destroyed by the economic revolution in the delivery of mental health services. The length of stay plummeted and the total number of long-term inpatient beds dramatically decreased. Managed care redefined intensive inpatient treatment for the treatment-resistant patient to a very short stay for diagnostic work, stabilization, and medication management.

Yet, we felt that the tried and true principles we utilized in this intensive work should be documented and shared in the belief that intensive inpatient treatment will always be necessary for many of the seriously disturbed adolescents, even with the most severely rationed fiscal resources. It is for this reason that we offer this volume.

In this book, the term "inpatient" is applied to both hospital and residential-based facilities that provide intensive diagnostic and therapeutic services. We feel that the knowledge and principles described in this book are not only applicable to inpatient facilities but also valuable to practitioners in day hospitals, group homes, and outpatient practice, especially the material in Chapters 3 to 11 and 13 to 17.

Adolescents are admitted to a psychiatric inpatient setting for a variety of reasons. The clinician's task is to ensure that only those adolescents who meet the criteria for inpatient treatment are admitted. Upon admission, the adolescent, his/her family, and the treatment team should begin the process of determining the setting and therapies that are required to address their problems. In Part I, we focus on indications for inpatient treatment, types of inpatient settings, and the treatment process.

It is interesting to note that adolescents who are admitted to inpatient programs, as well as their families, are both similar to others and unique in their presentation of problems and backgrounds. A good treatment program must address the general needs of the adolescent inpatient as well as the needs of each individual patient. Over the years, programs have developed on the basis of length of stay and a philosophy of treatment. Often, the length of stay is determined by the financial considerations and the philosophy of treatment depends upon the orientation and interest of the staff. We believe that the essentials of an adolescent inpatient treatment program should ideally include: (a) enough flexibility to provide for the treatment needs of an individual patient and also set the necessary priorities; (b) a realistic appraisal of the needs of the patient and the provision of the necessary treatment modalities; and (c) a treatment plan and length of stay that depend upon the patient's needs and are not determined just by financial considerations or by hospital philosophy. In Part II, our emphasis is on various treatment modalities utilized in inpatient work with adolescents.

Part III of the book covers special treatment issues encountered in inpatient settings. This includes adolescents with special problems, such as eating disorders and drug abuse. There is also a chapter on the use of seclusion, ECT, and hydrotherapy. These are controversial but at times much needed interventions. It is critical to address developmental issues in conceptualizing and implementing a treatment program for adolescents, as described in the chapter on developmental considerations. A chapter on limit setting is also included since we believe this is one of the important aspects of inpatient treatment.

Inpatient treatment is a group effort. Treatment outcome depends upon how well the staff is able to work together; thus, the critical issue of leadership within the team and in the institution is discussed. Part IV addresses issues related to teamwork and the administrative aspects of inpatient treatment. Also included are a variety of medicolegal issues, including patients' rights, parental rights, abuse and neglect, to name but a few. There is also a chapter reviewing research on various aspects of inpatient treatment, and the author has made suggestions regarding future research directions.

The remainder of Part IV is focused on the issues of funding and dealing with the third and fourth party reviewers. While there is seldom formal teaching on this subject at the graduate and postgraduate level, the practice of modern medicine requires, with ever increasing frequency, that the clinician be experienced in handling fiscal issues in order to continue to provide good clinical care. The impact of the current economic pressures on inpatient programs is discussed, and some speculation about the future of adolescent inpatient programs is ventured.

Most of our authors are clinicians from The Sheppard and Enoch Pratt Hospital, but we are delighted to have experienced authors from other institutions share their expertise on special topics. Our aim is to provide readers with an understanding of adolescent inpatient treatment and to stimulate them to put forth additional questions and answers so that all clinicians involved in inpatient programs can improve their work.

ACKNOWLEDGMENTS

Every book is a labor of love from conception through gestation, to delivery. The editors have labored through the entire process, but many important people helped, nourished, and pushed along the way. This acknowledgment is dedicated to those people who were so very helpful to us and without whose help this book could never have been possible.

We both give thanks first and foremost to our patients who have taught us so very much and to the entire staff of the Division of Child and Adolescent Psychiatry at The Sheppard and Enoch Pratt Hospital, who have helped us learn. We are very grateful to you all.

Special appreciation goes to Dr. E. James Anthony for training one of us (H.S.G.) and for his encouragement and guidance in preparation of this book. We are grateful to Ms. Eloise Liberty, Dr. Pal Pandher, and the Kubie Library staff for their help in preparation of chapter manuscripts, and to all our contributors for their participation, their significant efforts, and their tolerance for numerous editorial rewritings. We thank Steven S. Sharfstein, M.D., Medical Director, President and CEO of The Sheppard and Enoch Pratt Hospital, for his encouragement and support for this project. Sincere thanks are also extended to Ms. Natalie Gilman, Editorial Vice President, Brunner/Mazel, Inc. for supporting this book. A very special feeling of gratitude and appreciation must be extended to Ms. Loretta Jones who typed and retyped, sorted, organized, mailed, called, and labored above and beyond the call of duty to help us with this project; we could not have succeeded without her.

Finally, we wish to express our deepest gratitude and love to those people who have really sweated this out with us: our loving wives, Jaswinder Ghuman and Lois Sarles, and our children, Avniel Ghuman, and Kristen and Karen Sarles. Thanks to you all.

FOREWORD

Those of us who undertake the inpatient care of adolescents have, with experience, acquired "grounded" theories and practical approaches that serve us fairly well but are scarcely impartible, even to our immediate associates with whom we work. It is not an easy task to bring together the diversity of knowledge that accrues around sequestered human living, particularly when the beings composing it are disturbed, disturbing, and impetuously youthful. It is to the credit of the two editors, Ghuman and Sarles, that they have assembled a wide range of solid contributors who have specialized in their own area of the field and are skillful at bringing salient issues together in a logical format. The Sheppard and Enoch Pratt Hospital, unquestionably one of the leading therapeutic institutions for teenagers in the country, provides the setting for the enactment of the caring, containing, and controlling activities depicted in the book, bringing them to life in a picturesque and private ambience that must play a significant role in the success of the treatment program.

Before dealing with the particular features presented, I would like to speak briefly on the timeliness of the volume. It is being published in a period when the question of the psychiatric hospitalization of the adolescent over longer periods of time has been vociferously debated in the medical and general press with resulting restrictions in third party, state, and federal funding. A few decades ago, the adolescent admission rate reached such a crescendo that adolescent hospitals and units sprang up like mushrooms almost overnight with a corresponding demand to fill them. As a result, relatively benign cases found themselves unexpectedly hospitalized and maintained in hospital until their insurances or private monies dwindled to nothing, whereupon they were precipitately discharged. If some were unqualified for admission when admitted, there were others who were unfit for discharge when discharged. None of this was in accordance with the Hippocratic tradition aimed at helping and doing no harm. What is important about this publication at this time is that it not only will help to render such flagrant abuses less likely, but also it should orient the practitioner (psychiatric, psychological, social, or psychoeducational) toward the best interests of the emotionally sick patient.

If patients of this age need to be removed from the provocations of a severely dysfunctional family, the precepts incorporated in this book should see to it that they receive a comprehensively devised interlocking system of treatment; that the program works through their understanding and with their cooperation; that they be allowed to recover step-by-therapeutic-step from the turbulences that beset them and not hastily cast adrift before they are ready to re-engage with the outside world; and that they should not be maintained in a state of a protracted clinical moratorium until a forced, unplanned termination takes place. Inpatiency, in its best use, does not rob the adolescent of the precious birthright of the adolescent experience but, in skillful hands as depicted in these clarifying pages, allows for the restoration of normative development with all its developmental privileges and processes.

There is no doubt in my mind, after years of practice, that a sufficient period of intensive inpatient care away from a pathogenic home environment can help aimless teenagers, lost in a meaningless and mindless mode of existence, to discover a purpose for living and living decently both for their own benefits and for the benefits of others closely associated with them; in this way they can resolve at least some of their ingrained narcissism and self-centeredness to the point of a reasonable altruism. It is the inpatient milieu that this book teaches us that these adolescents can learn to share, to be considerate, to empathize with the feelings of others, and to realize that they are not all alone in their problematical world. Best of all, they can learn again to enjoy learning and learning for the sake of learning, which is what the inpatient school imparts to them.

One can therefore embark upon this valuable book with the assumption that there are adolescents who need and profit from this type of treatment program in this type of specialized milieu, in conjunction with a professional staff who have acquired the sophistication contained in these pages and who have the inner and outer resources to respond in keeping with the carefully formulated therapeutic philosophy. But how can we identify these patients? And how can we ensure that they will be able to make the most profitable use of this gift of therapeutic time? The answers are for the most part within this comprehensive compendium, which should enable you to do what you do better and to understand better what you do. It is every clinician's guide to the overall treatment of adolescents biologically, psychologically, socially, recreationally, educationally, and psychotherapeutically in a holding environment. It reviews in detail the responses required to deal with the helplessness and destructiveness of patients who claim that they have nowhere to go but down but who want to be saved from themselves in spite of themselves. The wide array of caregivers and caretakers involved in the total process include administrators, educators, nurses, houseparents, psychotechnicians, individual, family, and group psychotherapists, medicating physicians, and recreational personnel; they are all there to provide sanctuary, useful peer interactions, privacy when needed, heart-to-heart talks when self-reflection is not sufficient, and appropriate medications, which put together programmatically may allow the personalities to be restructured in healthier ways.

In brief, the inpatient world of the adolescent, in the terms of Aaron Antonovsky, *Health, Strength and Coping, 1979,* will become truly "salutogenic"or health-promoting, bringing life experiences and "generalized resistance resources" together to effect a better sense of coherence and a better capacity to manage both expectable and unexpectable stresses. In sum, the adolescents should go out as better copers than when they were admitted. Prevention should always be considered an integral part of the complete program.

E. JAMES ANTHONY, M.D.
Director of Child and Adolescent Psychotherapy
Chestnut Lodge Hospital, Rockville, Maryland

CONTRIBUTORS

JOSEPH T. COYLE, M.D., is Chairman, Department of Psychiatry; Eben S. Draper Professor of Psychiatry and Neurosciences, Harvard Medical School, Boston, Massachusetts.

HARINDER SINGH GHUMAN, M.D., is Associate Clinical Professor of Psychiatry and Behavioral Sciences, George Washington University, Washington, D.C.; Teaching Staff, The Sheppard and Enoch Pratt Hospital, Towson, Maryland.

WELLS GOODRICH, M.D., is Clinical Professor of Psychiatry, Georgetown University School of Medicine, Washington, D.C.; Consultant, Chestnut Lodge Hospital, Rockville, Maryland.

ERIKA GRANT, M.A., A.T.R., is Art Therapist, The Sheppard and Enoch Pratt Hospital, Towson, Maryland.

LOUISE RENAN HOPKINS, M.A., L.C.S.W., is Senior Social Worker, Child and Adolescent Psychiatry, The Sheppard and Enoch Pratt Hospital, Towson, Maryland; and Lecturer, Smith College School of Social Work, Northampton, Massachusetts.

STEVEN L. JAFFE, M.D., is Associate Professor of Psychiatry, Emory University School of Medicine; Clinical Director of Child and Adolescent Programs, Brawner Psychiatric Institute, Atlanta, Georgia.

JANICE J. JASKULSKI, M.S., O.T.R./L., is Psychiatric Occupational Therapy Supervisor, Johns Hopkins Medical Institute, Baltimore, Maryland.

PARAMJIT TOOR JOSHI, M.D., is Director of Inpatient Services and Associate Professor of Child and Adolescent Psychiatry, Division of Child and Adolescent Psychiatry, Johns Hopkins Medical Institute, Baltimore, Maryland.

GREGORY KEARNEY, M.A., C.T.R.S., is Recreational Therapist, The Sheppard and Enoch Pratt Hospital, Towson, Maryland.

BURTON H. LOHNES, Ph.D., is Director of Education, The Forbush School, The Sheppard and Enoch Pratt Hospital, Towson, Maryland.

DANIEL J. MOORE, J.D., is counsel to The Sheppard and Enoch Pratt Hospital; Partner, Semmes, Bowen & Semmes, Towson, Maryland.

THOMAS R. PENTZ, Ph.D., is Senior Psychologist, Child and Adolescent Psychiatry, The Sheppard and Enoch Pratt Hospital, Towson, Maryland.

DAVID ROTH, Ph.D., is Director, Weight Management and Eating Disorder Program, The Sheppard and Enoch Pratt Hospital, Towson, Maryland; and Adjunct Assistant Professor, The Johns Hopkins University School of Medicine, Baltimore, Maryland.

VERA ROTH, M.A., C.R.C., is Vocational Counselor, The Sheppard and Enoch Pratt Hospital, Towson, Maryland.

DONALD H. SAIDEL, Ph.D., is Senior Psychologist, Child and Adolescent Psychiatry, The Sheppard and Enoch Pratt Hospital, Towson, Maryland; Clinical Assistant Professor of Psychiatry, University of Maryland School of Medicine, Baltimore, Maryland.

RICHARD M. SARLES, M.D., is Clinical Professor of Psychiatry and Pediatrics, Director of Child and Adolescent Psychiatry, University of Maryland School of Medicine, Baltimore, Maryland.

STEVEN S. SHARFSTEIN, M.D., is President and Medical Director, The Sheppard and Enoch Pratt Hospital; Clinical Professor of Psychiatry, University of Maryland School of Medicine, Baltimore, Maryland.

FEREIDOON TAGHIZADEH, M.D., is Senior Psychiatrist and Service Chief, The Sheppard and Enoch Pratt Hospital, Towson, Maryland; Clinical Assistant Professor of Psychiatry, University of Maryland School of Medicine, Baltimore, Maryland.

JOHN T. WALKUP, M.D., is Director, Residency Education Program and Assistant Professor of Child and Adolescent Psychiatry, The Johns Hopkins Medical Institute, Baltimore, Maryland.

D. HEIDI WALTOS, R.N., M.S., C.S., is Clinical Specialist, Gundry-Glass Hospital, Baltimore, Maryland.

ELIZABETH A. WILLIAMS, Ph.D., is Clinical Psychologist, The Sheppard and Enoch Pratt Hospital, Towson, Maryland.

ERIKA E. WILMOTH, R.N.C., is Nurse Manager, Adolescent Units, The Sheppard and Enoch Pratt Hospital, Towson, Maryland.

HANDBOOK OF ADOLESCENT INPATIENT PSYCHIATRIC TREATMENT

PART I

General Considerations

Chapter 1

INDICATIONS FOR INPATIENT TREATMENT AND TYPES OF SETTINGS

Harinder S. Ghuman
and Richard M. Sarles

"Mental Hospital Chain Accused of
Much Cheating on Insurance"
The New York Times, November 24, 1991.

"Bounty Hunting"
Networker, July/August 1990.

Recent criticism of adolescent inpatient hospitalization by the media, public, and some professionals has had a profound effect on hospital programs and a somber effect on the hospital staff. It is, therefore, even more imperative that the hospital staff working with adolescents clearly document the necessity for inpatient treatment, what occurred throughout the hospitalization, and what was accomplished. A look at the chain of events leading to the present state of affairs may help to put the current criticism into perspective.

It was not until the late 1970s and continuing to the mid-1980s that proliferation of inpatient adolescent settings took place. However, this was preceded by other significant and fundamental changes in health care and funding for this care. In fact, 50 years ago there were limited hospital beds, not enough physicians, and very few people covered by health insurance. The medical model of care was a two-payer system—patient and doctor.

During the 1940s and 1950s, employers began to provide health insurance to employees as part of their "benefits" for working for a particular company. A new medical model of reimbursement was introduced, a third-party payer system. American medicine witnessed a "new" resource for funding health care, making possible an increase in the number of people being able to afford health care, which led to an increase in the number of physicians and to the number of hospital beds for treatment of these "new" patients. Coincidental with these increases in health care providers, funding, and facilities was the beginning of a technological boom.

During the 1960s and 1970s, technology exploded and government and industry made an open-ended commitment to comprehensive health care. Health care became a right for most Americans. In 1965, Title 18 established Medicare Part A & B and Social Security Amendment PL 89-97 was initiated.

By the 1980s, a clear increase in the incidence of adolescent suicide, and abuse of drugs and alcohol was evident. DSM-III (American Psychiatric Association, 1980) included child and adolescent depression as a bona fide diagnosable disorder. Manic-depressive illness was diagnosed with increased frequency during the adolescent years, there was an increased number (incidence-reporting) of sexual abuse cases, and runaways, family breakdown, and adolescent aggressive behavior all seemed to be increasing.

The Diagnosis Related Grouping (DRG) prospective pricing system initiated by the Federal government in the 1980s placed greater constraints on medical-surgical hospital treatment. As hospitals were forced to downsize these areas, these beds were converted to psychiatric beds, which were still unrestricted, or unregulated by DRGs. Thus, in a regulated-restricted DRG, cost-containment climate, which reduced growth, a new market was developed and the growth industry for hospitals became psychiatric beds, especially for chemical dependency and adolescents. The number of psychiatric admissions for children and adolescents under 18 years of age rose from 10,764 in 1980 to 48,375 in 1984. In geographic areas where psychiatric beds were unrestricted or deregulated with certificate of need removed, there was an explosion in the number of new psychiatric beds and hospitals. In Florida, it was reported that 456 new beds opened, with over a million dollars spent on lobbying.

During the 1980s, for-profit national chain hospital corporations capitalized on the burgeoning child and adolescent market and opened thousands of beds in hundreds of newly constructed inpatient facilities. This enormous increase in hospitals often led to intense competition for market share. Aggressive advertising "scare" techniques were introduced, unfortunately leading to, in some instances, unnecessary hospitalizations and unreasonably long lengths of stay. Even so, some hospitals operated at only a 40% to 50% occupancy. A more egregious example of "profiteering" was the practice of offering "bounties" to school personnel and other counsellors for referral of young patients for hospitalization.

The tremendous overbedding and the outrageous abuses in some hospitals made it painfully clear that business and government could not afford to and would not continue to pay. After a brief fling at Preferred Providers Organizations (PPOs), Health Maintenance Organizations (HMOs), Independent Practitioners Associations (IPAs) and Diagnosis Related Groupings (DRGs) that proved to be ineffective in containing costs, managed care became the dominant mechanism for controlling mental health costs. At the same time, most states tried to initiate plans to control escalating mental health costs. In the state of Maryland, for example, the State Health Plan for Children, Youth and Families clearly articulated the vision of child and adolescent mental health services as home-based and community-based, with all inpatient care to be "reduced and restricted." In 1992, Maryland had 800 children and adolescents in out-of-state residential and hospital facilities at a cost of $40 million per year. The aim of the health plan was to return these children and adolescents to Maryland and to reallocate these dollars to the least restrictive, least costly setting. The major emphasis was to restore the family unit and to "empower" families and communities to house, treat, and educate these children and adolescents in the community with the reallocation of monies from the out-of-state placements and in-state inpatient settings.

The net result of these events is that many adolescent inpatient treatment programs have been left in chaos. According to Lewis (1991, p. 165), "A combination of these forces has resulted in more beds, more empty beds, more competition among hospitals and practitioners, shorter lengths of stay, more hospitalizations, less control over treatment programming for the admitting psychiatrist, and a less secure, confident, and predictable context for inpatient psychiatric treatment of youth."

Rinsley (1990, p. 9) wrote, "Excellent programs for severely disturbed juveniles have suffered along with purely or basically custodial ones characterized by neglect or even abuse."

It may appear that the public, insurers, and professionals, who never appreciated the value of inpatient treatment or who may have had bad inpatient experiences, have written an "obituary" for inpatient treatment. As a result, large numbers of adolescents and families experience great difficulty in accepting the need for hospitalization now. When parents hear reports that inpatient treatment is unnecessary, not helpful, or even harmful, they are unlikely to accept inpatient treatment. The present confusion and turmoil of adolescent inpatient treatment may engender a sense of pessimism. However, it is vital for professionals working in inpatient settings to look inward and rectify any responsibility they may have for creating this negative picture. In fact, this publicity may provide an opportunity to weed out the growth of opportunistic facilities, where staff and administrators are more concerned with profit than with treatment of adolescents. Concurrently, opportunities exist for professionals to explore alternative methods of assisting adolescents by developing more creative, less restrictive treatment approaches and modalities. Lastly, a word of caution: Before discarding "older ways of treating adolescents" and starting new approaches, treatment programs and professionals must make sure these new programs are not again solely based on monetary gains from deceptive new sources of funding.

With this background and caveat, we believe it is most important to examine indications for inpatient treatment and to discuss various treatment settings.

INDICATIONS FOR INPATIENT TREATMENT

Various authors have described indications for inpatient treatment of adolescents (Potter, 1934, 1935; Petti, 1980; Harper & Geraty, 1989; Weintrob, 1975; Wardle, 1974; Kester, 1966; Barker, 1976; Silver, 1976; Rinsley, 1991). The American Psychiatric Association (1989) issued a statement regarding appropriate hospitalization for adolescents, and the American Academy of Child and Adolescent Psychiatry (1989) and the American Society for Adolescent Psychiatry (1990) have published guidelines regarding adolescent inpatient admissions. In general the indications for adolescent admission may be summarized in the following manner:

A. *Dangerous Behavior*
Most clinicians would agree to the hospitalization of an adolescent when his/her behavior is dangerous to self or others regardless of the diagnosis. For example:

A 16-year-old male had been intermittently threatening to kill his mother for several months. The night prior to admission, he held his mother's head in a headlock and tried to cut her throat with a knife, but stopped at the last moment, saying that he could not do it.

A 14-year-old female took an overdose of her antidepressant medication and required treatment in the intensive care unit of a general hospital. She continued to express suicidal ideation and was involved in cutting herself after discharge from the general hospital.

A 15-year-old male with a history of truancy, and aggressive and impulsive behavior made sexual advances toward his sister. The patient's level of intelligence was borderline. He stated that he heard voices telling him to touch his sister in "her private parts" and to have sex with her. The patient also had a history of making sexual advances towards other younger girls.

B. Disorganized Behavior Interfering in Daily Functioning

These behaviors include excessive withdrawal, agitation, rituals, disorganization in thinking and perceptual disturbances. In such cases, the adolescent may not be able to take care of basic needs or be involved in social interaction or education. Also, admission may be necessary when there is deterioration despite outpatient psychiatric interventions and/or as a result of noncompliance with treatment. For example:

A 13-year-old female required admission because she was talking to herself, hearing voices, isolating herself in her room, refusing to go to school, and refusing to eat. Her condition had deteriorated despite outpatient treatment that included the use of psychotropic medications.

A 16-year-old female who had history of obsessive/compulsive behavior became preoccupied with her menstrual period, visited the bathroom every few minutes, and spent inordinate time cleaning herself. She was in outpatient treatment receiving moderate dosages of Anafranil and Ativan.

A 14-year-old became extremely agitated and confused, was unable to sleep, and broke household articles after inhaling glue.

C. Severe Out-of-Control Behaviors

These behaviors include frequent runaways, inappropriate sexual behaviors including promiscuity, prostitution, exhibitionism, and molestation, and frequent fighting, stealing, robbing, breaking/entering, and fire-setting. For example:

A 17-year-old female was admitted to the hospital after a three-week runaway episode. The patient's parents were able to arrange, with the help of the police, to bring her to the hospital from the detention center. She had a history of runaways starting at age 15 and was involved in abusing various drugs and alcohol. Additionally, she was involved in severe risk-taking sexual activity with multiple males to support her drug habit.

A 16-year-old male was referred to the hospital for psychiatric evaluation and treatment by the juvenile court after having exposed himself to a female. He also had a history of stealing, breaking and entering, and drug abuse.

D. Miscellaneous Indications

These are indications which do not fit in the categories described above and may include court referrals or combinations of individual adolescent problems with severe family psychopathology. For example:

A 17-year-old female was brought to the hospital by a social service caseworker. The patient had not been out of her room for three months, except to go to the toilet, and had not left her house for one and a half years. She had a long history of school refusal, numerous somatic complaints, and various symptoms of anxiety. The patient and her family, particularly her mother, were quite enmeshed, with the patient's mother sleeping with her at night.

It may be useful to define indicators as either absolute or relative. Of the previous indications, (A) dangerous behavior is the only absolute indication for hospitalization, whereas the rest of the indications depend upon severity and chronicity of the problem. Before an adolescent is admitted to an inpatient setting, a thorough psychiatric evaluation should be completed to ascertain if and why the adolescent requires hospitalization. The evaluation can be done on an outpatient basis or during a preadmission interview. In case of acute emergency, one may have to do the assessment in the emergency room.

Issue of Diagnosis and Inpatient Admission

The adolescent's need for hospitalization is usually based upon the presenting behaviors, problems, and symptomatology, and not necessarily on the diagnosis. Occasionally, adolescents are referred for hospitalization so that a diagnosis may be substantiated or clarified. This should not be a valid criterion for admission unless the adolescent's behavior/ symptomatology is severe and dangerous enough that evaluation and treatment on an outpatient basis is not possible. In such instances, the advantage of admission is the opportunity for observation of the adolescent in a secure, safe environment where clarification of the diagnosis and an outline for treatment are formulated.

Silver (1976) tried to correlate diagnosis to inpatient admission and length of stay. An adolescent can have the same diagnosis whether an inpatient or outpatient, whereas the severity and chronicity of the problems dictate the need for hospitalization and length of stay required.

TYPES OF INPATIENT SETTINGS

There has been much confusion in the psychiatric literature regarding what constitutes inpatient treatment—for example, hospital vs. residential setting, the advantages and disadvantages of different approaches to inpatient treatment, and the influence of funding on setting and treatment. It should be noted that most inpatient settings offer a combination of all of the following approaches. We will attempt to discuss various inpatient treatment facilities from the following perspective:

1. TIME-ORIENTED APPROACH
    ultrashort stay
    short-term
    intermediate term
    long-term

2. TREATMENT-ORIENTED APPROACH
    medical model
    behavioral
    psychodynamic
    family-oriented
    goal-oriented

3. SPECIFIC PROBLEM-ORIENTED APPROACH
    forensic
    substance abuse
    eating disorder
    borderline personality
    organic

4. SETTING DEPENDING UPON AFFILIATION AND
   FUNDING
   university
   private for profit
   private not-for-profit
   public
   combination

TIME-ORIENTED APPROACH

Most inpatient facilities define themselves in relation to time frames. It is not clear how this came about. Most often, settings are divided into short-term (1-4 weeks), intermediate (1-6 months), and long-term (6 months plus). Recently, some short-term settings have turned into ultrashort programs with length of stay measured in days, not weeks. Intermediate and long-term hospital treatment is rapidly becoming extinct with the severe managed-care and cost-containing environment. However, the time-oriented approach is useful because it informs the adolescent and family of the amount of time available for treatment and the financial investment they need to make. For similar reasons, third-party payers question whether the treatment approach of the facility is short-term/acute care or long-term/chronic care, which is a critical factor in treatment planning and funding.

Conversely, this time-oriented approach may be viewed as putting the cart before the horse. Unfortunately, some adolescents are admitted to one or the other "term" settings without a proper evaluation, thus perpetuating the endless debate of which "term" treatment is better than the other, short vs. long. The severity, chronicity, and intensity of the problems, including the level of progress in outpatient and inpatient treatment, should be the deciding factors when one is determining the length of stay. Ultrashort treatment is relevant for acute crisis, short-term treatment for mild to moderate degrees of pathology, and intermediate and long-term settings are suitable for moderate to severe chronic pathology, as well as for the patient who has failed to respond to all previous outpatient treatment modalities and to repeated hospitalizations.

TREATMENT-ORIENTED APPROACH

Adolescent inpatient facilities invariably describe their treatment philosophy as one of a combination of approaches. The term "eclectic" is often used to imply an all-inclusive comprehensive program and to avoid controversy. The following are some of the approaches, basic principles, and advantages and pitfalls to each.

Medical (Medication) Model

This approach is often used in a university hospital or affiliated hospital. The adolescent is admitted for a short duration, often to assess the need for medication and/or to determine which medication would be most beneficial. Emphasis is primarily upon determining a DSM III-R diagnosis, and investigating brain pathology and organic/systemic etiology. The physician (attending) collects pertinent data regarding the patient's progress and behavior from other professionals involved, such as nursing, social worker, etc. This model is most effective with adolescents who have those diagnoses that respond well to medication—for example, the patient who is suffering from severe endogenous depression and has a family history of affective illness, or a patient who is suffering from psychosis. The problem with a medical-medication approach is that there are a large number of disturbed adolescents who do not respond to medication; meanwhile, developmental and family dynamic issues may not be optimally addressed.

Behavioral Model

Most, if not all, adolescent inpatient facilities use a behavior modification approach in the treatment program. The patient's maladaptive behaviors are identified and various behavior modification techniques are used to assist the patient to recognize these behaviors and adopt the necessary methods to change. This approach can serve to develop a program for the individual adolescent that incorporates his/her specific needs, along with the needs for the patient community as a whole who are collectively involved in milieu therapy. Common behavior interventions include the use of points and level systems, quiet-room programs, behavioral contracts, and passes (see Chapter 5 on nursing services for detail).

The advantage of this model is that it can be simple, direct, and concrete. Adolescents with limited intellectual and verbal skills may respond to behavioral interventions that can be particularly helpful if used as a part of comprehensive treatment for the adolescent with various psychopathologies. However, the difficulty with this model surfaces if it is used exclusively without consideration being given to the adolescent's level of cognitive and psychosocial development and the family situation. There have been reports of misuse/abuse within some behavioral modification programs, for example, when the patient is kept in isolation for prolonged periods of time.

Psychodynamic Approach

The basic emphasis in the psychodynamic approach is on helping severely disturbed adolescents make necessary changes in their personality structure and not limiting changes to symptomatic relief. As personality structure is developed over the life span of an adolescent, it is understandable that change in this structure will require a longer time frame. The psychodynamic approach is applied in the inpatient milieu in conjunction with a variety of therapies, including individual, group, and family. Bettelheim and Sylvester (1948, 1949), Rinsley (1967, 1968, 1990), Nosphitz (1962), and Reidl (1952, 1959) are some of the pioneers involved in conceptualizing this approach. Central to the psychodynamic approach is psychoanalytically oriented therapy in which the deeper conflicts of the patient are worked through and structural personality changes are made (Anthony, 1991). This treatment approach is often indicated for severely disturbed, treatment-resistant, psychotic, and personality-disordered adolescents. Using DSM III-R guidelines, most clinicians are hesitant to diagnose personality disorders in adolescents; instead, they use diagnoses such as oppositional, conduct, and identity disorders.

The inpatient milieu provides a "holding environment" (Winnicott, 1965) or "ego support" (Nosphitz, 1962). Gunderson (1978) described the essential elements of the inpatient milieu as containment, support, structure, involvement, and validation. One can conceptualize milieu functions into three categories:

1. *A Safe Environment*: A safe environment is required for anyone to function. Severely disturbed adolescents often have major problems with aggressive behavior and sexual drives. Violence and aggression must be controlled. This can be accomplished with limit setting, physical holding, using force, separation from milieu, medication, seclusion, restraints, or hydrotherapy.

2. *A Growth-Promoting Environment*: This includes: (a) helping the patient to become more adept in verbal expression of thoughts and feelings; (b) encouraging the development of a trusting, honest, close, and supportive relationship with peers and adults; (c) helping adolescents understand their conflicts and the reason for their behavior; and (d) taking care of basic needs and education needs.

3. *A Supportive Environment*: A milieu is created in which adolescents can get support to deal with upsetting feelings, stresses, and anxieties while accomplishing various tasks. This support can be from staff and/ or other adolescents on the unit. The support can be in the form of

talking to others, getting directions, nonverbal interaction such as playing pool, and observing or discussing how others deal or have dealt with similar situations.

Family-Oriented Approach

Some inpatient facilities have admitted the entire family or mother-child unit (Lynch, Steinberg & Oursted, 1975; Nakhla, Folkart & Webster, 1969; Main, 1969). This was done in keeping with a family system approach that does not focus on any one family member, but rather views the whole family as the pathological agent. This approach helped the adolescent to continue as a member of the family and not be scapegoated. It also allowed close observation of the family; accordingly, interventions were directed to modify disturbed family relations. The problem with this approach was that it was usually not practical to admit an entire family. The costs were prohibitive and the adolescent's individual needs were not always addressed. In most inpatient facilities today, family therapy and parent groups are provided as part of the program to deal with family problems.

Problem-Oriented Approach

Recently, due to economic pressures, emphasis on inpatient hospitalization has been on defining main problems (Nurcombe, 1989) or one main "focal problem" (Harper, 1989). Setting goals, organizing treatment to stabilize problems quickly, and discharging the patient from the hospital rapidly have become the primary focus. Nurcombe (1989) described various advantages and disadvantages of goal-directed planning. The advantages are in the area of education and communication for staff and in record keeping for regulatory and medico-legal reasons and research purposes. Nurcombe claims that goal-directed planning enhances efficiency, but he does not provide good research data to support this claim. The disadvantages include difficulty of framing psychodynamic and family objectives in goal-directed planning. Harper (1989) defined the focal problem as "not everything deviant in the patient's functioning, rather it is the one problem that requires hospitalization." Accordingly, the goal of hospitalization is to evoke sufficient change in the focal problem so that the patient no longer needs hospitalization. He emphasizes the need to write treatment plans in clear and easily understood language that also strengthens the treatment alliance.

SPECIFIC PROBLEM-ORIENTED APPROACH

There are some psychiatric inpatient facilities that provide treatment for specific disorders or problems. During the 1980s, while adolescent inpatient facilities were proliferating, there was a trend toward having specialty and subspecialty units. This was due to a number of reasons, including increased knowledge about specific disorders, society's preference to seek treatment from specialists, and financial profit. These specialty units included Eating Disorder, Borderline Personality, Multiple Personality, Brain-Injured Adolescents, and Drug Abuse, to name but a few. Most of these subspecialty units were developed in private hospitals; the units for adolescents with legal problems developed mainly in public sector facilities.

The advantages of specialty units include the capacity for a thorough and comprehensive evaluation of the adolescent's problem, a more intense focus on the specific problem, a specially trained staff self-selected and motivated to deal with the special problem, and a decrease in stigmatization of "special patient" on the unit. Potential disadvantages include the adolescent's further isolation, the possibility of negatively identifying with a diagnosis or symptom, adolescents feeding into each other's pathology, and often limited gains due to an overemphasis on symptomatic relief and inadequate attention to underlying psychopathology.

SETTINGS DEPENDING UPON AFFILIATION AND FUNDING

Adolescent inpatient psychiatric settings are extremely heterogenous, ranging from small units in general hospitals to large state hospitals, and from lavish for-profit facilities to functional university settings. Staffing patterns run the gamut from open professional staff to closed academic staff, from variable nursing staffing dependent on census to fixed numbers but irregularly rotating personnel. Types of patients treated are largely dependent on the geographic location. Sources of funding and treatment philosophy are probably the most variable of all.

The heterogeneity of adolescent inpatient settings derives in part from the affiliation, mission, and funding source. University settings are dedicated to training young professionals and creating new knowledge through research; funding is derived only partly from patient care with most from state-university revenues.

Private for-profit facilities are dedicated to delivery of patient care to generate revenue in order to create a level of profit to satisfy shareholders in the company; thus, financial gain is the major mission. In contrast, private, not-for-profit facilities, although equally dedicated to delivery of patient care to generate revenue, are limited to the amount of profit allowed by law. In both types of settings, reimbursement is obtained from indemnity insurance benefits. Since this is a service delivery system, research and teaching are not primarily emphasized.

Public facilities are also dedicated to patient care delivery, but are funded by state and local sources out of tax revenue. Historically, these facilities have been the most poorly funded, staffed, and maintained while they have had to treat the most recalcitrant, treatment-resistant, chronic patients. In such settings, teaching and research are generally minimal to absent.

Describing treatment setting in such a broad, inclusive fashion clearly negates the individuality of some settings. It is not unusual to find combinations of settings today: corporate for-profit university hospitals, excellent not-for-profit training and research facilities, and public hospitals totally integrated with university teaching and research programs. Each unit must be evaluated on its own merit, on the basis of the mission of the unit, the level of professional staffing, types of treatment modalities employed, the reputation of the facility, and the outcomes for the patients treated.

SUMMARY

Inpatient psychiatric treatment is at a critical juncture. Many old and new questions must be addressed. If inpatient treatment is necessary, does it help, what should be the optimal length of stay, and which treatment approaches are most helpful? Clinicians who work in inpatient settings have clearly seen positive outcomes with adolescents who are suicidal, homicidal, psychotic, and otherwise nonfunctional. There is clearly a need to systematically study inpatient treatment programs (Goodrich, this volume) to determine what treatment is indicated for each patient. Present changes in inpatient treatment do not seem to be based on any scientific advance or changes in social support systems; rather, they are driven entirely by economic factors. These changes demand the need for a comprehensive system that provides not only various hospital-based treatment modalities, but a continuum of care, including residential, day hospital, outpatient services, group homes, after-school programs, specialized foster homes, and intensive in-home services.

REFERENCES

American Academy of Child and Adolescent Psychiatry, Inpatient Hospital Treatment Of Children and Adolescents, Policy Statement, June 1989, pp. 1-4. Washington, D.C.

American Psychiatric Association (1987) *Diagnostic and Statistical Manual of Mental Disorders, 3rd Ed.,* revised. Washington, D.C.

American Psychiatric Association, 1989. Statement on Psychiatric Hospitalization of Children and Adolescent. Washington, D.C.

American Society for Adolescent Psychiatry (1990). Hospitalization, marketing guidelines proposed. Summer *Newsletter,* pp. 3-5.

Anthony, E.J. (1991). The therapeutic matrix in the inpatient treatment of the adolescent. In R.L. Hendron & I.N. Berlin (Eds.), *Psychiatric Inpatient Care of Children and Adolescents: A Multicultural Approach* (pp. 195-206). New York: John Wiley & Sons, Inc.

Barker, P. (1976). *Basic Child Psychiatry,* 2nd ed. London: Crosby Lockwood Staples.

Bettelheim, B. & Sylvester, E. (1948). A therapeutic milieu. *American Journal Orthopsychiatry,18,* 191-206.

Bettelheim, B. & Sylvester, E. (1949). Milieu therapy indications and illustrations. *Psychoanalytic Review, 36,* 54-67.

Gunderson, J. G. (1978). Defining the therapeutic processes in psychiatric milieus. *Psychiatry, 413,* 327-335.

Harper, G. (1989). Focal inpatient treatment planning. *Journal American Academy Child Adolescent Psychiatry, 28,* 31-37.

Harper, G., & Geraty, R. (1989). Hospital and residential treatment. In J. O. Cavenar (Ed.), *Psychiatry* (rev. ed.; vol 2, chap 64, pp. 1-20). Philadelphia: Lippincott; New York: Basic Books.

Kester, B. C. (1966). Indication for residential treatment of children. *Child Welfare, 65,* 338-340.

Lewis, J. M. (1991). The changing tales of adolescent inpatient psychiatric treatment. *The Psychiatric Hospital, 22,* 165-173.

Lynch, M., Steinberg, D., and Oursted, C.: Family unit in a children's psychiatry hospital. *British Medical Journal, 2,* 127-129, 1975.

Main, F.T.: Mothers with children in a psychiatric hospital. *Lancet, 2,* 845–847, 1969.

Nakhla, F., Folkart, L., and Webster, J.: Treatment of families as inpatients. *Family Process,* 8:79-96, 1969.

Nosphitz, J. D. (1962). Notes on the theory of residential treatment. *Journal of the American Academy of Child Psychiatry, 1,* 284-296.

Nurcombe, B. (1989). Goal-directed treatment planning and the principles of brief hospitalization. *Journal American Academy Child Adolescent Psychiatry, 28,* 26-30.

Petti, T. A. (1980). Residential and inpatient treatment. In G. P. Sholevar, R. M. Benson & B. J. Belinda (Eds.), *Emotional Disorders in Children and Adolescents: Medical and Psychological Approach to Treatment* (pp. 209-228). New York: NY, SP Medical and Scientific Books.

Potter, H. W. (1934). A service for children in a psychiatric hospital. *Psychiatric Quarterly, 8,* 16-33.

Potter, H. W. (1935). The treatment of problem children in a psychiatric hospital. *American Journal of Psychiatry, 91*, 869-880.

Reidl, F. (1952). *Controls from Within: Techniques for the Treatment of Aggressive Children*. Glencoe, IL: Free Press.

Reidl, F. (1959). The concept of a "Therapeutic Milieu." *American Journal of Orthopsychiatry, 29*, 721-736.

Rinsley, D. E. (1967). Intensive residential treatment of the adolescent. *Psychiatric Quarterly, 41*, 135-143.

Rinsley, D. E. (1968). Theory and practice of intensive residential treatment of adolescents. *Psychiatric Quarterly, 42*, 611-638.

Rinsley, D. E. (1990). The severely disturbed adolescent: Indication for hospital and residential treatment. *Bulletin of the Menninger Clinic, 54*, 3-12.

Silver, L. B. (1976). Professional standards review organization: A handbook for child psychiatrist. Washington, D.C.: American Academy of Child Psychiatry.

Wardle, C. J. (1974). Residential care of children with conduct disorder, in P. A. Barker (Ed.), *The Residential Psychiatric Treatment of Children* (pp. 48-104). New York: Wiley.

Weintrob, A. (1975). Long-term treatment of the severely disturbed adolescent: Residential treatment vs. hospitalization. *Journal of The American Academy of Child Psychiatry, 14*, 436–450.

Winnicott, D. W. (1965). *The Maturational Process and the Facilitating Environment: Studies in the Theory of Emotional Development*. New York: International Universities Press.

Chapter 2

EVALUATION AND TREATMENT PROCESS

Harinder S. Ghuman

The evaluation process and the treatment process of an adolescent in an inpatient setting occur simultaneously from admission to discharge. Most clinicians like to divide the inpatient stay into an evaluation period and a treatment period. Depending upon the setting, the assessment period may consist of the first several days, or even weeks, of the inpatient stay. Often, the very admission of the adolescent to an inpatient setting may be therapeutic as the disturbed adolescent is surrounded by hospital staff who provide both support and supervision. This support may be in the form of empathetic listening and clearly defined and enforced rules, regulation, and limits, with the possible use of psychopharmacological intervention to treat specific disorders such as depression or to control dangerous behaviors. In addition, the treatment team actively plans for discharge throughout the inpatient stay. One can divide inpatient stay into the following steps or stages: preadmission/intake; admission proper; diagnostic procedures and conference; treatment intervention; and discharge.

During inpatient treatment, the adolescent and the family go through various emotions and reactions. It is important for the inpatient team to recognize and work with these emotions in order to reach the most successful outcome possible. Due to recent developments in adolescent inpatient treatment (Chapter 1), the emotional reactions of the adolescent and of the parents have become even more complicated. In addition, the inpatient staff have experienced their own set of emotions and reactions in response to the dramatically shortened length of stay and intensive managed care review.

This chapter is devoted to describing various stage of inpatient stay, the adolescent's and the family's reactions to these stages, and the impact of economic factors on patients and staff.

PREADMISSION/INTAKE

Preadmission/intake is essential to: (1) ascertain that the adolescent needs admission to an inpatient setting; (2) determine what kind of treatment needs are there, and if the inpatient facility provides these needs; (3) assure that the family, social, and financial resources are available to complete the task of an inpatient setting; and (4) answer the adolescent's and the family's concerns and queries, and assist them to develop a clearer understanding of the need for admission. Criticism of inpatient facilities and programs and poor outcome of inpatient treatment may often be attributed to not addressing these initial questions with care.

Due to the increased pressure from third-party payers and managed care companies to limit inpatient care in favor of less restrictive, less costly care, inpatient facilities have been spending less and less time on preadmissions/intake, often focusing more on getting the adolescent into and out of the hospital as quickly as possible.

Ideally, the admission office, in collaboration with the treatment unit, should set up a procedure for preadmission/intake. This procedure should be sufficiently flexible to permit addressing the above questions adequately and yet to be responsive to the urgency of an admission. For example, a patient in acute crisis, waiting in the emergency room for transfer to a psychiatric facility, is seldom able to wait for a thorough Intake/Preadmission. Therefore, a well-trained admission staff in consultation with the unit director must obtain as much information as possible to make a decision by phone. When an adolescent is already in a short-term evaluation unit and is referred for longer-term treatment, a more elaborate preadmission/intake procedure may be done. In this case, it may be useful for the adolescent and/or parents to visit the unit for a preadmission meeting with the treatment team prior to the transfer.

During this preadmission meeting, the treatment team informs the adolescent and the family about the unit, the various treatment interventions offered, the treatment team's expectations, and some of the common issues that may arise during treatment. At this time, treatment team members can explain their role in the treatment program and answer the adolescent's and the parent's questions. The patient and family can relate their understanding of the reason for referral and discuss their expectations from treatment. A visit to the unit, educational facilities, and recreational areas should be arranged. It is useful to have a patient handbook describing the unit's schedule, rules, and expectations, a list of unit staff members, and visiting time, for example, to be given to the patient and family. If there is agreement regarding the need for the adolescent's admission, the unit director or designee can schedule the date and time, and begin the explanation of the admission procedure. This preadmission meeting can prepare the patient and parents for the hospitalization and may help to avoid or to resolve some of the problems that may arise during hospitalization. Sometimes, for the sake of expediency or due to distance, the preadmission meeting may need to take place immediately prior to and continuous with the admission.

Another important aspect of the intake/preadmission procedure is the involvement of the referral source. Depending upon the situation, contact with the referral person may be by phone or actual presence at the time of the preadmission meeting. This is especially important with adolescents referred by juvenile services. The close involvement of the referral source is a necessity to ascertain the referral source's expectations and to gain their support in implementing treatment and discharge plans.

The admission office usually evaluates insurance coverage or other funding sources (MA & JSA) for hospitalization, as well as family financial resources, before admitting the adolescent; often, insurance companies require precertification authorization for admission. Generally, parents need to meet with the financial office of the hospital to formalize pay and co-pay arrangements.

ADMISSION

The adolescent and parents should meet with a staff member from the admission office to go over various forms, including applications for admission, patient rights, medical power of attorney, release of information from referral source, and any other authorization that may be necessary, with signatures as required. This process takes place either in the admission office or on the unit. However, it is often helpful to have the admission process occur in close proximity to the unit as some intervention from the unit staff may be required should the patient become violent and/or pose a runaway risk.

After the admission paperwork is completed, the psychiatrist and social worker should meet with the adolescent and parents. It is important for the admitting psychiatrist to ensure that the adolescent and parents understand the patient's rights, three-day notice requirements for removal of the adolescent from the treatment program, and under what circumstances the hospital staff may ask for involuntary certification. The admitting psychiatrist must obtain a present history and medical history, and elicit information regarding significant events in childhood. After obtaining this information, the social worker may continue to obtain additional history from the parents depending upon time availability. The social worker obtains the family history, including any history of mental illness, and the patient's developmental and school history. The social worker may also wish to see the adolescent and parents together to assess family dynamics, communication, areas of conflicts, strengths, and weaknesses.

The psychiatrist performs the psychiatric diagnostic interview with the adolescent to get his/her view of the problems, do a mental status, to assess the risk of violence and/or suicide, make a preliminary diagnosis, and develop the initial treatment plan. The psychiatrist also performs a physical exam with special emphasis on the neurological examination and writes orders regarding responsibility level, special precautions if necessary, lab work, and medication as indicated. It is advisable to keep the adolescent confined to the unit for 24 hours to assess his condition and to enable him to become more familiar with the new surroundings, peers, and staff.

The nursing staff orients the patient to the unit, introduces him/her to the staff and peers, and explains the schedules, rules and expectations. Nursing staff evaluates the patient to identify problems and develops the initial nursing plan.

Adolescent and Family's Initial Reaction

Adolescents and their families demonstrate a variety of responses toward admission. In some cases, it may have taken several months or even years to finally decide upon inpatient treatment. Important questions to ask the adolescent and family are: When was the first time inpatient treatment was considered? What was their reaction at that time and how have they dealt with and arrived at the current decision for admission? There are times when the adolescent and the family have to make a decision in a very short time and are left emotionally numbed by the events leading up to the admission. In such cases, the treatment team must assist and support both the adolescent and the family to deal effectively with the various emotions as they unfold.

The treatment team must also consider the parents' reaction to the separation resulting from the hospitalization (Mandelbaum, 1962; American Association for Children's Residential Centers, 1972). One of the frequent emotions the adolescent and family experience is the sense of failure. It will be difficult to treat these adolescents unless they and their families are able to deal with this issue in a realistic manner. Feeling too much guilt, or defending against this, can result in acting out by both the adolescent and the family by premature termination of treatment.

Occasionally, parents use the threat of putting their adolescent into a mental institution in response to various intolerable behaviors. These parents are then vulnerable when they find themselves in the position of actually needing to admit the adolescent, for although many adolescents express their feelings of being "punished" or "jailed," parents who have used the threat in the past often have to deal with their own confusion and guilt.

Adolescents and parents often experience fear of a hospital or residential setting. They are concerned about safety and what influence other adolescents may have. These adolescents and parents need extra reassurance and information about the program. Additionally, adolescents and parents who use extreme denial, externalization, or projection may be equally difficult to reassure. The treatment team may need to seek outside support in treating these adolescents, such as social services, juvenile services, or the use of certification.

Parents who experience extreme anger and are totally fatigued by their adolescent's behavior may feel relieved and be somewhat distant from the adolescent on admission. The treatment team may have to help them deal with their feelings and encourage participation through patience and support. Failure to involve the parents is a common factor in the treatment failure in intermediate length of stay hospital and residential treatment settings (Petti, 1980).

DIAGNOSTIC PROCEDURES

The diagnostic process begins with the preadmission/intake and continues for several days after admission. A complete diagnostic workup includes an assessment of the following: (a) emotional status and cognition, (b) daily functioning, (c) family, (d) education, and (e) physical status.

A. Assessment of Emotional Status and Cognition

The adolescent's emotional status and cognition are primarily evaluated by a psychiatric diagnostic interview with the therapist and, when indicated, by psychological testing.

It is useful for the therapist to interview the adolescent over two to three sessions and to assess general behavior and motor activity, speech, affect, thought process, perceptions, orientation, attention, concentration, memory, general knowledge, intelligence, insight and judgment. The therapist must pay particular attention to the intensity of depression and suicidality, the risk of violence, psychosis, and organicity. In order to conduct psychotherapeutic work during an inpatient stay as well as to make recommendations for outpatient care, one needs to assess the adolescent's psychosexual development, defenses, object relationships, and development of self in order to determine which psychotherapeutic approaches would be most beneficial.

Psychological testing can be a useful tool in the diagnostic process when administered by an experienced clinician. Most commonly used psychological tests include the WAIS (age 16 and above), WISC-R, Bender Gestalt, Benton Revised Visual Retention Test, Sentence Completion Test, TAT, and Rorschach. The Luria-Nebraska Neuropsychological Test is indicated in patients with known brain damage and when cognitive deficits are suspected.

B. Assessment of Daily Functioning

Nursing staff and activity therapy staff assist the patient in activities of daily living, which include taking care of basic needs and hygiene, as well as recreation and various work groups. The staff assesses the adolescent's ability to relate and to express thoughts and feelings, the level of impulse control, and the ability to participate in physical activities. (For details see Chapters 5 and 8.)

C. Assessment of Family

The social worker, along with input from other treatment team members assesses family functioning, including communication among family members, family dynamics, strengths and weaknesses in the family, and the family structure. (For details see Chapter 6.)

D. Educational Assessment

The educational consultant for the unit contacts the adolescent's home school to gain information regarding his/her behavior in school, level of academic performance, any involvement in Special Education, and the school's experience with the adolescent's parents. The Woodcock Johnson Psychoeducation Battery and Wide Range Achievement Test (WRAT) is commonly administered to find the adolescent's level of academic functioning and any possibility of a learning disability. If there are indications that the adolescent is experiencing difficulty with speech and language a complete speech and language evaluation is mandatory.

E. Physical Assessment

A physical examination and comprehensive lab work are always indicated to rule out any organic reasons that may account for the adolescent's problems; this is necessary prior to initiation of medication. For example, it is important to obtain a baseline EKG before starting antidepressant medications and Lithium. A neurological consultation and EEG should be obtained if there are positive neurological findings on the physical exam or a history of seizure disorder, head injury, or episodic rage attacks are elicited. A CAT Scan and MRI is essential in first episode of acute psychosis with or without an organic component or when ordered by the neurologist.

It may also be necessary to request consultation from various specialists in cases where the adolescent presents specific problems and needs, such as alcohol and drug abuse, eating disorder, multiple personality disorder, and obsessive-compulsive disorder.

Diagnostic Conference
The diagnostic conference is the most critical event of the entire hospital stay. At this conference, the staff share their evaluation of the adolescent's problems, develop a five-axis diagnostic formulation, devise a treatment plan that includes setting goals, objectives, and interventions, and establishes a time structure to accomplish these goals congruent with discharge planning.

The adolescent and family usually anxiously await the outcome of the diagnostic conference. The adolescent's major concern is generally the recommended length of the hospitalization, whereas the parents primarily want to learn what is wrong with their child, the diagnosis, treatment, and prognosis. It is important to allow ample time to answer the adolescent's and parents' questions and concerns. They should be informed of the diagnosis in jargon-free, simple language that they can understand. A good therapeutic alliance with the adolescent and parents requires that they be educated regarding the diagnosis, diagnostic possibilities, and how the clinical team arrived at the diagnosis and treatment plan. This is also the optimal time to begin educating the adolescent and parents regarding any recommended medications and to enlist their permission to prescribe medications.

There are often confusion and feelings of guilt and hopelessness underlying many of these questions. It may be useful to discuss the etiology, prognosis, and present state of psychiatric knowledge and limitation in this knowledge regarding the adolescent's diagnosis and prognosis. The adolescent's and the family's strengths should be emphasized so that they may provide a balanced view and hope. It is generally not useful to attempt to totally alleviate the parents' anxiety or guilt; it is better to bring it to the optimal level necessary for them to continue treatment.

TREATMENT INTERVENTIONS

Treatment interventions can be divided arbitrarily into two categories: (1) interventions dealing with behavior and daily routine; and (2) psychotherapeutic interventions.

I. Interventions Dealing with Behavior and Daily Routine

These interventions are directed towards (a) bringing the adolescent's dangerous and destructive behavior under control by nursing-milieu interventions (Chapter 5), pharmacotherapy (Chapter 7), use of seclusion, restraints, ECT, and hydrotherapy (Chapter 12), and limit-setting (Chapter 14); and (b) improving the adolescent's ability to effectively deal with the daily routine, including caring for basic needs, interpersonal interactions, and school. This is accomplished by nursing milieu interventions (Chapter 5), activity therapy (Chapter 8), pharmacotherapy (Chapter 7), special education (Chapter 9), and limit-setting (Chapter 14).

II. Psychotherapeutic Interventions

These interventions are directed towards: (a) helping the adolescent and family to learn how to deal constructively with intense feelings and impulses, (b) helping the adolescent to reflect upon his behavior and how it affects his own life and the lives of others, (c) improving communication, and (d) providing hope, support, and encouragement.

Psychotherapeutic interventions include individual psychotherapy (Chapter 3), group psychotherapy (Chapter 4), family therapy and casework (Chapter 6), activity therapy (Chapter 8), and nursing talks and encouragement.

During the treatment process, the adolescent, parents, and staff go through the following phases:

1. Treatment-alliance phase
2. Working-through phase

Treatment-Alliance Phase

This phase is marked by issues related to trust and caring. Adolescents and families who have had traumatic, disturbed interpersonal relationships experience great difficulty in trusting when admitted for inpatient treatment. They demonstrate a need to test and retest the treating staff before establishing any therapeutic alliance. The following is an example:

> Mary, an 18-year-old female, was admitted to the hospital on an emergency basis after she made a serious suicide attempt by lying in front of an oncoming train. The patient had a history of severe emotional problems from age seven to eight. She had been hospitalized at age 11 and 16 for suicide attempts and had a history of repeated runaways and sexual promiscuity. The patient's mother was a teenager and a drug addict when her daughter was conceived and she abandoned her at eight months of age. Mary was adopted at age two years and from that time onwards was involved in a very intense conflictual relationship with the adopted mother, as manifested by Mary's extreme neediness and provocative behaviors.
>
> On the second day of hospitalization, the patient submitted a written request for her release from the hospital. But after two hours, encouraged by staff and her parents, she withdrew it. Over the following two to three days, the patient denied any self-destructive thoughts. But she continued to demonstrate lability in her mood, was defiant and demanding, and made frequent calls to her mother, following which she became very upset. Mary submitted another notice asking for her release. The patient's therapist talked with her several times to encourage her to stay. In addition, the therapist asked her referring psychiatrist and her mother to talk with her. The patient retracted her notice after her mother's encouragement and her promise to visit more frequently. In this case, the patient seemed to need to test both the therapist and her parents regarding their level of interest and commitment to her.

When the adolescent and parents both have difficulty developing trust, establishing any alliance can be cumbersome. They may inadvertently feed into each other's distrust.

> Another example is a 14-year-old female who was admitted to the hospital following an attempt to stab her mother. The

patient had a history of not following her mother's rules, running away, living on the street, drug abuse, and sexual acting-out. The patient had a great deal of difficulty trusting her male therapist who she said reminded her of a neighbor who had molested her. The patient often verbally attacked her therapist and avoided psychotherapy sessions. One day, the mother told the therapist that he reminded her daughter of the person who molested her daughter, and he, the therapist, "better watch himself" that he does not do the same thing. It thus became very clear that the mother's undermining of the staff's limit-setting was because of her own difficulty in trusting.

Treatment staff can help the patient and parents develop trust and form an alliance by making themselves available to answer their questions, by not overreacting to the patient's and parents' projections, and by developing a better understanding of the patient's and parents' disturbed past. The staff's verbal and nonverbal interaction play an important role in establishing trust and alliance. Adolescents and parents who are abusive, obnoxious, and sometimes violent towards staff present major obstacles to developing a therapeutic relationship. In these situations, the staff must emphasize that they are there to serve and assist the patient and family to overcome their difficulties, but will not tolerate such abuse. Such issues must be dealt with clearly, concisely, and consistently; otherwise, staff may act out their own feelings through verbal or nonverbal means. Forming a trusting alliance, however, may not always be possible, such as when the patient and parents come to the hospital under external pressure and are trying to avoid incarceration of the patient or other unpleasant consequence.

Working -Through Phase

The working-through phase is optimally to define and resolve the adolescent's and family's problems. The various treatment issues and modalities are described under Parts II and III of this book. The prerequisite to this phase is development of a treatment alliance, however rudimentary, between staff, adolescent, and family. This phase can be a long and complicated task when the adolescent's and family's psychopathology is long standing and severe. The present economic/political climate has made this a very difficult, if not impossible, task, especially in dealing with severely and chronically disturbed adolescents because of lack of support for long-term inpatient treatment. This working-through process usually takes place across a continuum of care, including inpatient, outpatient, and community settings. According to Gabbard (1988), any hospitalization, of whatever length, is really only a chapter in the "Book of Treatment." As a treatment alliance is established, the adolescent and family generally become more actively involved in the treatment process. The adolescent and family ideally begin to learn new ways of dealing with life situations and attempt to put their new knowledge into practice. Every time the adolescent and family practice and appreciate success in dealing with a situation, there is some internalization of the process. The end result is usually that the adolescent and family need less and less guidance and intervention from mental health professionals. Periods of relapse or regression may occur, however, and require professional interventions to work through old issues.

There are, however, always internal and external obstacles to change. Adolescents often fear losing their identity if they change, they fear becoming vulnerable or being taken advantage of by others. These internal obstacles to change affect the adolescent's attitude toward taking medications, trying new methods of dealing with conflict, exploring interpersonal relationship, risking success and failure, and complying with treatment. The treatment staff needs to consistently and repeatedly address these issues with the adolescent and family.

DISCHARGE

The treatment staff needs to address where the adolescent will reside after hospitalization, what outpatient psychiatric treatment will be necessary, and what the adolescent's educational/vocational needs are.

If the adolescent is to return home, staff need to work with the adolescent and parents regarding the necessary supervision and structure at home. Basic rules regarding expression of feelings, taking care of daily routine, and expectations of the adolescent and parents from each other must be clarified. It is essential that the adolescent and parents develop a written contract outlining expectations and rules for both parties to follow. Ideally, before the adolescent is discharged to home, it is important that a home visit and return to the community be scheduled as practice for dealing with various issues that occur while contract guidelines are followed. If the treatment team has come to the conclusion that the adolescent may require alternative placement, such as long-term hospitalization, residential care, or group home, the staff must actively work with the adolescent and parents to help them accept this decision, procure funding, and participate in the program. This process can be time-consuming and tedious. Staff need to be aware of the various sources of funding available, the procedures to follow, and the placements available in the community or other states. Visiting prospective placement alternatives will aid in increasing the parents' and adolescent's level of acceptance, confidence, and comfort.

If outpatient treatment following discharge is recommended, it should be arranged while the patient is still hospitalized. The adolescent may require referral to a Day/Evening Program. In the case of drug abuse, the staff should assist the adolescent and parents to locate AA/NA meeting sites. In all cases, it is of optimum benefit if the patient starts attending outpatient activities while still in the hospital.

Often, the onset of an adolescent's problems or the exaggeration in symptomatology can be traced back to a change of school, to entering middle or high school, or to the transition from special education class to regular classes. Many adolescents are already vulnerable due to cognitive deficits or emotional difficulties. The inpatient treatment staff must carefully assess these adolescents and determine what educational requirement they have after they leave the hospital. The need for input from teachers and special educators when one is performing diagnostic, therapeutic, and dispositional procedures is important (King, 1974; Alt, 1960). Staff needs to address if the adolescent can be educated in a regular class setting or requires placement in special education classes within or outside the regular school. Staff must also work closely with the home school and Board of Education to secure appropriate placement for the patient. With adolescents who have finished school or who have taken the GED exam, the staff should provide guidance for future education, vocational training, or entering the job market.

Adolescent and Parental Reaction to Discharge

Discharge of the adolescent from an inpatient setting is as significant an event as the admission. Some important factors that need to be considered in dealing with the adolescent's and parents' reaction to discharge include:
1. The length of stay on the unit.
2. Planned or unplanned discharge.
3. Living arrangements after discharge.

Length of Inpatient Stay

In general, adolescents who required longer lengths of stay are more likely to develop stronger attachments to peers and staff. Many of these adolescents have, for the first time in their life, developed meaningful relationships. Many such patients describe their inpatient experience as a "life line," and often comment to staff, "You gave my life back," "I might have been dead if I were not here." For these adolescents, discharge can be overwhelming, and can reactivate intense ambivalence, anxieties, and feelings related to separation or loss. Regression with reactivation of presenting symptoms often occurs in anticipation of discharge, this must be handled with reassurance, support, and a firm approach. Adolescents who have been inpatients for shorter length of stay, such as a few days to weeks, may show similar reactions, but usually with less intensity.

Planned or Unplanned Discharge

Unplanned discharges due to an adolescent's runaway, parents removing the patient against medical advice, and managed care denials of stay can cause confusion, defensiveness, and further acting out by the adolescent and family, often leading to a subsequent admission. For example:

> A 17-year-old adolescent with a long history of severe drug abuse was admitted due to suicidal and homicidal threats. After 12 days of inpatient hospitalization the patient's insurance company denied the need for continuing hospital stay despite the patient being agitated, depressed, and experiencing drug urges. Due to the insurance denial, the parents decided to take the patient home. However the patient was readmitted after only five days, precipitated by his feeling suicidal and snorting cocaine.

> Another example is a 16-year-old female with a history of severe self-destructive behavior, including cutting, overdosing, and burning herself. After three months of hospitalization, the patient continued to be self-destructive. Her parents had difficulty supporting supervisory limits placed on her and decided to take her home against medical advice. The patient required readmission after two days when she again became actively suicidal.

Unplanned discharges usually create a dilemma for the treatment team. On one hand, the staff needs to help the adolescent and family to seek appropriate outpatient follow-up. At the same time, they may clearly convey their disagreement with the decision to terminate inpatient treatment. The issue of prescribing medication to an adolescent who leaves an inpatient setting prematurely against medical advice needs to be carefully assessed on an individual basis. When there is lack of monitoring of medication by parents or a refusal of psychiatric follow-up, it may be advisable not to prescribe medication.

Reasons for unplanned discharge often influence the adolescent's and family's reaction. When there is an insurance denial or financial resources are depleted, the adolescent and parents may get angry, yet they often are able to work with the staff in establishing discharge plans.

Unplanned discharge due to parental decision to take the adolescent out of inpatient setting can be due to number of reasons, including failure to develop a trusting alliance with the staff, feeling of disappointment and hopelessness due to poor or slow progress, anger at the staff for not responding to their needs or demands, the adolescent's ability to manipulate and set up a split between the staff and the parents, and at times anticipation of major changes in the adolescent's and/or the family's situation. With the especially difficult adolescent and family, inpatient staff often experience their own feelings of hopelessness, disappointment, and anger. If unchecked, the staff's feelings can collude with the adolescent's and parents' feelings, resulting in unplanned discharge. Inpatient staff's awareness of their own and parental feelings often can prevent unplanned discharge. If parents continue to insist upon discharge and the adolescent still requires inpatient treatment, the only course left for the treatment staff is to either inform the protective services or initiate certification to continue inpatient treatment.

Living Arrangements After Discharge

Discharge and transition are smoother when the adolescent is able to finish treatment in one facility and is returning home. This is not always possible for many severely disturbed adolescents who have to continue treatment after discharge from the hospital in a residential setting or a group home. Many adolescents are often reluctant to go to the next facility, preferring to stay at one place and finish their treatment. Often, these adolescents have been moved from place to place, experiencing and reexperiencing the trauma of separation. One adolescent described this feeling as being a "Door Mat." These adolescents may become involved in acting out so as to prevent their next placement. Their parents also experience guilt, a sense of loss, and distrust; they are likely to act out if they are unable to work with these feelings.

ECONOMIC FACTORS AND THE TREATMENT PROCESS

Recently, economic factors have had a significant effect on inpatient treatment. With ever-increasing financial constraints being placed on inpatient care and resulting in very short lengths of stay, treatment teams accustomed to working with adolescent patients in an intermediate to longer-term unit are at risk of becoming demoralized, resulting in a "why try" attitude, avoidance of relationship, and giving up on the arduous task of adolescent treatment. Gabbard (1992), however, believes that relationships will develop, even in the briefest hospitalization. He states that these new attempts at relatedness encountered during inpatient treatment will be experienced again and again in partial-hospital settings, psychotherapy, and future hospitalizations until the cumulative impact leads to structural changes in the patient's internal world. It is, therefore, necessary that staff be encouraged to continue to do what they do best; hopefully, the adolescent will continue to experience these growth-promoting interactions.

Another problem the staff needs to be aware of is the danger of spending too much time focused on economic issues rather than on providing treatment. While it is essential that the hospital administration address the financial health of the institution in order to survive and to continue to provide treatment, the balance in dealing with both financial and clinical issues is the critical balance. Many inpatient settings have been forced to reduce the number of inpatient beds, realign staffing, and consequently make substantial changes in inpatient treatment programs. The treatment team should address their feelings regarding these issues and how this may affect their daily interaction with adolescents and families. There is a real danger that the adolescent, the family, and the staff may externalize and focus all problems on the insurance company, managed care reviewers, and utilization review, thereby potentially undermining the actual treatment process. Another danger is for the staff and parents to give in to the reviewers' unreasonable demands, due to constant pressure and even harassment, and initiate medication against the better judgment of the physicians or discharge the patient prematurely.

Another factor one needs to consider from an individual adolescent treatment basis to program basis is related to superego deficiencies and development. Treatment, it seems, is more and more dictated by economic factors rather than by clinical factors, often resulting in less than ethical behavior. Reviewers' superego lacunae often reverberate deficiencies in the inpatient staff, adolescent patients, and their families. For example:

> A 16-year-old female who was admitted due to a suicidal attempt, self-destructive behavior, and excessive drinking and sexual acting out, was responding to the inpatient treatment program by beginning to show some control of her behavior. However, she clearly was not ready for discharge. After 65 days of hospitalization, the insurance reviewer allocated one more week to plan for her discharge. When the patient was informed of this, she asked her therapist if he could tell the reviewer that she had cut herself and was suicidal, so that she could continue to stay in the hospital and finish the treatment.

There are patients who do act out and often prolong their treatment after hearing of the refusal of the insurance company and utilization reviewers. Thus, the reviewers play indirectly into patients' psychopathology. Treatment staff need to be aware of this and not become involved in acting out. A treatment plan developed just to placate the insurance companies and not based on any sound clinical reasons is dangerous to the patient, in addition to being unethical and even criminal.

The staff must, however, candidly address the issue of finances and how it affects treatment. Adolescents, and sometimes their families, often provoke by commenting that the staff is doing their therapeutic work because they are getting paid. When an adolescent has to be discharged due to insurance refusal or other financial reasons, this may cause heightened defensiveness on the part of staff.

SUMMARY

The evaluation and treatment process can be divided into various stages as described in this chapter. It is important for the inpatient staff to understand and pay adequate attention not only to these stages, but also to the adolescent's and family's reactions in order to have successful outcome. Economic factors have been playing an ever-increasing role in influencing the evaluation and treatment process. The inpatient staff must be alert in order to effectively deal with this reality.

REFERENCES

Alt, H. (1960). *Residential Treatment for Disturbed Child.* New York: Int. University Press.

American Association for Children's Residential Centers (1972). *From Chaos to Order: A Collective View of the Residential Treatment of Children.* New York: Child Welfare League of America.

Gabbard, G.O. (1988). A contemporary perspective on psychoanalytically informed hospital treatment, *Hospital and Community Psychiatry, 39,* 1291-1295.

Gabbard, G.O. (1992). The therapeutic relationship in psychiatric hospital treatment. *Bulletin of the Menninger Clinic, 56*, 4-19.

King, J.W. (1974). Teaching goals and techniques in hospital schools. In Feinstein, S.C., and Giovacchini, P.L. (Eds.), *Adolescent Psychiatry, Vol. III—Developmental and Clinical Studies* (pp.419-421). New York: Basic Books.

Mandelbaum, A. (1962). Parent-child separation: Its significance to parents. *Social Work, 7*:4, 26-35.

Petti, T.A. (1980). *Treatment of Emotional Disorders in Children and Adolescents.* Spectrum Publications, Inc.

PART II

Therapeutic Interventions

Chapter 3

INDIVIDUAL PSYCHOTHERAPY

Donald H. Saidel

BASIC CONCEPTS

The basic orientation to be followed in this chapter in discussing psychotherapy of the adolescent patient is derived from a psychoanalytic framework that includes theories of object relationship. It is important in this context to think of psychoanalytic theory as a developmental theory that provides a framework for the endeavor to understand patients engaged in the psychotherapeutic process. For purposes of this discussion, psychotherapy will refer to the process wherein the psychotherapist engages with the patient toward the goal of helping that individual to change aspects of herself or himself. The outcome sought by the therapist is improvement in the functioning of the adolescent and the development of more age appropriate relationships. More broadly, "Psychotherapy, coming out of psychoanalysis, is essentially to do with meaning; trying to construct some sense about a person's behavior and thoughts. It is something offered to another person, an opportunity...to find some sort of account of himself" (Wilson, 1986, pp. 109-110).

In the treatment of severely disturbed adolescents, the psychotherapist must be scrupulous in maintaining the focus on helping the patient to "change." It is also useful to keep clear the difference between therapy and psychotherapy. In the inpatient hospital treatment of adolescent patients, multiple therapies are used with hopes of relieving the distress and pain experienced by the patient and to help the patient to initiate important changes. However, these multiple therapies differ from psychotherapy in that psychoanalytically oriented psychotherapy makes use of the concept of transference and is based on the mediation of thoughts and feelings through the use of language. Indeed, one of the cardinal principles of this approach is to make use of the hospital structure to reduce the propensity of the adolescent to "act out" his conflicts.

It is important to keep in mind the distinction between inpatient hospital treatment and outpatient treatment. By the time the adolescent requires hospitalization, functioning has become severely compromised. Behavior has been evidenced that is bizarre, disruptive, or dangerous to the adolescent or to others, although the severity of the adolescent's symptoms is not necessarily reflected by diagnosis. Outpatient therapy has often been tried, but with no change noted, and generally the home, school, and community are unable to tolerate the adolescent's disruptions. In the hospital, the adolescent "... becomes the total responsibility of his therapist with respect to his behavior, his adaptive progress..., his safety, and the fulfillment of many of his affectional needs" (Holmes, 1964, p.88). O'Malley (1990, p.14) cites another important feature: "Adolescent patients who require... hospitalization... often fight against efforts to contain and confront their behavioral dyscontrol, and they avoid exploration of their personal pain and dysfunction because of character pathology, dynamic conflicts, and limitations in ego development." These patients then require a modification in the usual neutral position maintained by the therapist working with outpatients.

Much has been written of the advantages and disadvantages of the therapist/administrator split (Anthony, 1991; Errera & Levine, 1990; Holmes, 1964). In our view, when the psychotherapist assumes administrative responsibilities, different variables are introduced into the therapy process. These variables do not necessarily interfere with the process; in fact, it is recommended that the therapist be the patient's administrator when conducting longer-term inpatient treatment. The therapist then becomes an integral member of the treatment team rather than a peripheral part of the patient's world. In contrast, short-term hospitalization is generally focused on acute intervention to reduce the potential for harm to self or to others rather than on assisting the patient to make in-depth changes. Under these short-term conditions, either treatment model, therapist/administrator split or not split, would seem effective.

Further clarification is needed in considering open-staff vs. closed-staff hospitals. In general, it is our experience that treatment for disturbed adolescents is best organized and, thereby, most effective in a closed-staff facility. One of the important benefits derived is that the patient cannot use therapy as an escape from reality and responsibility. In the closed-staff facility, the therapist is continually informed regarding the patient's functioning outside of therapy sessions. The therapist is able, as needed, to use this "reality" during the psychotherapy sessions. This does not mean that the therapist allows this reality to interfere with the therapeutic endeavor. Rather, the patient can be better understood and helped to achieve more accurate approximations of the real world.

It is most essential that the therapist have a consistent conceptual framework of understanding, such as a psychoanalytic model, that governs his responses to the patient and allows him to conceptualize and better understand observations about the patient. In assessing ego functions, object relationships, superego development, and internal conflicts, for example, the therapist makes considered judgements not only about how he will respond to the patient, but also about how to assist others in their therapeutic interactions. All patients do not require the same treatment, but they do require the commitment of the therapist to a conceptual model that includes the concept that they can be understood. Therefore, while the orientation of the therapist may differ from that espoused here, as long as it is consistently maintained, the patient has the potential of benefitting from the efforts of the therapist. The therapist must believe and thereby help patients believe that it is possible, with therapy, to make better sense of their feelings, thoughts, perceptions, and life.

In the psychotherapeutic process, the therapist needs, at times, to "educate" patients on how to work in therapy. Patients need to understand that all their communications can be used by the therapist to assist them in learning about themselves and to work toward making changes. Following a psychoanalytic orientation, Wilson (1986, p.100) notes, "In that model, certain procedures and conditions were established to facilitate free association and the uncovering and interpretation of unconscious conflicts." While these procedures are not applicable to many adolescent patients seen in a hospital setting, patients can be helped to understand that there is much that is hidden from them in their minds. The therapist can assist patients to learn how to reach that hidden part of themselves and the potential value in doing so.

Patients particularly need reassurance regarding the value of expressing their feelings toward the therapist as part of the treatment process. It is especially important that the patient be provided with a therapeutic atmosphere where anger can be expressed toward the therapist. Some therapists may have difficulty in tolerating the adolescent patient's anger. This difficulty can be a major interference in the psychotherapeutic work due to countertransference implications and because the therapist has implicitly disavowed the value of honesty in the process. If anything, the therapist must be scrupulously honest if the patient is to be able to develop trust in the therapist and the process. If the patient is to accept our "education" about how to work in psychotherapy, we must help the patient feel safe regardless of what may emerge, even if it is rage toward the therapist.

It is especially important in the treatment of adolescents in a hospital setting, that the safety of all members of the community be maintained. A cardinal principle of all inpatient treatment is that it cannot go forward if the patient experiences fear of being harmed or poses a threat to the physical safety of others. The primary responsibility for maintaining a safe milieu usually rests with the nursing staff. However, it is essential that the psychotherapist clearly communicate to the patient that threats to the physical safety of anyone are unacceptable. The therapist must be clear not only in lending support and authority to the nursing staff in their endeavors to maintain a safe milieu, but also in taking any necessary action with the patient. This includes clearly stating the value and necessity for safety as well as providing the assessed level of external controls or restrictions. If the therapist expects patients to be able to engage in the painful and difficult work of relaxing their defensive armor to allow that which is hidden to be seen, the therapist must be an active participant in keeping the patients and all others safe.

TECHNICAL CONSIDERATIONS

Where and When

Structural issues are important in psychotherapy. A clear schedule of when therapy will take place and the length of each therapy session should be articulated. It is particularly important for the therapist to maintain the commitment to the scheduled appointments, making clear to the patient that the therapist will continue to be available for the designated time even when the patient refuses to attend or remain in the session. This communicates to the patient a commitment to him and to the value of the sessions and usually helps the patient who believes he will be rejected because of his feelings. This is of special importance with those patients who feel they have been rejected or abandoned by their parents and are left experiencing themselves as worthless or unlovable.

Whenever possible, a consistent setting should be used for all sessions. It is not advisable to see patients in their bedrooms on the unit as this represents a crossing of an important boundary. The patient's room, as it symbolizes the self, must not be used for therapy since the patient's right to privacy must not be compromised. The patient's right to withhold and keep secrets from the therapist must also be honored. This is not to say this behavior will not be addressed in therapy, but the integrity of the psychotherapeutic process is maintained when the therapist does not coerce the patient into revealing that which the patient feels unwilling to disclose.

> Kris was an 18-year-old hospitalized for the fifth time in one year. Each hospitalization was precipitated by violent outbursts, including uncontrolled rage and destruction. Her current hospitalization was precipitated by her breaking the door to her room, doing significant damage to her belongings, and by a suicide gesture of cutting her arms. Her adoptive parents needed the help of the police in order to get her to the hospital. Kris was adopted, along with three younger siblings, when she was seven years of age. When she was three, she was removed from her mother's custody due to physical abuse by her stepfather and she lived in a Catholic shelter until she was adopted. A prior adoption was unsuccessful when the potential adoptive parent was unable to deal with the then six-year-old Kris's out-of-control behavior.
>
> During this hospitalization, the first several therapy sessions followed a repetitive pattern. Kris was seen in an interview room on her unit. Soon after the therapy session began, Kris would become enraged, scream at the therapist, dart out of the room, run down the hall and enter the Quiet Room. Her therapist would follow her to the Quiet Room and, while standing outside the room, advise her that this was still her therapy time and he would remain in the interview room if she chose to return. Despite multiple expletives directed to the therapist by Kris, he expressed his hope that she would change her mind and be able to resume her therapy. Several minutes later, Kris would return to the therapy session. After several repetitions of this pattern, Kris was able to maintain herself throughout the therapy session. Interestingly, she repeated the same process during her last session prior to discharge from the hospital.

There are times when the reality of hospital work introduces emergencies that interfere with a therapist being available at the scheduled therapy time. It is important that the therapist make up these times. Patients should be given the opportunity to discuss feelings about the cancellation. The therapist need not feel defensive or guilty, even when patients defend against their own feelings by attempting to induce guilt in the therapist. At these times, it is important to make clear that the therapist is there to help the patient make changes, but this does not mean that the therapist relinquishes reality in order to do so. In this instance, the reality is that the therapist and patient are part of the hospital system and that there are requirements that the system places on both. These are times when the therapist can make use of here and now experiences to bring feelings from the past into the therapy process and thereby make these feelings available for the work at hand.

Resistance

Resistance is a normal part of psychotherapeutic work with adolescents. O'Malley (1990, p.16) notes that there are ". . . three distinct sources of resistance to forming an alliance. . .(1) the adolescent's perception that hospitalization is coercive because it is empowered by adults, (2) the normal adolescent revulsion against passivity and dependence, and (3) the psychopathology of the disturbed adolescent which heightens the reaction to separation from the parents and containment in the hospital." Holmes (1964, p.204) states, "The theoretical purpose of the analytic interpretation is to help the patient understand how, and why he protects himself from becoming aware of certain unconscious wishes, what they are, and how they affect his life. In general, his need to keep them out of his mind stems from the loss of self-respect which would result from his acknowledging them as belonging to him." Rinsley (1980, p.7) discusses the severely disturbed hospitalized adolescent's resistance maneuvers as an ". . . attempt to neutralize efforts. . . to engage him in a therapeutic process."

Rinsley also describes a number of resistance mechanisms including: "*Identification with the aggressor.* The patient in various ways attempts to imitate the adults' behavior, in an 'as-if' effort to ward off the latter. *Leveling.* The patient attempts to make siblings or peers of the treatment figures . . . . *Flirtatiousness and seductiveness.* The patient attempts to sexualize the relationship with treatment figures. *Persistent avoidance.* More frequent among the most seriously ill adolescents, persistent avoidance includes frank negativism, muteness, seclusiveness . . ., and the like. *Scapegoatism.* Includes such phenomena as denigration or vilification of ward peers . . . and efforts to manipulate wardmates into proxy roles by which the peer acts out for the subject . . . *Elopement.* Running away is a complex, overdetermined phenomenon, connected with all sorts of aggressive, erotic, rescue and reunion fantasies" (Rinsley, 1980, p.115-117).

It is important for the psychotherapist to respect the patient's resistances. These resistances, while often experienced as mobilized against the therapist, serve as defenses for patients against discovery of their internal world. The general opposition of the disturbed adolescent against adults serves well as part of the resistance evidenced in the psychotherapeutic process. The responsibility of the therapist is to recognize the characterologic defenses manifested in the specific resistances used by the patient and to assist the patient in recognizing these mechanisms. The therapist's work is to help the patient reduce externalizations and begin the arduous process of recognizing internal conflicts. We would then think of resistance as the mechanisms the adolescent patient uses to keep repressed feelings and thoughts not out the therapist's consciousness but, out of his own. It is important that psychotherapists recognize the painful and difficult work asked of the patient. Treatment and change are not easy, particularly since many of these patients have already experienced severely disturbed relationships within their own families. If we consider that, regardless of diagnosis, we are asking patients to relinquish behaviors, attitudes, feelings, and thoughts they have maintained for long periods of time, we can better respect and understand their resistances.

> Fourteen-year-old Mary had had multiple hospitalizations. All were precipitated by increasingly dangerous self-destructive behaviors, including alcohol abuse, runaways from home, and overt suicide attempts. Her father had made two suicide attempts, had been hospitalized, and was currently in outpatient treatment. He reported to his therapist his continuing suicidal feelings, as well as feeling he should kill Mary so she would not have the same unhappy life he had experienced. In the hospital treatment milieu, Mary constantly manipulated the rules and continually kept herself focused on everything except her feelings about and fear of her father. This process continued until one therapy session when she entered the office and sat in the chair usually occupied by the therapist. When questioned about this, her initial response was to minimize the significance of her behavior. She then became righteously indignant and asked if the therapist would prefer her to sit on the floor. Finally, she acted as if the therapist were upset himself because he preferred the chair in which she was sitting.
>
> The therapist did not directly respond to these evidences of her resistance but, instead suggested that there was something that could be learned from her choice of chairs. After a brief

silence, the therapist wondered if perhaps she would feel more comfortable if she were the therapist and he the patient. Mary's therapist next suggested this situation might be analogous to how she was managing her treatment in the hospital by actively keeping her attention on many external issues so that she could keep away from the feelings that were upsetting her. In later sessions, Mary was able to discuss feeling responsible for her father's suicide attempts and her fear that she would upset him further if she were to change how she related to him.

Reality in Treatment

Psychotherapy of the hospitalized adolescent, in contrast with outpatient work, brings two important issues to the forefront. First is the amount of information available to the therapist about the patient and second is the increased visibility of the therapist to the patient. Inpatient work provides the therapist a great deal of information about the patient from sources other than the patient or family. Unless the therapist uses this information carefully, it can result in a source of interference in the psychotherapeutic process. As noted earlier, the patient's right to withhold from the therapist needs to be honored. How and when material emerges in psychotherapy are important for the understanding of the development of transference and its manifestations in the therapeutic process. On the other hand, it is equally important that the therapist not hide behind a cloak of neutrality in the interest of the therapeutic process. For example, if the patient has tried to hurt himself or to run away from the hospital, he is well aware that his therapist has been informed. How the therapist uses this information when meeting with the patient is determined by the therapist's understanding of the patient's functioning. Generally, it is useful to wait and listen. If the patient does not introduce the event, then the therapist should, since it is reasonable and appropriate to discuss such important events. Not to do so conveys to the patient that the therapist and treatment team do not take him seriously. Reality needs to be registered if the patient is to see therapy as being valid and honest.

However, there are times when the patient uses reality as a defense, such as when the patient continually focuses on external events to provide a rationalization for his behavior and his difficulty in making changes. The therapist can easily become entrapped in the patient's clever manipulations, unconsciously colluding with the patient's defenses. This use of reality as defense is particularly resistive to the therapist's interventions and therefore the therapist must be especially careful in addressing this aspect of the patient's presentation. On the other hand, the therapist must frequently confront and clarify the patient's distortions of reality. While we generally look for improved functioning in work and the capacity to develop age-appropriate and mutually satisfying relationships as signs of improvement, we may also consider increasingly successful adaptation to reality as another measure of improvement.

A significant issue on inpatient units relates to the patient's frequent complaints about one or another member of the staff. Complaints may also be about an injustice the patient feels has been done to him. The patient may demand a response from the therapist regarding his complaint. Usually the patient will want the therapist to side with him against the staff or, sometimes, with the staff against the patient. The therapist need not respond to these demands. Furthermore, despite the patient's insistence, the therapist need not enter into discussion of the specific situation. This does not mean that there may not actually be some basis for the patient's feelings. Rather, the job for the therapist is to help the patient explore the meaning of this particular issue as it relates to his internal struggles. The work in psychotherapy is always to help the patient to learn more about himself. This does not deny the reality that, in fact, everything in the world is not perfect, including people. The problem for the patient is how to integrate this knowledge of reality with the ability to develop and maintain satisfying relationships. To place this concept in theoretic terms, there is the need to integrate the "good" and "bad" object as part of the development of mature object relationships. Translated into the work of psychotherapy, the therapist then needs to continually listen to the patient's communications as messages about himself, his perceptions of others, and his struggles to develop and maintain satisfactory relationships.

As noted previously, closed-staff, inpatient hospital treatment programs make the therapist more visible to the adolescent patient. This does not necessarily interfere with the psychotherapeutic process. It does require the therapist to be discreet in talking with other staff about personal matters, particularly in open areas on the patient unit. The therapist need not allow the patient to be unduly familiar, as this can encourage the use of "leveling" by the patient. The therapist should not, as in any psychotherapy, disclose personal information to the patient. However, it is usually best that the therapist act naturally while on the unit. Surprisingly, the quality and intensity of transferential feelings and thoughts develop in the hospital much the same as in outpatient psychotherapy.

Acting Out

The therapist must make clear to the patient the unacceptability of any acting out. Acting out is viewed as a means of discharging anxiety and tension. However, both are needed if the patient is to be able to engage in the treatment process. The therapist must confront, when necessary, the patient's acting out since it is a major source of interference to the psychotherapeutic process. The therapist needs to maintain a clear understanding of the patient's pathological behaviors, ideas, or thoughts. There cannot be implicit approval given to the patient by the therapist when these behaviors or thoughts are presented. The therapist must determine when interventions, that is, interpretations of the behavior, might best be made within the context of the psychotherapeutic process. However, acting out is most usefully confronted as it occurs. Only then will the patient ever be able to cease the repetition of the acting out and bring it under more conscious control. At these times, the psychotherapist, as a member and often leader of the patient's treatment team, needs to make use of the treatment milieu in setting limits and imposing restrictions. This is not contrary to maintaining a treatment alliance with the patient, but is essential to maintain the alliance, which has as its focus helping the patient to change.

A particularly difficult issue with many adolescent inpatients is their "need" to bang walls with their fists when they are angry, sad, or in some other way feeling intense affects. When confronted about this behavior, the patient's typical response is "At least I am not hurting anyone." Obviously, this is not true and the patient needs to be told that, in fact, he is hurting himself. This does not mean that the therapist can now safely assume that the patient will stop this behavior. It does mean that the therapist has made explicit expectations of change and that the safety of the patient is part of the therapist's concern for him.

> Richard was a 17-year-old admitted to the hospital because of continued deterioration in his functioning at school and at home. He was an adopted child and knew that his mother was a Native American and his father of Dutch background. He was also aware that his mother had abandoned him, which eventually led to his adoption. It was his belief that his mother had abused alcohol. While in the hospital, he disclosed his own alcohol abuse.
>
> As treatment progressed, he became able to show more feeling, but would do so by going into the Quiet Room to scream and beat the walls with his fists. After this behavior had

occurred several times, Richard entered a therapy session and advised his therapist that he was feeling hurt because his girl friend had rejected him. He continued to tell his therapist he would need to use the Quiet Room that night to get out his feelings. Richard was expecting praise from his therapist but was both surprised and angry when he was told that it was not necessary for him to do this. He was told we could know he was feeling hurt without his further hurting himself. Richard was able to express his anger at the therapist as well as his wish to strike him. He was then able to relate his anger to his feeling that he could never please his father. Richard did not use the Quiet Room that night.

This case illustrates an important aspect for the rationale for confrontation and disapproval of the adolescent's acting out. Children are dependent upon adults and, save for the minority with the most severely disturbed object relationships, want to do what they feel will meet with parental approval. As psychotherapists, while we respect the patient's freedom to reject our help and we endeavor to maintain the appropriate therapeutic neutrality, we must also present patients with reasonable expectations for their behavior. This is not so they will know how to please us, but ultimately to allow them to please themselves as they are able to achieve their goals.

Transference and Countertransference

With adolescents, and especially with those who require hospital treatment, the complications inherent in transference and countertransference may be difficult for the therapist to manage. In contrast to the adult outpatient with contact limited to the therapist's office, the adolescent inpatient has frequent contacts with the therapist outside of the designated psychotherapy sessions. This leads to both greater familiarity and to the increased reality of the patient's dependence on the therapist for privileges of one sort or another. For the patient to see the therapist as someone who has power is not of necessity a representation of a transference from feelings toward a parent. Generally, adolescents have difficulty in acknowledging their feelings about their therapists. This is particularly true for positive feelings because these patients often have great fear of closeness. The troubled adolescent, however, is generally more comfortable displaying rage and anger.

In general, the therapist needs to be judicious in making transference interpretations, but should not be reticent in recognizing when the patient is evidencing transferential feelings and thoughts. Often, the therapist needs to allow the patient to be rageful and angry and simply observe for the patient the expression of these affects without seeking to interpret the transferential meaning. The therapist should establish the rule early on in defining the treatment contract that the patient can say anything about the therapist, but attempts to harm the therapist or himself or to do damage to the office will not be allowed. It does not of necessity move the treatment forward when the patient is told that anger toward the therapist has to do with feelings about a parent. In fact, it is quite important that feelings be part of the psychotherapeutic process. Often, creating a feeling of safety for patients, where they discover that their anger and rage do not drive the therapist away, that their words do not destroy the therapist, and that the therapist does not retaliate, is more important then interpreting the transferential source of these feelings.

> Sarah was 15 when admitted to the hospital following a drug overdose suicide attempt. She had been abusing alcohol and drugs for some time and had been truant from school for about five months. Sarah had been adopted soon after birth and shortly after that her adoptive mother gave birth to a son. When Sarah was five, her adoptive parents separated, with the two children remaining with the mother. Her adoptive father maintained active involvement with his former wife and children. Sarah described him as passive, particularly in response to her mother, who was by this time abusing alcohol and engaging in abusive relationships with men. On one occasion, when Sarah was seven, she observed her mother being strangled by her drunken boyfriend. Mother had two psychiatric hospitalizations following suicide attempts, had remarried and separated, and was in recovery and active in Alcoholics Anonymous.
>
> For the first month of her therapy, it seemed all Sarah could do was rage at her therapist. She complained there was no need for her to be in the hospital and it was her therapist's fault that she had to stay. She insisted that she was not depressed as her therapist had diagnosed her and that, in fact, she had not made a suicide attempt. She bitterly complained when the therapist would look at her during sessions. The therapist usually listened and made a few observations about how angry she was, but did not acquiesce to her demands for discharge nor change the diagnosis. Gradually, the rage subsided as Sarah continued to work in psychotherapy. As she was nearing discharge from the hospital, she shared with her therapist how much it had

helped her to have her initial anger tolerated. Sarah felt she would not have been able to move forward in her treatment if she had not felt safe and reassured when her therapist did not retaliate nor even seem upset by her rage.

Therapists may be more vulnerable to countertransference issues in their work with hospitalized adolescents than with other patient groups. Sometimes, therapists identify with the anger and rebelliousness of the adolescent and their failure to address the patient's opposition to authority seriously compromises their value to the patient. In some cases, the therapist has difficulty saying "no" to the patient because of the belief that this would interfere with the therapeutic process. In fact, failure to provide adequate supervision interferes with the process as the patient may lose trust in a therapist who approves of the patient doing anything he wishes. The other side of this issue is that the therapist needs to be aware of the adolescent's need for gratification. The therapist must carefully assess when and to what degree he should gratify the patient, keeping in mind that too much gratification leads to tension reduction, while too little leaves the patient feeling that he cannot please the therapist. However, withholding from the patient may for the therapist be dynamically related to the countertransferential inability to say no.

Adolescent patients often defend themselves by trying to induce guilt in others. Therapists need to be particularly alert to this dynamic and sensitive to their own feelings. Therapists need to alert themselves when they begin to feel guilt or anger toward a patient. Usually, this means the patient has struck a sensitive chord and it behooves the therapist to engage in some introspective work to prevent any acting out of the countertransference. Besides asking oneself why this is happening, it is also helpful in learning more about the patient to not only recognize the defense but also to consider why it occurs at this time in the treatment process. That is, the therapist begins with the hypothesis that the patient intended the therapist to experience the particular affect. The next question would be why? What does this tell me, for example, about the nature of the patient's object relationships? Or, is the patient trying to create distance in the service of defending against insight or an interpretation? In short, the therapist's feelings are then considered not solely as reflecting countertransference, but also as part of the therapeutic process.

Another potential source of countertransferential difficulty for the therapist is when the patient does not seem to be improving or the rate of improvement is not within the expectations set by the therapist or the third-party payor. When the therapist feels there is a limited time to accomplish long-term treatment goals, his frustration may be directed at the patient. The therapist must be aware of this and not try to do in one month what would otherwise require a year. Psychotherapists need to sense that they are valued and appreciated and are competent in their work. If the therapist relies on receiving this approbation from the adolescent patient, he is in trouble and it may be wise for the therapist to consult a colleague, obtain supervision, or enter psychotherapy.

Meaning and Hope

The severely disturbed adolescent has particular difficulty in believing there is meaning to his behaviors, words, thoughts, and feelings. A major feature of the therapeutic process is the therapist's continued efforts to demonstrate to the patient that it is possible to find meaning. The patient defensively denies but also truly see no meaning to his or her angst. The therapist observes and makes observations and interpretations, but even the most benign of these are usually rejected. At times, the therapist may get into an argument with the patient in the effort to demonstrate that there is significance and meaning to the patient's words, thoughts, and behavior. This by no means represents a breakdown in the therapeutic process. The therapist's give and take with the patient conveys not only respect, but also the message that the therapist cares enough to put this energy into the therapeutic process with the patient.

The therapist continually works to understand the patient's communications. Despite the patient's denial, the therapist must operate from the position that everything that is said or done has meaning. The therapist may help the patient learn where to look for answers. For example, whenever a feeling or attitude is expressed that represents one extreme of a continuum, it is useful for patient and therapist to look at the opposite end, for that is often where the conflict may well reside. Whatever the patient says or does not say in therapy needs to be understood, although the meaning may not be immediately available. Sometimes, the meaning may relate to aspects of the personality organization, the patient's defenses, and/or the nature of the patient's internal conflicts. The meaning may also relate to the dynamic issues with which the patient struggles and/or to the content of the patient's thoughts and fantasies. Often, the meaning may touch on all these variables.

The pursuit of understanding and meaning in the patient's communication is not merely in the service of the therapist's intellectual curiosity. As stated earlier, it is to help patients make sense of themselves. Adolescent patients, in particular, seem to be afflicted with nihilism. It seeps through their pores and contributes to their anger and dread of life. They continue to act as if life has no meaning or value, compounding each self-destructive act with another. They deny their fear of living by putting their lives in danger in both subtle and obvious ways. By the time they enter the hospital, many are full of hopelessness. The first challenge the therapist faces is to help the patient to believe that entering into the treatment relationship may bring him hope once again. The therapist cannot promise that the work will be without pain just as the therapist cannot promise that the future will be without pain. What the therapist can offer is the hope that the patient will be able to make some sense of himself and thereby feel more in charge of his life and, therefore, of himself.

SUMMARY

Basic concepts in the psychotherapy of the hospitalized adolescent were presented from a framework of psychoanalytic and object relations theory. The focus was on understanding the role of therapy in assisting patients in making change. Emphasis was placed on the therapist maintaining a consistent framework of understanding in determining treatment interventions. The need for safety in the treatment milieu was stressed, as well as the need for the therapist to participate in maintaining a safe milieu. Technical considerations included discussions of where and when, resistance, the role of reality in treatment, acting out, transference and countertransference, and the importance of meaning and hope for the adolescent patient.

REFERENCES

Anthony, E. J. (1991). The therapeutic matrix in the inpatient treatment of the adolescent. In R. L. Hendren & I. N. Berlin (Ed.), *Psychiatric inpatient care of children and adolescents: A multicultural approach.* (pp. 194–206). New York: John Wiley & Sons, Inc.

Errera, P. & Levine, I. (1990). Teaching residents to recognize administrative issues in clinical situations. *Psychiatric Quarterly, 61,* 87–95.

Holmes, D. J. (1964). *The adolescent in psychotherapy.* Boston: Little, Brown and Company.

O'Malley, F. (1990). Developing a therapeutic alliance in the hospital treatment of disturbed adolescents. *Bulletin of the Menninger Clinic, 54,* 13–24.

Rinsley, D. B. (1980). *Treatment of the severely disturbed adolescent.* New York: Jason Aronson, Inc.

Wilson, P. (1986). Individual psychotherapy in a residential setting. In D. Steinberg (Ed.), *The adolescent unit* (pp. 97–111). New York: John Wiley & Sons.

Chapter 4

GROUP PSYCHOTHERAPY SETTING, STRUCTURE, AND PROCESS

Harinder S. Ghuman
and Erika E. Wilmoth

Adolescence is a stage in which the peer group exerts high, if not maximum, influence on an individual. Often, adolescent peer groups exert negative influence resulting in a variety of destructive behaviors. A vital task of the inpatient staff is not only to channel group influence in a constructive manner, but also to curtail negative-destructive acting out. Methods employed to accomplish this include various verbal interventions, such as group psychotherapy, community meetings, and identity groups, to name but a few. Physical group activities, including therapeutic camping and recreational and occupational activities have also proven to be extremely beneficial in promoting a more cohesive community. The scope of this chapter is to cover group psychotherapy and to some extent community meetings. Various other group activities will be covered in other sections of this book.

INDICATIONS AND CONTRAINDICATIONS OF GROUP PSYCHOTHERAPY

Various authors have written about indications and contraindications to group psychotherapy. Buxbaum (1945) described the violent swings from rebellion to submission taking place in an adolescent group. In his view, giving the adolescent a chance to both submit and revolt alternatively is one of the characteristics that make the group therapy structure indispensable for the adolescent. Berkovitz and Sugar (1986, p.6) mentioned that group therapy may afford an opportunity to open an individual's mind to the fuller appreciation of, and, hopefully, reduction of blocks to warm, honest, nonexploitative relationships with others. These authors tried to quantify the degree of indications for group therapy into absolute, relative, or minimal. Under the absolute indications was included "adolescent so well defended against therapeutic relationship, that only in a peer group or network group can there be any significant confrontation, introspection or interaction with therapist or peers." The minimal degree of indications included adolescents who related to an adult therapist fairly well, but might defy or withhold at times. The relative indications lay somewhere in between the above two categories.

Rinsley (1972) discussed usefulness of group experiences in a hospital milieu. He noted that, attentively conducted and properly structured, a group that met directly in the patient living area served to minimize the clinical/administrative splits which an adolescence will often exploit for fear of self-revelation, and may thus supply a motivation for treatment. Blaustein and Wolff (1972) found that friction decreased between adolescents and staff, and adolescent and adult patients after a small group therapy for teenagers was conducted on a mixed (adolescent and adult) ward. Groups helped to lessen stress related to intimacy and enabled group members to communicate without the use of drugs as a crutch. Grold (1972) described a decrease in destructive behavior and testing of limits as a positive result of group experience. Mordock, Ellis and Greenstone (1969) wrote how group therapy experience improved interpersonal relationship to a greater extent than did individual therapy. Berkovitz and Sugar (1966) emphasized how groups were useful in maturing sexual attitudes and how group therapy was a way of increasing therapeutic contact with patients who were resistant in individual casework.

It is possible, that, at any given time, a patient or number of patients can be excluded from the group on a temporary basis. For example, a severely psychotic or violent patient who is constantly disruptive or who clearly demonstrates the potential to be a danger to the group may be excluded from participation until better control is achieved. However, even in such cases, sometimes a group experience can be very useful to the patient as he has the opportunity to hear peer reactions, experience confrontation, and receive needed support. The authors have seen acutely disturbed, violent, or self-destructive patients attend group therapy sessions while restrained in a cold wet-sheet pack. On these occasions, the patient was able to hear what peers had to say without the fear of losing control. Additionally, the peer group felt safe in providing their input regarding the patient's condition without fear of harm due to the patient's retaliation.

GROUP THERAPY SETTINGS AND STRUCTURE

All inpatient therapies, including group therapies, are currently in a state of flux due to a tendency toward shorter hospital stays governed largely by financial considerations rather than by clinical needs. Nevertheless, group therapy continues to be an important treatment modality. Group therapies can arbitrarily be divided into three categories:

1. *Short-term groups* are run on hospital units in which the average length of stay is up to two or three weeks. The group goals are limited and the focus is directed toward behavioral correction, problem-solving enhancement, use of peer pressure to control acting out on the unit, quick abreaction of traumatic events, and crisis intervention.
2. *Long-term groups* are conducted in long-term hospital units or residential inpatient treatment centers. The adolescent may be in this group for one to one and a half years or longer. Here, group goals are more intrapsychically focused. In addition to many goals similar to those for short-term groups, there are observable stages of group development (Powles, 1959 a,b; Westman, 1960). Although some of the above goals under A are also included in this type of group, the focus remains on issues of resistance, transference, and development of insight. The desired outcome in this setting is to have the individuals in the group make needed changes in their personality structure.
3. *Intermediate groups* lie between A and B. These group settings are largely in hospital and some residential inpatient settings. The adolescent is in group for three to six months and has specific goals pertaining to areas mentioned in both A and B.

Various authors have written about group therapy structure and setting. Some of the questions that have been raised are related to: (1) age; (2) sex; (3) number of patients and therapists in a group; and (4) where and how often to hold the group, and what, if any, rules and limits are enforced in the group.

Age

Age ranges can be divided into early (13-14 years), middle (15-16 years), and late adolescence (16-19 years). If there is a large enough population and a sufficient number of treatment units to be divided according to these age ranges, one can have three different age groups. For practical purposes, it may be useful to have two age-range groups, one from 13-16 and another from 15-18; those 15-16 years old can be placed in either group, depending upon maturity level. These age ranges are not completely arbitrary, and should serve as a guideline. Strict adherence to a specific chronological age is not necessary, as each adolescent situation should be individually assessed. For example, in a co-ed group it may be useful to have older boys along with females a year or so younger when one takes into consideration the developmental differences of adolescent males and females. However, the purpose of grouping patients according to age is based on different developmental tasks and activities. Younger adolescents are more activity-oriented and less verbal. If a 13-year-old is placed in a group of 18-year-olds, the 13-year-old may not be able to adjust to the current peer group. Additionally, staff may set unreasonable and unrealistic goals and expectations for the patient. Sugar (1986) states that adolescent groups should be designed so as to have no more than a three year gap between two members. Younger adolescents may require a nonverbal style of communication and may, for example, be encouraged to bring their writings or drawings to group for the purpose of exploration and communication enhancement.

Sex

Sugar (1986) suggested that 12- to 14-year-olds be placed in groups of their own sex. At this stage of adolescence, the inclination is to avoid the other sex because of a revived oedipal conflict with incestuous fears and wishes; these adolescents needed to figure out what was going on with themselves. The middle and late adolescents can be grouped together as far as gender issue. Ackerman (1955) and Boenheim (1957) suggested that the presence of both sexes provokes material otherwise dormant or latent. Schulman (1959) thought that the adolescent's ability to handle sexual problems is enhanced in mixed groups. It is our opinion that a mixed group sensitizes the adolescents toward each other's needs and helps them deal with sexual prejudices and stereotyping.

Number of Patients and Therapists

It may be useful to involve all the patients on an adolescent unit in one group to develop cohesiveness on the unit and work out interpersonal conflicts. Limiting the group to eight to 10 may also prove more beneficial so as to provide sufficient time allotments in which to discuss the individual members' agenda. Combining patients from two units can result in a more objective overview in addition to enabling the patients to look beyond their individual unit's particular issues (Ghuman & Sarles, 1989).

Several authors have written on the usefulness of having multiple therapists in group therapy for adolescents. Kassoff (1958) stated that the tremendous emotional demands of such deprived boys are really too great for one therapist. Adler, Bermen and Slavson (1960) reported the use of dual leadership which combined authoritative and nonauthoritative representation as a key factor in their project. Ghuman and Sarles (1989) emphasized the importance of multiple therapists and several nursing staff participating in an adolescent group while simultaneously incorporating the three phases of group work on an adolescent unit. However, Yalom (1983) wrote critically of the use of multiple leaders for an adult inpatient group.

Where to Hold Group; Rules and Limits

It is most beneficial to conduct the group in a room on the unit with ample space, sturdy comfortable furniture, sufficient lighting, and minimal sound distractions. If group is held away from the unit, highly disturbed patients may not be able to attend due to potential for violence and safety risks in returning to the unit. It may also be difficult for nursing staff to attend sessions away from the unit due to limited number of staff. Rules regarding eating, drinking, and smoking during the group, or leaving the group to go to the bathroom must be articulated. In general, it is useful to keep these activities to a minimum. With younger adolescents, one may need to take a more flexible approach; however, it is useful to encourage the group to take care of personal needs prior to or after group therapy.

There are various views regarding the management of authority issues. Thorpe and Smith (1952) suggested that the therapist's role should be characterized by warmth, understanding, and permissive disidentification from institutional authority. In contrast, Shellow, Ward and Rubenfeld (1958) emphasized the need for limit-setting by the therapist. They recommend the dismissal of members or the entire group for a session if their acting out reaches disruptive proportions and they write disciplinary reports for destruction of property or violation of rules. It is our opinion that, in general, it is useful to state expectations that group members respect each other and that abusive, threatening behavior is unacceptable. If a group member is extremely agitated or disruptive, he/she has the option to go to the quiet room in an effort to help de-escalate and regain control. Along with the group expectations, consequences for violating group rules, such as losing a permission level, losing points, or receiving a fine, should be articulated. Punctuality and confidentiality should also be emphasized to encourage an environment more conducive to goal achievement and building of trust.

Enhancing group participation is essential. Bardill (1977) has described a successful behavior contracting program of group treatment for early adolescents in a residential setting. Behavioral approaches that include a point system and privileges can be useful in attracting the adolescent's attention to promote active participation in group therapy. Beitel et al (1983) wrote about experiences with the "Hub" group which utilized a merger of behavior, psychodynamic, and humanistic approaches.

ON GROUP THERAPY PROCESS AND TECHNIQUE

The observations discussed here are derived from the opportunity to conduct group therapy on an adolescent inpatient setting for over 12 years. The group met three times a week for 50 minutes and used a psychodynamic approach. Some of the issues that we believe occur frequently in group therapy are discussed in the following sections.

Issues of Trust and Confidentiality

Experienced therapists are aware of the important role trust plays in group therapy. In an ongoing inpatient group, issues of trust and confidentiality invariably arise. These include, but are not limited to, the addition of a new patient or therapist to the group, disclosure of some important events by group members, and, at times, the issue of trust or confidentiality being used by group members to derail or stop the group process. It is the therapist's duty to evaluate issues of trust as they surface and to explore and discuss methods of enhancing or regaining trust in a time-effective manner. There are times when even after long exploration a member or members may continue to be unable to trust sufficiently to talk about themselves. The therapist and the group may then need to identify the concern at all times, respect the group member's wish for confidentiality, and wait until a level of comfort exists to allow disclosure. Prior to moving on, however, the reluctant members should be informed by either the group or the therapist that the expectation is that eventually they will be able to discuss their issues in group. Reluctant members continue to bring up issues but refuse to explore them. The group should be encouraged to exert their influence on any group member to not make a habit of withholding information or delaying progress by using confidentiality or trust as an excuse.

Issues other than trust must be considered. For example, some patients do not want to experience painful affect and seek to avoid disclosure. Issues of distrust may also arise when members are fearful of others' reaction to information they may offer. In an inpatient setting, especially with the admission of a new patient, group members are often fearful of the extent to which a new patient may act out. For example, the admission of a very large, male patient with a history of physical and sexual violence increased the level of anxiety and distrust within the patient group and members expressed concern regarding their own safety, given the uncertainty of the new group member. A small female who had a history of sexual abuse cautiously asked this new patient if he would hurt her. The new patient denied any intention to hurt anyone and was also able to talk about his fears related to joining the group. This interaction proved to be very helpful to the new patient, as well as to other group members as it allowed the group to discuss their individual concerns and fears that would have potentially delayed group trust and cohesiveness. In addition, group members were given the opportunity to verbalize their concerns rather than acting them out in other ways such as negativity, open hostility, avoidance, withdrawal, and/or lack of attendance.

Silence and Overactivity

Ongoing groups go through periods ranging from very quiet to overly stimulated, depending upon the mix of patients and their progression in treatment. The therapist's role is to assist the group in providing an optimal therapeutic environment so that the work can continue. Often, silence and overactivity in group are observed when a difficult issue creates significant anxiety and intense affect. Once the polarity of these behaviors is pointed out, the therapist may enlist the group to effectively deal with the issue. Occasionally, patterns may develop in which vacillating periods of increased withdrawal/silences occur after several depressed and/or schizoid patients have entered the group at the same time. The therapist must actively engage these patients to help them emerge from their "shell" by directly asking them to participate or by focusing the group's attention toward them. In extreme situations, it may be useful to go from one member to another and ask that they share issues and goals they are working on for that day. At other times, the therapist may introduce an issue regarding a group member that has been noticed during the daily routine on the unit.

A group of patients we refer to as "paranoid narcissist" and "passive aggressive" may contribute to the group dysfunction, not necessarily due to their silence. These patients become easily hurt and are often fearful that the staff and therapist may harm them. They are sarcastic and unable to trust. The therapist needs to assist these patients in exploring and verbalizing issues surrounding trust and their feeling of being attacked. If their behavior becomes too disruptive or destructive, the therapist may have to actively confront their interference in the group's ability to work. Their grandiose sense of self needs to be actively deflated, but, at the same time, they must be provided support in maintaining whatever healthy ego function they possess.

There are groups in which too much occurs. Such situations are generally easier for the therapist to deal with in comparison to ongoing silent sessions. In dealing with overactive groups, the therapist may assist group members in briefly describing and prioritizing their issues at the onset of the group meeting. The therapist may direct the group to focus on issues not completely dealt with in a previous group. In overactive groups, patients may often be very needy and will do or say anything to gain attention. These patients are often characterized as "monopolizers," but we prefer to view them as "narcissistic attention-seekers" as they have been deprived physically and emotionally throughout their life. The therapist and group must jointly assist this type of patient in order to insure that optimal attention is received by all. The therapist should direct and support such a group while encouraging them to express their feeling in relation to deprivation and to the elements of competition they may be experiencing with others.

Reality versus Feelings, Needs, Wishes, and Fears

Often, in an inpatient setting, a group is subjected to behavioral disturbance by one or more members of the group. It is important for the therapist and peers to confront inappropriate behavior, encourage the group to control this behavior, and encourage the offending person to explore reasons for his or her behavior. There is another side to the behavior in which a patient's needs, wishes, fears, and feelings are hidden. One may not be able to help until a therapeutic balance is achieved by addressing both sides of the issue. It is often easier for a patient or patients to focus on the behavior. They may feel too vulnerable to discuss feelings, wishes, needs, and personal experiences. Anxiety and the fear of embarrassment and ridicule usually decrease the patient's ability to be open and spontaneous. The following is an example in which group members were encouraged to deal with a patient's behavior, as well as to explore what had promoted the behavior.

> In group, Kate, who had not been eating, had fainted recently and required treatment at a nearby hospital emergency room. She opened group therapy by stating that she had been very upset and angry at the nursing staff for ignoring her and wanted to hurt one particular staff member. Shawn asked her if she could tell what happened over the weekend. Kate talked about not eating and fainting. Robin asked if she had learned anything from this. Kate stated yes, that it "messed up her electrolytes." One of the therapists questioned if she really had learned anything. Kate talked about how she knew she could get brain damage or hurt herself badly, and that is why she had resumed eating. Several peers stated that Kate needed to take responsibility for herself or else she was going to get hurt and that only she could help herself get better. The second therapist intervened at this point to note that Kate had been doing well until the past two or three weeks and wondered if there were other issues affecting her.
>
> Hearing no response from the patient or other group members, the therapist explored the patient's concerns about discharge and the effects of her therapist's recent vacation on her. Kate stated she missed her therapist but knew the therapist had to have vacation some time. Several of her peers reiterated how a therapist has to go on vacation and Kate needed to take care of herself. One therapist stated that even though this seemed logical, from time to time a person may have some thoughts and feelings that are not logical. Kate stated she was angry when her therapist came back and she began having a problem with eating and felt the therapist did not care about her when she was told it was up to her to decide what to eat or not to eat. Prior to the therapist's vacation, Kate had felt comfortable discussing issues and felt that her therapist was the only person with whom she could talk regarding her eating problems.

Several peers again focused on Kate's behavior and on how unrealistic she was to believe that staff would spoon-feed her. The therapist stated how important peer feedback was, but it would be useful for the group to explore some of these illogical thoughts and feelings since several members had recently required staff intervention because of their own attack on staff. Robin admitted feeling embarrassed because she was having some "stupid" thoughts about her therapist. Kate stated her previous therapist had been very supportive, had told Kate that she cared about her, and had given things to her. Kate wished the new therapist would do the same, but she knew that the new therapist's approach was different. Several of the group members talked about how they were angry at times with staff and the therapist for not being real and for analyzing issues too much. Thus, in assisting Kate in exploring reasons behind her behavior and how unrealistic she had become, the therapist encouraged other members to identify their own issues which reflected similar aspects.

Resistance, Defenses, and Ambivalence

It may be difficult for group members and the therapist to decide how to deal effectively with group members who present issues to the group in an ambivalent manner. For example, one patient states he wants to talk about an important issue but does not trust the group and therefore is not able. The group and therapist must then have a clear understanding of the group process and decide whether there is really a trust issue in the group or if the patient is using this as a defense mechanism or a combination of both. If there is a trust issue, the therapist needs to help the group explore this. However, if the patient is using this as a defense, the therapist may need to push the patient toward further exploration of the defense and why it was utilized.

A 15-year-old female patient became quite agitated just prior to group and required the use of quiet room. Shortly after the group session began, the patient decided to come in and the group asked the patient what had happened. However, some of the group members felt she should talk, while the other members felt it was best to wait and let the patient decide when she felt comfortable about talking. In these situations, it is not uncommon for the patient to feel uncomfortable and reluctant to talk. As a group therapist, one can choose to push the patient and group members in a certain direction. It is possible that if the therapist does not push, the opportunity may be lost for the group to effectively work on certain issues. As a group therapist, one has to be more in tune than in individual therapy because of the number of patients and issues and the limited amount of time.

With this patient, the therapist decided to emphasize to the patient and the group that it seemed to be a difficult issue for her and the group needed to help support her. The group was also told that the therapist's observation or conclusion was derived from the patient's behavior, and that although she was upset in the quiet room, she had chosen to come to the group and, therefore, she must want to talk about this issue. The therapist's intervention enabled the group to address and clarify their collective ambivalence and achieve an effective resolution. The patient was then able to admit that she did want to talk, but was uncomfortable about what the group would think about her. Group members provided her with support and reassurance. The patient talked about an incident in which she had been sexually taken advantage by her cousin when she was eight years old. This issue had been suppressed due to its sensitive nature, but with increased trust and support by the therapist and group she was finally able to address it openly and begin the healing process.

It is useful for the therapist to ask the patient to be more specific about what he/she is talking about or to provide examples to enhance clarification and understanding. This can provide additional material and feelings to explore. The therapist needs to be aware that there are layers of resistances and memories. Often, a new therapist may be satisfied with the patient saying that he/she is upset, or depressed. There are patients who use defenses of intellectualization as well as psychiatric jargon to avoid painful issues. Crying and sometimes showing anger dramatically can be used as a specific defense, with the patient knowing that the professional often thinks this is an expression of feelings. The authors have seen patients who have used tissue after tissue to wipe their tears as if to show their feelings, yet inwardly nothing has changed. They may be trying to please other group members or the therapist, and at the same time distract others from their issues.

Acting out is a common defense mechanism used by adolescents in group therapy to avoid what may be frightening or uncomfortable. Group therapists need to be a mixture of authority figure and traditional therapist. One of the common defenses in group is for one member to start an argument with another. When a particular patient does not want to talk about sensitive issues, he may utter a provocative remark like, "I don't like anyone here; you're all jerks." If the group is not in tune or consists of too many narcissistic patients who act out defensively, the therapist needs to assist the group in redirecting and focusing on what the patient is trying to achieve by the provocative remarks. The therapist may also help the group focus on the group members' method of defense and resistance.

> For example, Lisa, a 16-year-old adopted female with a history of thyroid cancer, was in the hospital after demonstrating self-destructive behavior. During the hospitalization, the cancer reoccurred. Lisa became withdrawn and depressed, but didn't want to talk in group. She and the other group members had a great deal of difficulty dealing with this issue. She often provoked group members by saying she didn't trust them or want to be around them and would rather go to another place. She was defending feelings of hopelessness, abandonment, and fear of dying. The therapist had to consistently explore with the group what she was doing and what the group was doing with her. This enabled the patient and the group members to focus on her very intense, upsetting feelings.

As already mentioned, the group therapist has to remain an active leader, sometimes in the area of confrontation, but other times in setting limits on acting-out behavior in the group. At the same time, the therapist has to continue to encourage a particular patient or a number of patients to take a more active role in exploring their behavior.

> In a recent group meeting, Michael, who had been previously quite psychotic, again regressed. He demonstrated his difficulty by becoming confused and expressed suicidal jokes (thoughts). To add to this patient's stressors, his mother had broken her arm and his therapist was away on vacation. The group members tried to ask him what was going on. He started calling his roommate a faggot, thus provoking him to anger. The group members were quite perceptive about the issues involved. When they pointed out that his behavior might in some way be related to his mother's sickness, Michael again started calling his peers names.
>
> The therapist intervened to "fine" this patient for abusive language and at the same time made a comment that Michael had been able to handle things much better in the past and

seemed to be experiencing a great deal of difficulty at this time. The patient was encouraged to try and verbalize what was making him so upset now. He called the therapist names and was again "fined." The group had to end. In the next group meeting Michael apologized for his behavior and was able to talk about how he felt sad about his mother and abandoned by his therapist. The group members, at first, were very anxious and made remarks like, "Why do we have to have group," but when it was pointed out that perhaps they might be experiencing some uncomfortable feelings from the last group meeting, they were able to talk and encourage Michael to focus on his issues.

Adolescents often look up to therapists for support in confronting each other's problems. This support may be necessary due to the adolescent's inexperience, negative peer pressure, and as a face saving device. It is also useful to visualize group therapy going through three phases, i.e., acting out, working through, and resolution (Ghuman & Sarles, 1989). One can observe these phases at times in one group session and at other times it may take several sessions.

For example, in one group meeting three patients reported having a very difficult day. One of them, James, looked very angry and sullen, reporting he was having a "shitty day." Chris, who had missed the last group session because she was in seclusion at the time, asked these three patients how they were doing and moved from one to another. At last, she asked James what was going on with him. James continued to pout, and several of his peers who were sitting next to him stated James was not ready to talk and everyone knew why he was upset. The therapist, as well as some peers, questioned this, but their questions were ignored.

Later, James stated he was upset because his girlfriend and his best friend were "screwing" each other, and if he was out of here he would slash them. He went on to say, in a threatening tone, if he were not in the hospital everything would be all right and his stepfather would not be in jail. The therapist pointed out to the group that it seemed to be a very difficult issue for James to talk about. Ross sitting next to James became more friendly toward him and accused the therapist of causing problems, always analyzing and making a big thing out of nothing. James became more threatening and talked about what would happen if he were to throw the table at the therapist's head. The patient was warned by the therapist

about his threatening behavior and was told that if he continued to threaten, he might have to leave the group and go to the
quiet room until he could regain his control.

James was encouraged to look at what specifically was
bothering him. The group members were also encouraged to
express their feelings about James' behavior. Kerri, who had
been abused in the past, stated James would never hurt his
peers. James mimicked what she said. The therapist asked
Kerri does it mean that James would hurt others, like the
therapist or staff. Kerri again stated she was not worried about
getting hurt, and if James did hurt staff that was something they
deserved. The therapist confronted Kerri about her asking
James to act out, and wondered if she, too, was angry at staff
for other reasons. Kerri said people who work with mental
patients should expect this to happen. The therapist informed
the group that the safety of patients and staff is of the utmost
importance and no treatment can go on if patients and staff do
not feel safe. This statement seemed to reassure some of the
group members who had been fearful of James. Some of the
peers were then able to confront James and talked about their
fear of him. They also talked about times in the past when they
had acted out because they didn't know how to express their
fears and hurt feelings openly. Chris looked anxious and stated
that it was hard for her to hear about hurt feelings, and she
would rather go off.

In the second session, one of the group members started
talking about how he liked to talk about some issues but felt no
one would support him. He also felt that everyone was selfish
and centered only on themselves. Two other peers from the
group joined in saying how they recently had been trying to
keep themselves away from others. One of them stated that
since new peers had joined the unit, she had more friends
outside the unit than on the unit. Kerri, who had been negative
in the last group meeting, then said things were going such that,
if not talked about, no one would be able to get any help.
James, who had been threatening in the last group, got up and
said he knew what this peer was saying and wanted to bring
something from his room. James returned from his room with
a great deal of contraband and placed it on the table in the
middle of the group. Ross, who had been sitting next to James
and had been supportive of him in the last group, pulled
contraband from his pants pocket and also placed it on the
table. The group looked very tense and shocked into silence.
James looked at the therapist and stated that he was not worried
about the restrictions he would get. Group members and the

therapist supported James. Several group members stated that James bringing contraband to the group made them respect him more. James looked embarrassed but happy at the response. Group members talked about how they knew what was going on but were afraid to confront James and Ross as they did not want to lose their friendship. The group seemed much closer and less tense.

COMMUNITY/HALL MEETINGS

Community meetings, also referred to as hall meetings, can provide an additional opportunity to explore feelings, solve problems, resolve conflict, and enhance group cohesiveness. In addition, the community utilizes the meeting time to make plans for hall-related activities, define expectations of each other, request feedback, assistance, or support from peers and staff, and clarify policy or rules. Collectively, group members and a skilled group leader can develop trust, define both group and individual goals, and be instrumental in developing and maintaining a safe and therapeutic milieu in which work can be successfully accomplished. Although community meetings and group therapy show some similarity, their specific purposes are quite different. Community meetings are held more frequently and are of much shorter duration due to the nature of their purpose.

A community meeting is usually held daily for about 15 to 30 minutes and will include all the patients and two or three staff members. Although the specific agenda for the meetings may differ from day to day, the dynamic remains the same. Emphasis on punctuality and attendance for all patients and staff promote a sense of value and importance for all members. Although the meetings may appear less formal and somewhat casual, the same expectations of respect for others and controlling behavior is strictly enforced. Staff members may request a patient to leave the meeting if there is a reluctance or inability to participate in a productive manner. The status of the milieu is often demonstrated quite clearly in the group's ability or inability to address issues in an appropriate and mature manner. At times, issues discussed can become too sensitive or intense to explore in community meetings and may be "shelved" and referred to as a group therapy issue or one that may be more successfully dealt with in individual therapy.

Confidentiality in this meeting is strictly enforced as it is of extreme importance for the building of a trusting relationship with those with whom you share a communal living space. The hall meetings provide an excellent media for newer members to feel "at home," depending, of course, upon their individual reason for admission and the status of the patient group's functioning ability. Additionally, these meetings provide an excellent opportunity to meet with the patients collectively and for the staff to give additional support, guidance, recognition, and direction to ensure the group's motivation and investment in treatment.

Several issues that may decrease the productivity of the group and thereby increase counterproductivity regardless of motivation include violence, scapegoating, lack of active staff participation, lack of closure, and lack of limit setting/rule enforcement.

The degree to which the hall meeting succeeds is dependent upon participation of both patients and staff. Although the level of success varies from one meeting to the next, an increased success rate can be anticipated where there is consistency, task adherence, and skillful direction by the staff. Success is also dependent upon the maturity level of the patient group, their level of investment in treatment, and the quality of leadership.

In addition to the regularly scheduled meetings, impromptu meetings may be called by either the patient or staff group. The purpose of these additional meetings is to impart specific pertinent information or to quickly address an issue that is impairing the group's functioning as a whole. Thus, patients or staff may decrease the amount of conflict, confusion, or misinterpretation by clarifying issues and achieving resolution in a more timely fashion. The patients or staff may also elect to increase the number of daily meetings when the patient group demonstrates some difficulty in cohesiveness or goal attainment. Regardless of the type of community meeting (regularly scheduled or impromptu), all are treated with the same value and level of importance.

Similar to group therapy, patients must feel safe in these meetings. Acts of violence or "scapegoating," or episodes of threatening behavior impair the ability of the members to participate, often leading to increased absence and must be terminated as soon as possible. Frequently, these behaviors are used by group members to avoid or delay discussion of painful, frightening, or uncomfortable issues. Staff needs to quickly and clearly address these incidents and their impact on the group in order to redirect the patients in a more productive manner.

Generally, it is valuable to have at least two staff members participate in community meetings. It is particularly important when a newer, less experienced staff member is present to have additional staff members available to provide guidance and support. Adolescents often tend to intensify their behaviors and escalate quickly when limits are not set or are set too late. An inexperienced staff member may become over-whelmed in a meeting where members are extremely verbal, negative, and noncompliant. In such instances, the meeting may become too disruptive and may need to be terminated and reconvened at a later time when more guidance, direction, and support are available. Strict task adherence is advisable to maintain patients' boundaries and to enhance their opportunity to experience success.

SUMMARY

Group psychotherapy in an inpatient setting provides an important growth-promoting experience for an adolescent. Adolescents learn how to communicate their thoughts and feelings to each other, how to resolve conflicts while living together, how their problems are similar, and how they can help each other and themselves. As the group becomes cohesive and trusting, adolescents are able to share their traumatic experiences, fears, and wishes, appraise their strengths and vulnerabilities realistically, confront each other, and overcome their need to present a false image to themselves, their peers, and adults.

The group therapist needs to carefully monitor composition of the group, establish ground rules for the group members to follow, and provide necessary structure. An adolescent group goes through various stages while the therapist helps the adolescents in developing trust, decreasing their defensiveness, exploring reasons for their behavior, and learning new ways to dealing with both internal and external conflicts. Each inpatient group session can reflect what is occurring on the unit with either the adolescents or their caretakers.

REFERENCES

Ackerman, N.W. (1955). Group psychotherapy with a mixed group of adoles-cents. *International Journal of Group Psychotherapy, 5*, 249-260.

Adler, J., Berman, I.R., and Slavson, S.R. (1960). Residential treatment of delinquent adolescents: V. Multiple leadership in group treatment of delin-quent adolescents. *International Journal of Psychotherapy, 10*, 213-226.

Bardill, D.R. (1977). A behavior-contracting program of group treatment for early adolescents in a residential setting. *International Journal of Group Psychotherapy, 27*, 389-400.

Beitel, A., Everts, P., Boile, B., Nagel, E., Bragdon, C., Mackesson, B. (1983). Hub group: An innovative approach to group therapy in a short-term inpatient adolescent unit, *Adolescence, 18*, 2-15.

Berkovitz, I.H. & Sugar, M. (1986). Indications and contraindications for adolescent group psychotherapy. In Max Sugar (Ed.), *The adolescent in group and family therapy* (pp. 5-7). Chicago and London: The University of Chicago Press.

Berkovitz, I.H., Chikahisa, P., Lee, M.L., & Murasaki, E.M. (1966). Psychosexual development of latency-aged children and adolescents in group therapy in a residential setting. *International Journal of Group Psychotherapy, 16,* 344–356.

Blaustein, F. & Wolff, H. (1972). Adolescent Group: A "Must" on a Psychiatric Unit—Problems and results: A reparative superego experience. In I.H. Berkovitz (Ed.), *Adolescents Grow in groups* (pp.181-191). New York: Brunner/Mazel.

Boenheim, C. (1957). Group psychotherapy with adolescents. *International Journal of Group Psychotherapy, 1,* 398-405

Buxbaum, E. (1945). Transferences and group formation in children and adolescents. *Psychoanalytic study of the child, 1,* 351-365.

Epstein, N. (1960). Recent observations in group psychotherapy with adolescent delinquent boys in residential treatment: Activity group therapy. *International Journal of Group Psychotherapy, 10,* 180-194.

Ghuman, H.S. & Sarles, R.M. (1989). Three group psychotherapy settings with long–term adolescent inpatients: Advantages and disadvantages. *The Psychiatric Hospital, 19,* 161-164.

Grold, L.J. (1972). The value of "youth group" to hospitalized adolescent. In I.H. Berkovitz (Ed.), *Adolescents grow in groups* (pp. 192-196). New York: Brunner/Mazel.

Kassoff, A.L. (1958). Advantages of multiple therapists in a group of severely acting out adolescent boys. *International Journal of Group Psychotherapy, 8,* 70-75.

Mordock, J.B., Ellis, M.H. & Greenstone, J.L. (1969). The effects of group and individual therapy on sociometric choice of disturbed institutionalized adolescents. *International Journal of Group Psychotherapy, 19,* 510-517.

Powles, W.E. (1959a). Group management of emotionally ill adolescents in a Canadian mental hospital. *Can.: Psychiatric Association. J., 4*(2), 77-89.

Powles, W.E. (1959b). Psychosexual maturity in a therapy group of disturbed adolescents. *International Journal Group Psychotherapy, 9,* 429-441.

Rinsley, D.B. (1972). Group therapy within the wider residential context. In I.H. Berkovitz (Ed.) *Adolescents grows in groups* (pp. 233-242). New York: Brunner/Mazel.

Schulman, I. (1959). Transference, resistance and communication problems in Adolescent psychotherapy groups. *International Journal of Group Psychotherapy, 9,* 496-503.

Shellow, R.S., Ward J.L. & Rubenfeld, S. (1958). Group therapy and the institutionalized delinquent. *International Journal of Group Psychotherapy, 8,* 265-275.

Sugar, M. (1986). The structure and setting of adolescent therapy groups. In Max Sugar (Ed.) *The adolescent in group and family therapy* (pp. 42-43). Chicago and London: The University of Chicago Press.

Thorpe, J.J. & Smith, B. (1952). Operational sequences in group psychotherapy with young offenders. *International Journal of Group Psychotherapy, 2,* 24-33.

Westman, J.C. (1960). Group therapy with hospitalized delinquent adolescents. *International Journal of Group Psychotherapy*, *11*, 410-418.
Yalom, I.D. (1983). *Inpatient Group Psychotherapy*. New York, Basic Books.

Chapter 5

NURSING SERVICES
COACHING THE PATIENT TO IMPROVED MENTAL HEALTH

D. Heidi Waltos

Nursing staff are the primary caregivers within a psychiatric inpatient setting. They are participators in and providers of corrective growth producing experiences. Nursing's role with the patient is multifaceted, since the intensity and types of interventions vary with the patient's needs. Historically, nursing staff have relied heavily on the use of the therapeutic relationship in their work with patients; however, with diminishing resources, shorter patient stays, and increasing severity of illness, nursing has needed to reconceptualize its role to include more directive and educative approaches. Describing nursing's role in the adolescent inpatient setting as one of "coach" incorporates these instructing, training, and goal-directed functions while still emphasizing the importance of the one-to-one relationship. Additionally, "coach" speaks to the role of nursing in a language that is easily understood and perhaps more easily tolerated by the adolescent patient.

The concept of teams within psychiatric inpatient settings is not a new one. Similarities have previously been illustrated between nursing management functions and coaching functions.

Brooks (1990) stated that the manager is expected to set realistic goals for the nursing team, balance the strengths and weaknesses of the players, work with administration to secure needed resources, and produce a winning record in the delivery of patient care. This chapter will examine the various coaching activities utilized by direct care nursing staff.

CHARACTERISTICS OF AN EFFECTIVE COACH

A nationally recognized coach, Lou Holtz, stated that there are three universal questions all players should ask their coaches and expect to be answered. They include: "1) Can I trust you? 2) Do you care about me as a person? and 3) Are you committed to and capable of achieving excellence?" (Brooks, p. 108).

Not surprisingly, adolescents often address these same issues: "Staff should communicate to me like any other human being should—with understanding, honesty, and with a genuine feeling so that I can give back what I'm getting."—Suzanne, age 17. "Adults can communicate better with me if they approach me in a more caring way. I like to feel like I'm being confronted because the adult cares about me and isn't just doing their job. Another way I like staff to communicate with me is to try and relate to me with similar experiences."—Mike, age 16.

However, in order to convey these qualities effectively, staff must also be attuned to the transference issues and preconceived notions regarding authority figures which enter into the staff-patient relationship. Jones, Pearson and Dimpero (1989) discuss nursing staff as frequently being the "targets of the adolescent's hostility, the subject of his conflictual anxiety, or objects for his instinctual wishes (resulting in the development of close, warmly toned attachments)" (p. 489). They point out that, for these reasons, a part of treatment takes place primarily in the context of the relationship between the adolescent and the nursing staff. Establishing parameters of this relationship by viewing it in a coach-player context allows nursing staff to comfortably blend authority and caring, without being seen purely as authority figures or, at the other end of the spectrum, as friends to the patients. It also allows the adolescents to feel that the staff is on their side, providing guidance and direction without getting on the field to play the game for them.

An ability to achieve and commit to excellence is the third expectation players place upon their coach. An effective coach does not tell team members how he would carry out the play, but instead draws on his own past experiences, experiences of others he has coached, a thorough knowledge of the game (rules, tactics, and proven strategies), awareness of his coaching style, and an understanding of the abilities, strengths, and limitations of individual players. Emotions are expressed during the course of the relationship, but a good coach remains objective and avoids becoming emotionally reactive or involved with the players. Fortunately for the athletic coach, the boundaries of the playing field are physically drawn, making it virtually impossible for the coach to enter the game. Nursing staff does not have this luxury and must constantly work to draw their own boundaries, thus preventing the subtle intermingling of staff and patient feelings. Knowledge and appreciation of normal adolescent development as well as an understanding of their countertransference issues will assist staff in maintaining boundaries and therapeutic relationships with the patients.

UNDERSTANDING THE COACHING EXPERIENCE

Nursing staff working within adolescent inpatient settings may need to face their own unresolved conflicts surrounding independence-dependence and identity issues. It is not unusual for novice staff to experience a range of conflicting emotions when setting limits with the adolescent patient. This can result in either refraining from setting limits or becoming overcontrolling. Through careful supervision, the novice staff can recognize that limits are set to facilitate independence and that the two are not mutually exclusive. New staff may also personalize the "pull-me, push-you" behaviors of patients and seek to remedy perceived rejection by inappropriate nurturing. And finally, in response to the regressions many patients frequently demonstrate prior to discharge, staff may experience a sense of failure, disappointment, loss or abandonment.

With guidance, support, and experience, staff develop the "capacity to love and empathize with teenagers and their families and the ability to let go of attachments when care is completed" (Hogarth, 1991, p. 8). They learn to assume flexibility in their approach in order to meet the individual needs and fluctuating moods of the adolescent. Eventually, the ability to relax and have fun with the patients emerges as a natural part of the work. As patients stumble and have setbacks, these staff adeptly help patients to understand that managing losses and learning from errors are all part of the "game." Interactions with patients promote acceptance of realities while conveying optimism, much like the coach who guides and cheers his players on to success.

PLAYER ASSESSMENT AND GOAL-SETTING STRATEGIES

The assessment process begins treatment and continues to shape interventions throughout hospitalization. A multidisciplinary approach is most commonly utilized, with each discipline contributing a component of the diagnostic formulation. The typical nursing assessment includes a systems review, a food and drug history, a developmental history, a sexual history, a mental status review, problem areas identified by the patient and family, identification of strengths, abilities, and limitations, and preliminary goal-setting.

With increasingly shorter lengths of stay, clinicians must streamline assessments without sacrificing necessary information and must initiate discharge planning at the time of admission. Ney, Adam, Hanton, and Brindad (1988) recommend that assessments be completed in the prospective patient's natural setting prior to hospitalization. This is both time-effective and a source of data more applicable to developing discharge plans for the patient. However, this method does not account for emergency admissions and may require a conceptual shift from current procedures. To aid in the rapid yet comprehensive assessment for the short-term patient, Nurcombe (1989) devised an intake format identifying six "p's" of assessment.

1. physical and/or psychosocial factors *predisposing* the patient to developing future psychiatric disturbances;
2. stresses which may *precipitate* future psychiatric disturbances;
3. factors which occasioned the patient's *presentation* to the hospital.
4. factors which *perpetuate* the current disturbance;
5. biopsychosocial *patterns*, i.e., physical or neuropsychological dysfunctions, recurrent symptoms, regularly utilized coping mechanisms, pathogenic dispositions, family patterns of functioning, and social functioning (including school and community);
6. patient *potentials*—strengths and resources that could be fostered in such a way as to circumvent or compensate for psychopathology.

This format clearly focuses on discharge planning needs and serves to prioritize problem areas.

During the initial assessment period, many adolescents feel frightened, defensive, and distrustful, and may believe their viewpoint has been minimized or misunderstood. As a counterbalance to this, the adolescent can be encouraged to complete a self-assessment form. This allows the adolescent age-appropriate autonomy, removes the direct power struggle with authority, reinforces the importance of the patient's input into treatment, and affords the adolescent time for self-reflection. Staff gain additional diagnostic information while establishing the foundation of treatment as a collaborative effort. Because of nursing's 24-hour-a-day patient accountability, they are in a unique position of being able to observe, assess, and report patient behaviors occurring in a wide variety of situations within the milieu (the playing field). Interventions are designed to be proactive and preventative, as well as reactive. Nursing staff are often the first to detect the effects of medications or see prodromal signs of illness, etc. The frequency and intensity of these assessments and observations are increased for patients who present a risk to self or others.

Following the initial assessment, a treatment plan is devised which incorporates objectives with short- and long-term goals. Establishing priorities becomes essential when hospitalization is time-limited. In addition, the adolescent is encouraged to set *daily* goals which are monitored and reviewed with nursing. These goals should be behaviorally oriented and focused on the patient's development of specific cognitive, psychological and social skills. The adolescent is assisted with the following steps of skill building: identifying the problem itself, identifying the feelings, thoughts and situations associated with it, identifying alternative behaviors, and practicing alternatives (Hogarth, 1991). Goals and steps that are clear and achievable become strong motivational forces. If one can imagine a player on the field without goals or game plans, one can begin to appreciate what a lack of realistic goals and behavioral objectives does to the patient's ability to utilize treatment.

OUTLINING THE RULES AND BOUNDARIES OF THE PLAYING FIELD: THE MILIEU PROGRAM

Establishing and maintaining a successful milieu is, by and large, the responsibility of nursing staff. It is a safe environment designed to promote appropriate interactional skills while discouraging inappropriate ones. It is where practice takes place—learning new ways of relating, new behaviors, new coping strategies. Corrective emotional experiences can occur with the guidance and support provided through positive and negative reinforcements and through trusting, alliance-building relationships with staff (Dalton, Bolding, Woods & Daruma, 1987).

Within a milieu, there are structured and unstructured elements. Both are contingent to the success of the program.

Unstructured Elements

Unstructured elements include a system of human interactions (Peplau, 1979), and a shared vision regarding the philosophy and functions of the milieu. The unwritten norms or culture of the unit are established by these elements which are intangible, yet central to determining the productivity, quality, and success of the milieu. This can be seen when one compares two units with the same patient population, same policies, etc., but which have vastly different rates of quiet room and seclusion use. The difference lies in the groups' norms for managing behavior—the philosophy or team spirit embodied by staff.

Gunderson's (1978) description of the functions of the milieu has become a standard to many inpatient units. These include *containment*—the unit's ability to contain patients' unacceptable impulses and behaviors; *support*—lent by empathic and caring attitudes; *structure*—the organization of the patient's day in a protective fashion; *involvement*—the unit's ability to engage patients and to observe these patterns of relating; *validation*—the exploration of intrapsychic events and their relationship to current realities.

Woven further into the philosophical fabric of a successful milieu are basic beliefs/tenets which staff share regarding children and adolescents. Rolfe (1990) identified several useful operating principles in working with this population. He emphasized: 1) the innate ability and desire of children to do well, given positive expectations and healthy environment, 2) the need for children to receive positive validation of their importance, which includes disallowing something that will be harmful to them, 3) the child's propensity to observe and interpret everything and the expectation they have that others will do the same for them, 4) the tendency for children to hear abstract messages prior to concrete ones, especially when limits are placed on them (i.e., hearing that no one wants them around as a response to being sent to their room for misbehavior), 5) the resulting need to employ referencing techniques when working with children (referencing them back to the more concrete level, i.e., "People want you around but expect your behavior to improve"), 6) the child thriving on allowance and guidance to do what is right rather than on the use of force and control, 7) the child's strong response to fulfill expectations whether they be positive or negative, 8) the child's heavy reliance on imitation as a learning method, and 9) the child's adoption of certain behavior patterns in order to meet needs (negative behaviors may have been the only means available to meet a need). Finally, Rolfe emphasized that children are basically receptive to genuine communication. It is essential that the importance of these intangible elements be recognized in the process of streamlining programs to meet fiscal requirements. Each coach plays by the same rules and has access to the same playbooks. However some have winning records and some never make it to the playoffs. A deciding factor resides in the coaches ability to generate this intangible "team spirit."

Structured Elements

In a study on treatment characteristics of effective psychiatric programs, Collins, Ellsworth, Casey, Hickey, and Hyer (1984) identified four items that were statistically significant in determining a successful program as defined by patient posthospital adjustment. These are: 1) a moderate level of *order and organization* on the unit, 2) the provision of *multiple activities* for the patients rather than large spans of unstructured time, 3) *stability of assignments* for nursing staff, allowing staff to play a predictable and responsible role in the patients' treatment, and 4) a *lower reliance on medications* to control anxious and acting out behaviors.

Order and Organization

Order and organization apply to the players as well as to the coaching staff. It is necessary for coaches to establish an organizational framework that promotes clear communication among team managers and financial backers, and that establishes a forum for reviewing previous games and developing new strategies. The following meetings and communication mechanisms are suggested for inpatient settings:

a. Treatment Planning Conferences.
b. Program Evaluation and Planning Sessions—to review, revise and improve treatment approaches and to assimilate administrative changes.
c. Staff evaluation and supervision sessions.
d. Nursing Staff Meetings—to discuss administrative, patient-care, and staff-related issues. A review of any major patterns of patient acting out must always include an examination of staff dynamics first.
e. Shift Change Reports—to provide treatment continuity.
f. Staff Assignment Sheets and Patient Assignment Sheets.
g. Bulletin Boards—centrally located for staff, patients, and families to announce schedules, orientation information activities, treatment resources, educational sessions, etc.
h. Communication Books—to record minutes of meetings, messages, announcements, and patient care-related issues that require team knowledge.
i. Orientation Programs and Manuals—for patients, families, students, volunteers and staff.

For the patients, units are "typically structured around actions that must be accomplished as part of a daily routine such as wake-ups, meals, meetings, school, and activities and the degree of supervision to be provided for the patients" (Benfer & Schroder, 1985, p. 455). The patient's ability to accomplish these activities of daily living is monitored

and incorporated into a point system (Table 5.1) which partially determines what responsibility level the patient is capable of maintaining.

Responsibility or privilege levels allow the patient to move along a
continuum of staff observation and supervision, from a highly structured
set of expectations and activities to self-determined structure. Rules, or
community expectations, constitute the guidelines for maintaining order
and organization and are similar to the boundaries and penalties occurring on a playing field. A player automatically knows when he has
stepped out of bounds or when there is "interference"—only on occasions are these issues disputed. Rules and consequences on the unit should
be clear and consistently enforced. Thus, staff are allowed the freedom to
give attention to positive behaviors rather than focusing on misbehavior
by cajoling, clarifying, or nagging the patients regarding behavioral
expectations (Rubin, 1986). In general, a well-functioning unit should
limit the number of rules. Eight to ten major rules that pertain to socially
responsible behavior such as safety, sexual conduct, substance abuse,
privacy, confidentiality, and physical destructiveness are adequate (Table
5.2).

All staff should be consistent when managing patient behaviors.
Children and adolescents will test limits and need to know that if they
push against this structure it will not weaken or falter. Written policies
on time-outs, aggression management, consequences, etc. should be
available to reinforce consistency. Interventions that are carried out with
a respectful yet firm tone and that seek to shift control back to the
patient's internal resources as rapidly as possible are optimally effective.

A pre-established set of "Patient Group Responsibilities" to be instituted in the event of a fellow patient harming him/herself, harming
others, or running away (Lewis, 1969) is a useful treatment tool that
promotes patient accountability and responsibility, encourages positive
peer pressure and delineates a consistent plan of action for dealing with
a turbulent milieu. All rules and responsibilities should be clearly posted
and reviewed in the orientation received by patients and their families.

Multiple Activities
A coach develops a team through a set of established activities: warm-ups,
drills, practice, strategy sessions, and one-to-one guidance. Team members should have goals and be willing to put forth effort and to tolerate
sometimes grueling and tedious preparation in order to achieve these
goals. Patient goals can be viewed in the same light through the identification of those activities the patient needs to practice in order to cope
more successfully. The patient's individualized schedule includes a

Table 5.1: The Sheppard and Enoch Pratt Hospital Point Sheet

Name: Dates: Level:

A.D.L.s	Rate	M	T	W	TH	F	S	S	Wk. Tot.	M	T	W	TH	F	S	S	Wk. Tot.
Up on Time	1																
Goal Set	2						X	X							X	X	
Hygiene	1																
Room	1																
Breakfast and/or Lunch	1																
Group (on time, part.)	1																
Dinner	1																
School (a.m., p.m.)	2						X	X							X	X	
Homework	1						X	X							X	X	
Activity	1																
Hall Job	1																
Check-in	2						X	X							X	X	
Bedtime	1																
Laundry	1																
Quiet hour without interven.	1																
Courtesy 7-noon	1																
noon-6	1																
5-bed	1																
Appropriate peer interact 7-noon	1																
noon-6	1																
6-bed	1																
Appropriate staff interac. 7-noon	1																
noon-6	1																
6-bed	1																
TOTAL	28																
PERCENTAGE	%																

PERSONAL TARGET BEHAVIORS

Behavior	Rate	M	T	W	TH	F	S	S	Wk. Tot.	M	T	W	TH	F	S	S	Wk. Tot.
#1	√ 0																
#2	√ 0																
#3	√ 0																
TOTAL/3																	

Table 5.2: Community Expectations

1   *Confidentiality*: Your privacy is respected and will be protected during your hospital stay. Staff is not permitted to give your name, address, telephone number, or any information to anyone outside of the treatment team. No one is permitted to have tape recorders or cameras for recording any other patients. You are expected to respect other's privacy, and any personal information about other patients should remain on the unit. Violating another's confidentiality is a serious matter and will be responded to by staff.

2   *Threats and Aggression*: Threatening behaviors are not allowed at any time. Verbal threats toward anyone will result in quiet room or other limits. Any type of physically threatening behavior will be followed by external controls. (This includes slamming doors, hitting walls, etc.)

3   *Profanity*: Cursing is not acceptable. Use of foul language will be fined and will result in time-out.

4   *Radios and Stereos*: Be considerate and maintain a moderate volume level. Your radio/stereo may be removed in the event of consistent loudness.

5   *Telephone*: Phone calls are permitted before school, at lunch, and after school. Phones will be turned off during groups, meetings, study hour, quiet hours, and quiet night. There is a 15-minute limit per call.

6   *Dress*: Shoes must be worn. No revealing clothes.

7   *Peer Interaction*: Going into one another's room is not allowed.

8   *Health and Safety*: All sharp objects must be kept in the nurses station. No food in patient rooms. No horseplay.

9   *Substance Abuse*: This is a substance abuse free environment—you owe it to yourself and others to maintain this. Any infraction will result in loss of privileges and will impact discharge planning. (This is also a smoke-free environment.)

combination of cognitive, physical, social, and psychological activities such as self-appraisal, goal-setting, skill-building, psychoeducation, discharge-planning, individual, family, and group therapy, school, visitation, exercise, socialization and meeting basic needs of rest, nutrition, and hygiene. Many adolescents complain that this is a grueling and tedious schedule. However, their behavior and goal achievement indicate that they thrive in the structure and in the expectation that they are capable of doing the work.

In sports, players must concentrate on their individual performance as well as on their functioning as a team player. This combination of individual and group work is also emphasized in the adolescent milieu as it is so uniquely suited to the developmental needs of this group. The patient profits from a balance of learning to rely on the feedback and support of others, as well as developing a higher degree of self-awareness and self-reliance. Ideally, nursing staff should receive formal training and supervision in group theory and process.

Nursing staff regularly employ one-to-one talks with patients. Whatever the focus of the interaction, be it problem-solving, limit-setting, or supportive, staff should bear in mind that the end result is to enhance the patient's self-awareness, internal resources, and self-esteem. The tone and frequency of the interaction will depend on the patient's symptomatology. For example, an angry, paranoid patient requires a calmer, more distant approach, while a depressed patient benefits more from an active, friendly approach (Hogarth, 1991). Patients who experience difficulty with authority may be requested to attempt more interactions with staff, while patients who have difficulties with peers would be encouraged to interact more with peers.

Treatment may also include individualized behavior modification programs designed and prescribed by staff. Virtually all patients who require inpatient treatment benefit from a degree of this intervention. In essence, the "Responsibility Level System" functions as a behavior modification tool, encouraging positive behaviors with an increase in privileges and responding to dysfunctional behaviors by an increase in structure and observation. Specialized programs are developed for patients to address a gamut of issues, for example, communication skills, nutritional intake, and appropriate management of anger. Implementing behavioral programs without a solid philosophy to guide the process minimizes therapeutic effectiveness. Developing these programs requires a great deal of proper assessment and a discussion as to what outcome is expected. All too frequently, behavioral paradigms are unwittingly developed to benefit staff instead of the patient, or standardized formats are utilized that do not account for patient individuality. The following guidelines are useful in designing successful programs:

a. Introduce the concept of behavior modification as a useful treatment tool early in treatment. If the patient regards this intervention as a last resort designed for especially difficult patients, adolescent may feel singled out and may operate with negative expectations.

b. Remember that "old habits die hard." A patient's failure to change behavior may be due to difficulties inherent in making changes, not to resistance or opposition.

c. Because patients need to trust that staff are looking out for their best interest, adequate rapport is necessary for program success.

d. Properly assess and understand the targeted behaviors. There should be a knowledge of the antecedent and consequent event—what triggers the behavior and what is the outcome.

e. Clarify the specifics of the program: What is the goal? What specific behaviors need to be performed to receive the reward or incur the consequence? What will the reinforcers and consequences be? What are the time dimensions? Who will monitor the behavior and how?

f. Take into account the normal developmental issues and tasks of adolescents. The adolescent needs to maintain a sense of competence and control and should be very involved in self-assessment of the targeted behavior and in the design of the program. This can be accomplished through the use of behavior cards on which the adolescent marks down the behavior along with the trigger and outcome each time it occurs, and with videotaping or journals. The self-observation period may result in the patient agreeing that the behavior really *is* problematic or he/she may discontinue the behavior in order to avert a modification program. The patient should also be involved in choosing effective consequences and reinforcers.

g. Focus on increasing positive adaptive behaviors. Behavior modification programs frequently target negative behaviors without focusing on alternative behaviors. Behaviors are driven by need, consequently if the patient is expected to cease a behavior, a substitution for getting the need met should be available. For example, if a patient inflicts self-injury in order to express anger without fear of retaliation, then attention should be given to alternative methods of expressing anger appropriately.

h. Develop a program that has stages from more external, staff-provided controls to more internal controls, and begin it some-where in the middle. In this manner, staff give the patient the benefit of the doubt and establish a "safety net" for the patient in case more external structure is necessary.

i. Develop a program that can be transitioned to the patient's home environment. As patients near discharge, paradigms should be modified to include reinforcers and consequences that can be applied in the nonhospital setting. Instructing parents and signifi-cant others in behavior modification principles and soliciting their input for the "transitional" program are extremely important in preventing recidivism (Table 5.3).

The following guidelines are useful for implementing behavior modi-fication programs (B-Mod):

1. A major point is to stress the earning rather than losing of points and privileges. It is not uncommon to hear even the most skilled clinician say, "You did not achieve your request because you didn't get enough points," rather than, "You have 20 of the 30 points needed to reach your goal. What can you do to earn the remaining points?"

2. When the patient's goal is not achieved, it is necessary to reevaluate the B-Mod program itself. Is the target behavior too tough to reach for the patient? Should it be broken down to a portion of the desired behavior? Is the reward too remote for the patient's ability to delay gratification? Can the patient tolerate rewards or is self esteem so diminished that even desired rewards are sabotaged.

3. Emotionally disturbed youngsters may sabotage their own pro-grams, feeling uncomfortable with success and projecting that failure is imminent anyway. This highlights the rationale that Behavior Modification is a treatment approach and not a total treatment answer. It is in such instances that therapeutic commu-nication becomes essential to help the patient explore the behavior patterns, along with the issues of self-esteem and self concept.

4. Contracts should be very specific—the more specific the less room for differences in interpretation by staff and by patient. Target behavior should be limited to those areas that most negatively impact the patient so that the length and breadth of the program do not make it prohibitive. Depending on the patient's ability to maintain positive behaviors, reinforcers may be given at varying lengths of time, for example, every hour, every eight hours, or every

Table 5.3: Behavior Modification Program

TARGET BEHAVIORS	TIME							
	12–3am	3–6am	6–9am	9–12pm	12–3pm	3–6pm	6–9pm	9–12am
Short-Term Goals: The patient will remain safe for 3 hours with staff support. **Long-Term Goals:** The patient will develop self control, alternative coping skills, communication skills, self awareness regarding the problem behavior. 1. Will remain safe for 3 hours with staff support. No attempts to hurt self. 2. Verbalize one positive attribute about self once per shift. 3. State and describe one feeling per shift that precedes desire to hurt self (may use feelings list handout to help define and select feeling.) 4. Minimum 5 minutes 1 to 1 talk with staff every 3 hours: 9–3 and 3–9 (should identify problem behavior and should identify alternative behavior at least once per shift.) **Reinforcers:** Patient and team need to define not only the reward but how and when the patient receives the reward. Rewards need to be given not only for accomplishment, but also for trends (i.e., coping as well as mastery.) 1. Telephone time 15 minutes. 2. 1 to 1 time with special staff to play game/walk. 3. Select video for movie night. 4. Extra health food snack. 5. Extra 15 minutes free time. 6. Card game with peer. 7. Choice of reading from Library cart. 8. Extra 15 minutes of music at bedtime.								
Short-Term Goals: Patient will exhibit no aggressive behaviors per 8 hour period. **Long-Term Goals:** The patient will develop self control, alternative coping skills, communication skills, self awareness regarding the problem behavior. 1. No aggressive behaviors or verbal threats in 8 hours. 2. State a safe cue that alerts self to feelings or arousal (example: pacing; clenched fists, rapid speech). 3. Practice appropriate self expression of anger. 4. Practice relaxation strategy. **Reinforcers:** 1. 4 Checks = 15 minutes 1 to 1 with selected staff. 2. 3 Checks = 10 minutes 1 to 1 with selected staff.								

24 hours as the patient improves. Contracts, though helpful tools, must not change or replace the vigilance on the part of staff with the patient.

Formal and informal educational activities are part of the patient's individualized schedule and vary with the patient's needs. Relaxation training, sex education, nutrition education, and medication education are but a few examples of what may be provided. Patient-family coeducation is essential because of its significant impact on posthospitalization adjustment. Sessions are usually co-led by nursing, social work, and physician staff. Katma (1987) recommends that the following items be addressed:

a. Patient's diagnosis, definition of psychiatric illness or dysfunction, type of treatment the patient is receiving in the hospital, names and types of medication the patient will be on inclusive of proper administration, side effects, and compliance issues.
b. Relapse signs and symptoms of illness, along with concrete plans for what to do if they reappear.
c. Normal growth and development issues and tasks of the adolescent and family.
d. Parent effectiveness training.
e. Community resources and support available for both patients and staff.

The general topics are discussed within a multifamily group format of parents with patients, or parents alone, while more specific, confidential issues are reviewed with just the patient and family present.

Providing activities for an increasingly mixed population of longer- and shorter-term patients, with fewer staff resources, presents an interesting challenge. Self-study packages, consisting of selected activities and exercises, offer a partial solution. Staff can design and individualize these workbooks to address specific patient needs as well as allowing the patient to select items. Results are discussed with staff or peers, individually or within a group forum, and are integrated into the patient's therapy. This approach is adaptable to programs with varying lengths of stay and promotes introspection, ownership, and a sense of accomplishment for the patient (Table 5.4).

Stability of Staff Assignments

Stability of nursing staff assignments is the third structured element Collins et al. (1984) identify as correlating positively with patient

Table 5.4: Menu Tracking Sheet

1.	Self Esteem Checklist	—	—	—	—	—	—	—	—
2.	Self Evaluation Exercise	—	—	—	—	—	—	—	—
3.	Nursing Self Assessment	—	—	—	—	—	—	—	—
4.	Goal Planning Exercise — Short-Term	—	—	—	—	—	—	—	—
5.	Goal Planning Exercise — Long-Term	—	—	—	—	—	—	—	—
6.	Self Evaluation Time — Part I	—	—	—	—	—	—	—	—
7.	Self Evaluation Time — Part II	—	—	—	—	—	—	—	—
8.	Problem Assessment	—	—	—	—	—	—	—	—
9.	Feeling Awareness Exercise	—	—	—	—	—	—	—	—
10.	Feeling Responsive Awareness Exercises	—	—	—	—	—	—	—	—
11.	Stress Management Evaluation	—	—	—	—	—	—	—	—
12.	Stress Exhaustion Exercise	—	—	—	—	—	—	—	—
13.	Stress Management Exercise	—	—	—	—	—	—	—	—
14.	Communication Exercise	—	—	—	—	—	—	—	—
15.	Writing Assignment	—	—	—	—	—	—	—	—
16.	Arts/Craft Project	—	—	—	—	—	—	—	—
17.	Journal Writing	—	—	—	—	—	—	—	—
18.	Mood Chart	—	—	—	—	—	—	—	—
19.	Step Work	—	—	—	—	—	—	—	—
20.	Reading	—	—	—	—	—	—	—	—
21.	Videos (therapeutic)	—	—	—	—	—	—	—	—
22.	Physical Exercise	—	—	—	—	—	—	—	—
23.	Staff Talk	—	—	—	—	—	—	—	—
24.	Peer Talk — Social Issue Related	—	—	—	—	—	—	—	—

(Courtesy of Kim Weinert, Andrea Origoni, Jill Rowan)

outcome. Perhaps the best way to exemplify the importance of staff consistency is to again draw on the analogy of the coach. It is difficult to conceive of a team developing any degree of competence or cohesiveness in the absence of regular coaching staff. Suppose each day, as the players arrived for practice, they were greeted with a different coach who did not have a working knowledge of their strengths and limitations, an awareness of their history and progress, knowledge of which strategies they were working on, or a grasp of the team's philosophy. Improvements could still be made through practice of prescribed drills and maneuvers; however, gains would be limited.

In an inpatient setting, irregular assignment of staff has a similar impact. Continuity of care is disrupted, leading to poor follow-through on treatment plan goals, patients lose the benefits of interactions with familiar staff, and they may be exposed to varying philosophies of patient care. In many cases, inconsistency of caregivers has permeated the patient's history, and staff's duplication of this scenario is to be avoided. Patient incidents and acting out typically rise in response to a lessened sense of security and safety. Staff morale may also be negatively affected by irregular shift or unit assignment. In terms of adequate staffing numbers, Hogarth states that ensuring safety in a least restrictive manner requires at least a 1:4 ratio of direct-care staff to adolescents. She further cautions against inappropriate controls on staffing, citing that institutions ultimately incur revenue loss through staff and patient dissatisfaction.

LOWER RELIANCE ON MEDICATIONS

A lower reliance on medications to control anxious and acting-out behaviors was the final item found to be statistically significant in determining a program's success (Collins et al., 1984). Although medication prescription practices are not under the domain of nursing, this finding does serve to again illustrate the extent of impact that a unit's philosophy has on its structured elements. If staff subscribe to the beliefs discussed throughout this chapter, they will design and implement treatment interventions that foster patients' development of internal controls and their efforts will not be limited to merely controlling behaviors through external means.

SUMMARY

The coaching paradigm provides a useful model for conceptualizing the role of the nursing staff in psychiatric inpatient treatment. However, coaches differ in their ability to "put it all together" and their winning or losing record must be studied to best know what works and what doesn't. In the inpatient setting, this translates into a strong need for longitudinal outcome-oriented studies, based on patient condition before, during, and after treatment. Only then can we know which teams develop competent players and make it to the playoffs.

REFERENCES

Benfer, B., & Schroder, P.J. (1985). Nursing in the therapeutic milieu. *Bulletin of the Menninger Clinic, 49*(5), 451-474.

Brill, A.A. (Ed.) (1928). *The Basic Writings of Sigmund Freud.* New York: Random House, Inc.

Brooks, A.T. (1990) Overview and Managing For The Future. In A.T. Brooks (Ed.), *Team Building* (pp. 1-7, 99-108). Nurse Managers Bookshelf, Baltimore: Williams and Wilkins.

Collins, N., Ellsworth, R., Casey, N., Hickey, R. and Hyer, L. (1984). Treatment characteristics of effective psychiatric programs. *Hospital and Community Psychiatry, 35*(6), 601-605.

Dalton, R., Bolding, D.D., Woods, J., Daruna, J.H. (1987). Short-term psychiatric hospitalization of children. *Hospital and Community Psychiatry, 38*(9), 973-976.

Erikson, E. (1963). *Childhood and Society.* New York: W.W. Norton & Co., Inc.

Gunderson, J.G. (1978). Defining the therapeutic processes in psychiatric milieus. *Psychiatry, 41,* 327-335.

Havighurst, R.J. (1972). *Development Tasks and Education.* New York: David McKay Co., Inc.

Hogarth, C.R. (1991). Strategies for the therapeutic milieu and intervention strategies for adolescent psychiatric nurses: an overview. In C.R. Hogarth (Ed), *Adolescent Psychiatric Nursing* (pp. 215-245, 273-311). St. Louis: Mosby Year Book.

Jones, J.M., Pearson, G.T., Dimpero, R. (1989). *Long-term treatment of the hospitalized adolescent and his family; an integrated systems-theory approach.* University of Chicago.

Katma, A.Y. (1987). Discharge planning for psychiatric patients: The effects of a family-patient teaching programme. *Journal Of Advanced Nursing, 12,* 611-616.

Klein, M. (1975). *The Psychoanalysis Of Children.* New York: Dell Publishing Co., Inc.

Lewis, J.M. (1969). *The Development Of An Inpatient Adolescent Service.* Presented at Southern Psychiatric Association, Ashville, N.C.

Mast, L.A., Schoppe, L.R., and Hogarth, C.R. (1991). Development of the healthy adolescent and family. In C.R. Hogarth (Ed.), *Adolescent Psychiatric Nursing* (pp. 27-51). St Louis: Mosby Year Book.

Ney, P.G., Adam, R.R., Hanton, R.R. and Brindad, E.S. (1988). The effectiveness of a child psychiatric unit: a follow-up study. *Canadian Journal of Psychiatry, 33,* 793-799.

Nurcombe, B. (1989). Goal directed treatment planning and principles of brief hospitalization. *Journal of the American Academy of Child and Adolescent Psychiatry, 28(1)*, 26-30.

Peplau, H.E. (1979). *The psychotherapy of Hildegard E. Peplau.* W.E. Field (Ed.). New Braunfels: PSF Productions.

Paget, J. (1981). *Children and adolescents: Interpretive essays on Jean Piaget.* D. Elkind (Ed.). New York: Oxford University Press.

Rolfe, R.C. (1990). *You can postpone anything but love.* New York: Warner Books.

Rubin, R. (1986). Assisting adolescents towards mental health. *Nursing Clinics of North America, 21(3)*, 439-450.

Tanner, J.M. (1978). *Foetus into man; physical growth from conception to maturity.* London: Open Book.

Chapter 6

SOCIAL WORK SERVICES

Louise R. Hopkins

INTRODUCTION

Every adolescent exists in and interacts with a social environment. The task of the social worker who is working with adolescents in an inpatient psychiatric treatment program is to evaluate and to modify that social environment as is necessary and possible. The activities can range from the simplest case management tasks, such as assisting a family to apply for medical assistance, to the most sophisticated interventions, such as intensive family therapy. The social worker, then, needs to be very much a generalist. The social worker provides a wide range of services with the goal of modifying the environment and the adolescent patient's interactions with that environment so as to optimize the chances of recovery by the adolescent patient.

A key word here is interactions. It is important to remember that the patient is not only affected by the environment, but he or she also affects the environment. Many theories state that a sick child is always the product of a dysfunctional family. This clearly is not always the case. Bateson (1972) and other systems thinkers provide a model for understanding causality and change that is helpful to the social worker working with adolescent psychiatric inpatients. Bateson states that linear causality, such as A plus B equals C may be comfortable and easy to comprehend, but it is simply not how things really happen. Instead, A, B, and C are often dynamic, not static features which impact on one another through feedback systems. Systems also are rarely closed or as simple as three factors. Therefore, not only can A, B, and C change and be changed by one another, but also they can change and be changed by D through Z and more.

An example may be helpful. Many years ago, long before I had heard of Bateson or systems thinking, I was doing a family evaluation of a very active, out-of-control young boy. The boy moved constantly, challenging every limit given him, and seemed strangely disconnected. In retrospect, he was clearly suffering from a severe attention deficit hyperactive disorder. The mother was angry, rejecting, and confusing, saying at one moment that she was devoted to her child, later that she could hardly stand to be with him and longed to escape. I thought I understood the situation. It was A plus B equals C. A normal child plus an angry, rejecting, confusing (pathogenic) mother equaled a disturbed child.

I had opportunity to reevaluate the family a month after the addition of stimulant medication. The boy had a good response to medication. He was much less active and he responded to his mother and her limits. The mother was calmer and less exhausted, and was loving and supportive of her son. Where had the pathogenic mother gone?

Simplicity would state that the only error had been the selection of what A, B, and C were. Perhaps A was a pathological child, B was a normal mother, and C was a sick mother? But I then recalled reports that the child behaved much better, prior to medication, in nursery school than at home, so surely it was the mother? Systems theory provides an explanation that is not "either/or." Neither mother nor child is seen as static. Instead they impact on and change one another. This feedback system was synergistic, with mother and son bringing out the worst in the other, until the addition of D, the stimulant medication, which in this case interrupted the process and allowed the positive interactions to dominate.

This model is of particular importance to the social worker working with the inpatient adolescent, as it is necessary to appreciate not only how the adolescent is affected by the environment but also how the environment is affected by the adolescent, and how both affect and are affected by the adolescent's disorder and by the hospitalization. The more the social worker, using a systems model, is able to conceptualize factors that are interacting, the better the likelihood of bringing about positive changes in the patient's environment.

The adolescent patient's home environment can be divided roughly into three parts: 1) the family, 2) the educational system, and 3) health and social service systems. With each system, the social worker has three roles: 1) evaluation, 2) liaison, and 3) modification or treatment. With each of these roles, there are, of course, times that there is overlap between the social worker's role and that of other team members. For instance, the social worker shares responsibility with special educators for selection of the special education facility which may be needed for the patient after discharge. Often, however, the bulk of the mechanics of the referral rests on the social worker.

THEORETICAL BASE

Good clinical practice always works best from a sound theoretical base. However, because the social worker must be a generalist, a single theory is rarely sufficient to provide all needed direction for a single case, much less for all cases served. The social worker must be acquainted with a broad range of theories and must be eclectic in the best senses of the word (Lunde, 1974). There are a multitude of theories that are effectively used by social workers in adolescent inpatient facilities. The following is not inclusive of all useful theories, but is an exposition of those theories which I have found most useful in practice.

The social worker needs to know theories of individual development and behavior, in order to understand the adolescent patient and the parents, and to be able to interpret each to the other. Individual psychotherapy needs to be understood, even though the social worker may not be the individual therapist. Due to current economic pressures and shifting priorities, social workers are often called upon to interpret the treatment to the family and to maintain communication regarding therapeutic issues. The social worker, then, must be well versed in the therapeutic frameworks used by the attending psychiatrists and psychologists. This requires an understanding of psychodynamic theories, including drive theory, ego psychology, object relationship theory, and self-psychology.

The social worker needs to understand behavior modification. This is a major factor in the milieu treatment of adolescents. Each adolescent patient is on a behavioral program where privileges are earned both by producing specific positive behaviors and by eliminating specific negative ones. The social worker interprets these programs to the families. These programs are often a bone of contention between families and the treatment staff as parents, many of whom have had a very difficult time putting limits on their children, may experience behavior modification as harsh and punitive. "What do you mean he lost his privilege to go swimming? He's a growing, active boy. He needs exercise," said one parent. Other parents may find behavior modification too slow and weak. "What do you mean he's allowed to refuse to go to school and he only loses privileges? Make him go to school!" The social worker must be prepared to explain the reasons for the decisions. Behavior modification is also taught to the parents for use in the home. A large percentage of parents whose adolescents require inpatient psychiatric treatment report that they have lost control at home. Behavior modification provides a model for effective, nonpunitive limit setting.

It is also necessary for the social worker to be well acquainted with theories of adolescent development. In the liaison function with parents, the social worker is asked many times weekly: "Is it normal for an adolescent to . . . ?" or "Why has my child begun to do . . . ?" The social worker needs to be able to field such questions with confidence, not only so that the parent is educated and therefore able to understand and function better, but also so that the parents have confidence in the competence of the institution and staff. The parents who have turned over the care and treatment of their troubled child to an institution that may seem strange and harsh, in an age when television and press exposés of inadequate care and abuses of adolescent psychiatric patients are frequent, are understandably anxious. A calm and competent social worker can allay some of these anxieties.

In the previous example of the child with attention deficit hyperactive disorder, a change in the child's behavior had enough impact on the family system to enable the system to self-correct. Unfortunately, this is often not the situation with the families of adolescent psychiatric patients. The social worker is often confronted with a family that has entrenched maladaptive interactional patterns.

There are many theoretical frameworks for conducting family therapy. I find Bowen (1978) and Minuchin (1974) particularly helpful in working with symptomatic adolescents and their families. However, a social worker who is an exclusive follower of family systems theory would probably be miserable and ineffective working in an inpatient adolescent treatment program. Such programs demonstrate that dysfunctional children are not simply the result of dysfunctional families. The biopsychosocial model indicates that there are many factors, including genetic endowment, that contribute to psychiatric disorders in adolescents. Change in the family system is only one part of the treatment program.

Much of what a social worker does in the role of environmental evaluator and modifier might fall under the rubric of case management or discharge planning. The social worker needs to evaluate the adolescent's social environment, to decide what changes need to be made, and to have knowledge both of which social supports are available to a patient and family and of how to access these supports. Modifications may be as small as informing a family of a mental health center in their neighborhood, or as great as helping the family to select and find funding for a residential treatment center. This practice also needs to be guided by a theoretical base. Psychosocial theories (Towle, 1945; Hartman & Laird, 1983; Woods & Hollis, 1990) speak to the need to provide even the most concrete of social services in a way that is respectful and empowering to the clients. The social worker needs not only to access services for patients, but to teach patients and their families how to negotiate social systems so that they are able to receive services. At times, this process can have a powerful impact on the family system. A parent who has learned to battle for the services his or her child needs may receive a much needed boost to self-esteem, self-esteem which is often damaged by the experience of having an ill child.

Many adolescents who require inpatient treatment have substance abuse problems in addition to other psychiatric problems. The social worker needs to understand the treatment needs of such adolescents and to be aware of Twelve Step Programs, such as Alcoholics Anonymous, Narcotics Anonymous, Alanon, Naranon, Adult Children of Alcoholics, and Alateen.

The social worker also needs to have a knowledge and understanding of DSM-III-R. Although the training of many social workers emphasizes a psychosocial evaluation rather than a clinical diagnosis, the reality of psychiatric treatment today is that all patients are given DSM-III-R diagnoses. Patients and their families have questions about diagnoses that are often brought to the social worker. The diagnosis itself becomes a factor in the total system. It may be overidentified with or rejected, a source of relief or additional proof to the parents that their own sense of failure or badness was accurate.

PRACTICE: EVALUATION, LIAISON, AND MODIFICATION OF THE ENVIRONMENT

The Family

On the Adolescent Inpatient Service at Sheppard Pratt, the social worker contacts the family at the time of admission or as soon afterwards as possible. At that time, the social worker's task of liaison between the family and the treatment team begins, and it continues throughout the patient's hospitalization. The family is told, "If you have questions or concerns, and you don't know whom to call, you can always call the social worker." Also, with this first contact, evaluation and treatment begin. How the family reacts to the hospitalization is an early important issue. Some are devastated, feeling the hospitalization is proof that something is terribly wrong, without yet having any firm belief that it can ever be made right. Others are relieved, able to sleep for the first time in weeks, knowing their suicidal or acting-out adolescent is finally physically safe. Some are enraged, believing their willful adolescent has chosen to bring the situation to this extreme. Others are frightened and mistrustful of the hospital, wondering if their children will be hurt and abused. Some are hopeful, trusting, and confident they have made the right decision. Others are bewildered, confused, and in shock. In reality, most families manifest some combination of the above. The social worker uses evaluation of the meaning of the hospitalization as a beginning evaluation of the family. Helping them deal with the hospitalization often represents the beginning of treatment.

During the first week to 10 days of hospitalization, the social worker completes an initial evaluation of the family. This includes exploring the family of origin with each parent. What are the multigenerational issues for each parent? What is the sibling position? Are there emotional cutoffs (abrupt and unprocessed terminations of one or more intrafamily relationships) in the families of origin? How is the family functioning? Is it overanxious, enmeshed, detached? How do triangles function in the family? Why have they ceased to function, requiring the addition of a new triangle: patient, family, and hospital? Are there boundaries between individuals which are respected? Are generational boundaries respected? Is parental authority intact? Do parents have the knowledge and emotional capacity to set down clear behavioral expectations, enforce limits, and give consequences?

Out of all this comes the family evaluation and treatment plan which is designed by the treatment team at the diagnostic conference. Family treatment may take place while the patient is hospitalized. In this case, it is provided by the social worker. With shortened lengths of stay, it is often not possible to do the needed work while the patient is hospitalized. In this case, the social worker helps the family to see and accept what change is needed, and to find adequate family therapy in their community. The kind of family intervention needed, of course, depends on the needs of the individual patient and family. At times, it is apparent that a major change in family dynamics is needed for the adolescent to have a chance for recovery.

> Robert's admission to the psychiatric hospital at age 16 was due to suicidal ideation, violent, noncompliant behavior at home and school, and school failure. Robert was the only child born to his middle-class, Jewish, professional parents. Though this only marriage for both partners was intact and seemed stable, Mr. and Mrs. M. both reported unhappiness and dissatisfaction in the marriage. Both parents came from families of origin that contained illness, tragedy, and emotional cutoffs. The paternal

grandfather was a Holocaust survivor, the only surviving member of his family. Robert's father described his father as an angry, bitter man who regularly abused him physically as he was growing up. The paternal grandmother was described as nice, but powerless. Mr. M. found his parents' presence intolerable, saw them rarely, and grew up committed to the idea that when he was a parent he would not abuse his child as he'd been abused. As treatment progressed, he sadly realized he had not abused his son the same way, but he had abused him differently. Physical abuse was replaced by rages and humiliating verbal abuse.

Robert's mother grew up with a very impaired father. The maternal grandfather was an orphan who grew up in foster homes. He was an angry, confused man who lost job after job due to his inability to accept direction. Her mother was also a nice but powerless woman who stayed married to this impaired man as her religious duty. Mrs. M. grew up feeling unacceptable, inadequate, and stigmatized. She escaped to college and there met and married Mr. M. She had little contact with her parents. Once Robert was born, she experienced Mr. M. as impaired due to his rages at Robert, and she reported she would have left the marriage years ago had she not lacked the self-confidence to live alone. She had become a nice, but powerless mother.

Bowen tells us that emotional cutoffs make repeats, and clearly both these parents had replicated in their family pathological patterns they had tried to leave in the past. In family therapy, each was encouraged to explore his or her family of origin. Mr. M. was devastated when he realized he'd truly hurt his son with his rages. With enormous energy, he began to explore his roots. He read about the Holocaust and joined a support group for children of Holocaust survivors. Although his family lived thousands of miles away, he spoke by phone to his mother about his childhood. He tried to understand rather than just to reject his parents. In a particularly moving session, he told his son he realized he'd metaphorically been in the midst of a multicar accident. "The Holocaust hit my father. He hit me. Then I hit you." He was able to tell his son he forgave his father. Several sessions later, Robert was able to say simply and unemotionally that he too forgave his father, Mr. M.

Mrs. M., as her mother before her, played the overadequate member of the couple. As Mr. M. grew healthier, she became anxious. She was encouraged to look at herself and her roots. She focused on how inadequate she was at getting her own needs met, how she saw woman's role as caring for a damaged other. She began to take classes, working on a long wished for Masters Degree.

Mr. and Mrs. M. began to focus on their marriage. They realized they'd stayed together to help Robert, but that placed him in a triangle where his illness stabilized their unstable relationship. They considered divorce, then decided there was much beside Robert to keep them together. They began doing activities together, enjoying their couple relationship.

Robert, meanwhile, had been involved in intensive treatment in the hospital. He had explored his own sense of anger and alienation from parents and was more able to engage in a healthier, more differentiated relationship with them. After discharge, both Robert and his family continued with individual and family therapy. A year after discharge, Mrs. M. wrote to report they were all doing well. Both Mr. and Mrs. M. had made trips to visit their families of origins. The visits were experienced as powerful and healing. She reported that both she and Mr. M. were keenly aware of how much they'd grown since Robert's admission. She said, "His [Robert's] pain was the instrument of our salvation."

In this case, it was clear that Robert was the identified patient or symptom bearer in a dysfunctional family. When parental dysfunction and marital issues were addressed, Robert was freed from his role of identified patient and was allowed to heal.

In Margaret's case, however, she brought her own dysfunction to the family, and her parents' apparent pathology proved to be their attempt to deal with her illness. Margaret was 15 when she was admitted for her second psychiatric hospitalization following an outburst during which she grabbed a kitchen knife and tried to kill her parents. The T.'s, a middle class, well-educated family, seemed very anxious, suspicious, and uncertain when contacted by the social worker after admission. Their response was puzzling as they seemed clear that Margaret required hospitalization and they wanted our hospital. They had carefully researched and selected a hospital that was a long distance from their home, because they believed we provided the best treatment available.

Margaret's mother came from a confusing family where her mother had radical mood shifts and was at times physically and emotionally abusive. Despite this, Mrs. T. had maintained a relationship with her mother and many holidays were spent with her. Mr. T. was a recovering alcoholic whose father was also alcoholic. Several other relatives were alcoholic and/or mentally ill. Again, family relationships were maintained.

When asked about the marital relationship, the T.'s looked anxious and suspicious, saying they had thought it was good.

At the time Margaret became violent, she had recently begun treatment and was receiving an antidepressant medication. Because of this and because of the family history of alcoholism, mental illness, and violent mood swings, Margaret was diagnosed as suffering from a bipolar disorder. Her violent behavior was seen as a manic episode precipitated by the antidepressant medication. Lithium was added to Margaret's medication regime, and she slowly began to improve.

The family continued to be surprisingly guarded and distant until, following a particularly cold fall weekend, the social worker received a lengthy, confusing letter from Mrs. T. about how Margaret didn't have her coat, and saying that her mother was worried, but didn't want to do anything wrong, so she'd leave it up to the social worker. In the next family session, the confusing letter was explored, and finally, the mysterious suspiciousness was clarified.

During the previous hospitalization, the family was treated by a therapist who believed there were no biological mental disorders. This therapist told them Margaret was ill because they wouldn't let her grow up, and that they wouldn't let her grow up because they needed her to stabilize their marriage. This made little sense to them, but they were not certain. Perhaps Margaret *was* ill because they were bad parents. If that was true, they must be terrible parents, because Margaret was terribly ill. The letter was the result of the mother's concern because Margaret, who was very depressed, had not asked them to bring her coat, and it was growing cold. If they brought it without her asking, would they be making her sicker by not letting her grow up? They didn't bring it. Mrs. T. spent the weekend crying because it was cold and her sick child had no coat. Thus the letter, and thus the fearfulness and suspicion of the social worker. To the T. family, social workers had been parent blamers who made them feel awful.

After this disclosure, the family was educated about the biological basis of bipolar disorders. They were assured that whatever their shortcomings as a family, they were not the reason Margaret was sick. They were sent to a support group for families of patients with affective disorders. Their guilt and anxiety decreased, their fearfulness and suspiciousness disappeared, and their hope and sense of competence grew. The last contact was two years after discharge. Margaret was doing well, had begun college, and the T.'s continued to define themselves as, and to function as, a healthy family.

The Educational System

Often, the treatment plan for a particular adolescent will require modification of the educational setting. Public Law 94-142 requires that all states in the United States provide education to all children regardless of handicap until the child graduates high school or turns 21, whichever comes first. This dictates that the education system must provide special education services up to and including residential treatment if such services are needed to deal with a child's educational handicap. To be eligible, a student must have a specific handicapping condition such as a learning disability. Emotional illness is considered educated. Social maladjustment, however, is not considered a handicapping condition.

Many adolescents who receive inpatient psychiatric treatment will require special education services after discharge. These services can be very expensive. However, under Public Law 94-142, they must be provided if circumstances meet the criteria of the law. Depending on the resources and priorities of the patient's local educational system, accessing these services can vary from somewhat easy to very difficult. In psychiatric hospitals, special educators on staff usually provide guidance and leadership in accessing these services. However, it is often the social worker's task to support the family during the process, especially when problems arise. Learning to negotiate this system can be empowering and therapeutic to the adolescent patient and the family. This was the case with Sara's family, in the following example.

> Sara was 15 when admitted to the psychiatric hospital following a suicide attempt. She was a sad, angry, confused adolescent who was failing in school and was abusing alcohol and marijuana. Sara's parents were divorced, and she had been kidnapped by her noncustodial father at age three. Eleven years later she was returned to her mother by the Child Protective Services Department of another state. She had been physically and sexually abused by her father.
>
> The mother took Sara in and tried to parent her. With much guilt, however, she acknowledged she did not feel connected to her angry, substance-abusing teenager. The child she had lost was a cuddly three-year-old. Mrs. R., who had a history of depression and poor self-esteem, added this lack of a motherly bond to her already long list of "lacks." Sara perceived her mother's lack of connection and interpreted it as proof of her [Sara's] unlovableness. During the 11 years of separation, Sara had dreamed about and longed for an idealized mother to

rescue her. She finally had a mother, but the situation was far from her ideal.

Sara had only a month of insurance available. That was enough time to stabilize her acute psychiatric disorder, but she required long-term residential treatment to consolidate her gains and to receive educational services. Sara knew she needed long-term care and agreed to the plan. Application for educational funding was made and was denied by the school district. They indicated Sara was a socially maladjusted child. Sara's mother was encouraged by the staff to appeal the decision. She hired an attorney and, with renewed energy and resourcefulness, appealed the decision and won. Sara finally had a mother who could fight for her. Mrs. R. began to feel less a failure and less disconnected. Sara received funding for residential treatment and, following a nine-month stay, she remained in intensive therapy. She lives, not with her mother, but with another family in her mother's neighborhood. She cannot really experience her mother as a mother, but she describes her as a really good friend to whom she can turn. Both Sara and Mrs. R. experience the limitations of their feelings for each other as products of their 11 years of separation, not as proof of the badness of either or both of them.

Health and Social Services

Many of the adolescents who require inpatient psychiatric care are involved with one or more health or welfare systems in the community. These may include outpatient therapists, protective services, foster care services, juvenile services, and other services. The social worker provides liaison to staff from all these services.

In cases where services need to be initiated, a large portion of this task falls to the social worker. Reports of suspected child abuse and neglect are generally made by the social worker. This can be a very difficult and painful experience for parents and sensitive support by the social worker can often ease the situation. It can also be a painful time for the social worker, who sometimes receives full force the parents' rage over the necessity to report. Explanations of mandatory reporting laws and of limits to confidentiality in cases of child abuse sometimes do little to modify the parents' subjective experience of betrayal. In order to minimize the potential negative relationship of the parents with the psychiatric hospital, it is critical that the social worker personally inform them that a report must be made. It is also helpful for the social worker to keep in mind that even angry, abusive parents love and want to protect their child. Parents may be enraged by the report, but may also be grateful that someone is helping them control themselves in their desire to best parent their children.

Discharge Plans

A wide range of aftercare plans can be made. Most adolescents will return to their parents with a plan for outpatient therapy. For some, however, more extensive services are needed. Some adolescents will not live at home after the hospital because of their special needs, or problems in their families, or both. The most comprehensive out-of-home placement is residential treatment. For adolescents, this means a therapeutic boarding school with 24-hour staffing, structured living, and full clinical services. Most residential treatment centers are unlocked and require that the adolescent participate on a voluntary basis. Most are also very expensive. Therapeutic group homes are less expensive, less structured, and do not have schooling as part of their programs. Residents usually attend neighborhood schools. They are also unlocked and require voluntary participation.

Some adolescents will go into therapeutic foster care after discharge. Here, too, there is a range of services. Therapeutic foster homes have paid, professional foster parents. Some services are short-term and offer one-on-one care to unstable adolescents. These are generally more expensive. Others are longer term, require more stabilized adolescents, and are less expensive. All therapeutic foster homes are sponsored by social service agencies which provide support and case management services to foster parents and to the adolescents.

For the adolescent who cannot return home and who does not require extensive therapeutic services, regular foster care or group home placement may be an option. Such adolescents also sometimes go to boarding schools. For the adolescent who can return home but who requires more extensive therapeutic services, day hospital programs or therapeutic day school may be used. Therapeutic after-school programs are also available.

Most of these services are expensive and it is a rare family that can afford them without help. Other funding sources are generally needed and it is the social worker who helps the family explore possible funding sources. Areas to be explored include schools. Does the child qualify for services under Public Law 94–142? Medical insurance will sometimes fund such service if they are covered in the patient's policy or if the policy allows for flexibility, under a managed care program. With such programs, less expensive alternatives to hospitalization are funded. State funds may be available through Children's Services. All states will provide funds for services to abused or neglected adolescents as children in need of assistance. Some states have broader definitions of children needing services. State departments of mental health sometimes have funds for services. They sometimes sponsor services that are free or have a sliding scale. In some states, a child who has been in an out-of-home placement for at least a month becomes eligible for state medical assistance based on that child's own income and assets, regardless of parents' income or assets. Medical assistance funds then may be available. If a child has been involved in the juvenile justice system, juvenile services funds may be available. All these possibilities should be explored; this is usually the social worker's task.

Some of the most challenging and frustrating work of the social worker working with adolescent inpatients and their families involves discharge planning. With shortened lengths of stay, more ongoing treatment is almost universally needed after inpatient care. Many adolescents are leaving the hospital "quicker and sicker." The social worker must to be aware of all potential services available to patients and all potential funding sources for such services. Unfortunately, resources for many such services are limited and funding is elusive. Thus, patients who need residential treatment or other intensive programs after discharge are often not able to access them. The task of discharge planning has become for the social worker how to do "more with less."

For those adolescents requiring less extensive services after discharge, the task is easier. If the adolescent is admitted without an outpatient therapist, the patient and family are referred upon discharge to a private practitioner, mental health clinic, or family service agency in their area, depending on their needs and wishes. In those cases referred by an outpatient therapist, the patient and family are referred back to that therapist.

> Paul, age 14, was admitted for his first psychiatric hospitalization after he physically attacked his foster mother. This was Paul's third foster home and, as with the first two, this foster family had decided Paul was too difficult to manage and were unwilling to keep him. At admission, the social worker contacted the foster care worker who requested guidance from the hospital on how to meet Paul's needs. Paul's mother's whereabouts was not known and his severely mentally ill father, who had many times required psychiatric hospitalization, was not an option for Paul's placement. Paul adored and at times idealized his father.

Paul's foster care worker was invited by the social worker to attend Paul's diagnostic conference, during which the recommendation was made for a therapeutic group home following a two-week hospitalization. It was felt Paul could not be managed in a foster home and should not have to face further pain of failure by foster families potentially rejecting him. While Paul was in the hospital, the social worker held two family sessions with him, one with his foster mother so that they could say goodbye and one with his father, so that both Paul and the father could feel that the father was part of the planning. The social worker also arranged for a preplacement visit to the group home, which was funded by the state, since Paul was a ward of the state.

SUMMARY

The social worker as part of the treatment team working with psychiatrically hospitalized adolescent patients is responsible for addressing the social environment of the patient. The social environment includes the family, the school system, and other health and social services. The social worker's tasks include evaluation, liaison, and environmental modification or treatment. The social worker provides a wide range of services, which must be based on a sound theoretical framework. The social worker must always remember that the adolescent and the social environment interact as a system rather than through simple linear causality. The social environment not only affects but is affected by the adolescent patient, while both affect and are affected by the patient's disorder.

REFERENCES

Bateson, G. (1972). *Steps to an Ecology of Mind*. San Francisco: Chandler.

Blos, Peter. (1962). *On Adolescence*. New York: the Free Press.

Bowen, M. (1978). *Family Therapy in Clinical Practice*. New York: Jason Aronson.

Hartman, A. and Laird, J. (1983). *Family-Centered Social Work Practice*. New York: Free Press.

Lunde, D. (1974). Eclectic and Integrated Theory. In A. Burton (Ed.), *Operational Theories of Personality* (381-414). New York: Brunner/Mazel.

Minuchin, S. (1974). *Families and Family Therapy*. Cambridge: Harvard University Press.

Towle, C. (1945). *Common Human Needs*. New York: National Association of Social Workers.

Woods, M. and Hollis, F. (1990). *Casework: A Psychosocial Therapy*, 4th ed. New York: McGraw Hill.

Chapter 7

PHARMACOTHERAPY IN CHILDREN AND ADOLESCENTS

Paramjit T. Joshi, Joseph T. Coyle, and John T. Walkup

The use of pharmacotherapy in the treatment of psychiatrically disturbed children dates from 1937 when Bradley first introduced amphetamine in the treatment of a heterogeneous group of institutionalized children with behavior disorders. In 1942, Bender reported the improvement in children who had symptoms of short attention span, increased motor activity, and poor organizational skills when treated with Benzedrine. Nevertheless, over the next two decades, there was considerable controversy and negative public sentiment against the use of pharmacological agents in the treatment of behavioral and emotional disorders in children and adolescents. In the 1950's, phenothiazine neuroleptics became available and were used primarily in the management of institutionalized, severely behaviorally disordered and brain-damaged children.

In the ensuing 40 years, there has been a remarkable increase in the number and type of psychopharmacological agents available. However, the emerging field of pediatric psychopharmacology has been fraught with many difficulties. In addition to having a philosophical bias against using drugs to treat childhood psychiatric disorders, many of the early studies designed to assess efficacy have been limited in that the childhood psychiatric disturbances have often been poorly defined, diagnostic classifications have varied over time, and a relatively small number of subjects have been included in most clinical trials. Moreover, most studies have been poorly designed, with a paucity of empirical and scientifically designed double-blind crossover studies, compounded by methodological difficulties, including lack of standardized rating scales and outcome measures, and the lack of control groups in most studies. The high rate of placebo response, along with the lack of follow-up of children placed on medications beyond six–ten weeks, has led to even further difficulties in interpretation.

Notwithstanding all of these past problems, there has been over the last 10 years an enormous increase in the number and quality of studies examining the use of psychopharmacological agents in the treatment of psychiatric disorders in children and adolescents. Epidemiological studies have given a clearer picture of the prevalence of psychiatric disorders in children and adolescents. The development of a descriptively based diagnostic classification system has led to clinicians becoming more reliable in classifying childhood psychopathology. This has had a positive effect on the field of childhood psychopharmacology, which has expanded in diversity and methodological sophistication.

Psychopharmacological agents for the treatment of behavioral and emotional problems in children are characteristically first studied in adults. In fact, the Food and Drug Administration has provided explicit approval for only a limited number of medications for the treatment of psychiatric disorders in children and adolescents. To address this problem, a number of studies are under way using various pharmacological agents for the treatment of psychiatric disorders in children, including antidepressants, lithium, and anticonvulsants. We should be encouraged by these efforts to try to better understand the pharmacokinetics and efficacy of psychotropics and to delineate appropriate indications and contraindications of these drugs for children and adolescents.

Pharmacotherapy for children and adolescents is only one aspect of a biopsychosocial treatment model. Youngsters admitted to inpatient psychiatric facilities have usually failed outpatient interventions and often pose a danger to themselves or to others, thereby requiring the most restrictive mode of treatment. The majority of the patients who are admitted to such facilities are seriously disturbed and many have co-morbid conditions, making treatment complex and difficult. Pharmacotherapy is usually considered in the primary treatment of hospitalized children and adolescents with major depressive disorders, childhood schizophrenia, attention deficit disorder, anxiety disorders, obsessive compulsive disorders, and Tourette's syndrome. In other instances, medications are used to reduce symptoms such as aggression, anxiety, perseveration, and self-mutilation, as seen in children with pervasive development disorder. The reduction of aggressive and markedly disruptive behaviors with psychotropic medications perhaps attracts the most controversy in the field, since some view it as a "chemical restraint." Nevertheless, controlled studies are now providing evidence of the efficacy of certain medications in trials where severely disturbed children and adolescents are selected based on the presence of symptoms, rather than on diagnosis. This may reflect, in part, the current limitations of diagnostic nosology, but is also analogous to the effectiveness of antipsychotics on delusions and hallucinations, regardless of whether they occur in the context of schizophrenia or of psychotic depression.

The remainder of this chapter will be devoted to groups of medications commonly utilized to treat psychiatric symptoms and disorders in children and adolescents. Emphasis will be placed on indication for initiating treatment, dosage titration, measuring outcome, follow-up, and the identification and management of adverse side effects.

It is of utmost importance when undertaking pharmacologic treatment of minors to discuss, in detail, with the patient, the parents, or the legal guardian the purpose of treatment, expectations, potential risks, and side effects, as well as to address any fears that the patient and parents may harbor. It is perhaps advisable to obtain written consent from the parents, not only to increase their awareness of medication usage but also to decrease the potential for misunderstandings and future litigious actions. In general, a well-documented outline of the discussion in the medical record is critical for risk management. A discussion with the patient and the parents of the advantages and disadvantages of particular medications will not only enhance the communication between the psychiatrist and the care-giving adults, but also serve to improve compliance with the medication after discharge from the hospital. The poorer the understanding that parents have of medications, the greater the likelihood of noncompliance.

STIMULANTS

The psychostimulants are the drugs of choice in the treatment of attention deficit disorder with hyperactivity. These include the amphetamines (Dexedrine and Benzedrine), methylphenidate (Ritalin), which has structural and pharmacological properties similar to amphetamines, and magnesium pemoline (Cylert), which is dissimilar in structure but is similar in function to the amphetamines. All these drugs are prescribed orally with good absorption, easily cross the blood brain barrier, and cause significant central nervous systemic excitation.

With the amphetamines, peak plasma levels are achieved within two to three hours, with a half life of four to six hours in children (Brown et al., 1979; Cantwell & Carlson, 1978). Clinical response is usually seen at one to three hours, before achieving peak plasma levels. A steady state half life of 10 hours is usually achieved after the patient has been on the drug regularly for approximately six months (Greenhill et al., 1984). Methylphenidate remains the most commonly prescribed medication for ADHD because of the relatively low incidence of side effects. Peak plasma levels are reached in one to two hours with a half life of two to three hours. A long-acting preparation (Ritalin SR) is also available and fairly widely used, but treatment with Ritalin SR has been shown to have inconsistent effects over time (Greenberg, 1985). Magnesium pemoline reaches peak serum levels in two to four hours but has a much longer half life of 12 hours. Significant clinical improvement may not be noted for up to three to four weeks (Cantwell & Carlson, 1978; Weiner & Jaffe, 1977). With the current status and emphasis on brief hospitalization (i.e., 10 to 20 days) in most psychiatric facilities, it may be unrealistic to prescribe pemoline to an inpatient and expect an unequivocal response during the inpatient stay.

Despite the fact that stimulants have been shown to be quite effective in the treatment of ADHD, the decision to prescribe them is largely a clinical one. This is based on the severity of symptoms, the ability of the school and classroom teacher to manage the child's distractibility and short attention span, the degree of disruption that the symptoms cause, interference in learning, and the views of the parents and the child in taking medication. The decision is also based on the results of previous treatment modalities employed.

Before the institution of stimulant treatment, a careful psychiatric and physical examination is essential. In addition, baseline ratings of the patient's behavior on the Connors' Teacher Rating Scale should be compared to ratings obtained while the child's dosage is being titrated to the desired balance between optimal clinical response and adverse drug effects. Preferably, teachers should be unaware as to whether the child is on medication, to avoid bias as they make their observations on the rating scales. Parent rating scales are available as well. However, because of the relatively short duration of action, and end-of-dose exacerbation in some children, the desired clinical effect is rarely seen in the late afternoon after a noontime dose. Parents can get discouraged and demoralized about the lack of change in behavior at home. Therefore, they need to be educated and advised about the nature and timing of the effects of stimulants in their children to avoid noncompliance, based on unrealistic expectations. Because of the appetite suppressant effects of stimulants, consideration of restricting treatment to school days should be considered, depending upon the ability of the parent or caretaker to tolerate the behaviors at home.

The recommended dose of methylphenidate for children is 0.3 to 0.6 mg/Kg, usually given in two doses, morning and noon. However, it may be necessary to rearrange dosage schedules depending on the particular needs of the child as it pertains to time of onset, duration of effect, and schedule of classes and work assignments. There is evidence to suggest that the lower dosages selectively improve attention (0.2 to 0.4 mg./Kg) while higher dosages (0.5 to 1.0 mg./Kg) affect behavior and may not improve attention (Greenberg, 1985). Controversy exists whether stimulant treatment results in academic gain. A double-blind, placebo-controlled study found improved behavior as well as better cognitive and academic performance in children receiving 0.7 mg/kg of methylphenidate a day (Kupietz, Winsberg & Sverd, 1982).

The most frequent and annoying early, and usually temporary, side effects are gastrointestinal, which include anorexia, nausea, abdominal cramps or pain, thirst, and vomiting. Cardiovascular effects, tachycardia, and elevated blood pressure can sometimes persist after the first few weeks of treatment. CNS effects reported are insomnia, lability of mood, irritability, sadness, and dysphoria. Potential long-term consequences of stimulant treatment are inhibition in growth, both height and weight. Safer, Allen & Barr (1972) and Klein et al. (1988) in a controlled study observed a significant reduction in growth velocity during the time the children were receiving stimulants. However, an accelerated rate of growth or "rebound growth" occurred after the stimulants were discontinued. This phenomenon supports the utility of "drug holidays" on weekends and vacations. Some children are more vulnerable to these side effects of growth suppression than others (Hamill et al., 1976). Measurements of height, weight, blood pressure, and pulse rate should be done approximately every four to six weeks.

Stimulants can precipitate tics, especially in those who are predisposed to a tic disorder, and controversy exists over whether stimulants are totally contraindicated in such cases (Greenhill, 1992). Hepatotoxicity is of special concern with the use of pemoline and elevated liver enzymes have been reported in 1–3 percent of children treated with this drug. These abnormalities are reversed after the medication is discontinued. It is, therefore, essential to monitor liver function tests in children being treated with magnesium pemoline throughout the duration of therapy (PDR, 1991). In order to minimize untoward side effects, one should titrate the dosage schedule slowly, with the goal of achieving the most effective dose with the fewest untoward effects.

Stimulant dosages seem to have a "creeping effect" where at times children receive Ritalin dosages of up to 80 mgs./day. We often admit children and adolescents to the hospital whose dosages of stimulants have been gradually increased to such high doses. This has usually taken place after poor response to standard doses, in an attempt to get a therapeutic effect. It is uncommon to achieve a good effect at such high doses and unwanted drug effects of dysphoria, even delirium, are often seen, and appetite suppression is usually profound. In such cases, there are often co-morbid conditions, such as mental retardation or anxiety, which may indicate treatment with other drugs besides stimulants. It is important to remember that more is not always better.

A common myth that parents usually have is that stimulants will result in their children being more prone to substance abuse as adults. Without minimizing the severe problems and prevalence of substance abuse in youngsters with a history of attention deficit hyperactivity disorder, there is no evidence to date to suggest that children who have been treated with stimulants are at any greater risk than controls to become drug-abusing adolescents or young adults (Greenhill, 1992).

ANTIDEPRESSANTS

Three groups of antidepressants have been used in the treatment of children and adolescents for a variety of conditions. These include the tricyclics, the most widely used class, the monoamine oxidase inhibitors, and the serotonin selective re-uptake inhibitors.

Tricyclic Antidepressants

The most commonly prescribed tricyclic antidepressants are imipramine (Tofranil), desipramine (Norpramine), and nortriptyline (Pamelor or Aventyl). The newer generation of heterocyclic antidepressants, such as amoxapine (Asendin) and trazadone (Desyril), are seldom used in children. This section will focus only on the most commonly used ones.

It is highly advisable that patients have a physical examination, including an EKG and blood pressure and pulse rate recordings both in the prone and supine positions, before treatment is initiated with any of the tricyclic antidepressants. Informed consent is again desirable. Several studies on the cardiovascular effects of tricyclic antidepressants (Puig-Antich, Ryan & Rabinovich, 1985; Biederman et al., 1989; Schroeder et al., 1989) demonstrated that a slight but significant lengthening of the PR and QRS intervals occurs at doses of 5 mg/Kg. Saraf et al. (1978) reported that the greatest lengthening of the PR interval during imipramine therapy occurred among children with the shortest PR intervals to begin with and suggested that this effect perhaps may be protective. The results also indicated that relatively longer PR intervals is not a contraindication to receiving tricyclic medication.

Indications for Tricyclics

1. *Enuresis*: Pharmacotherapy is used in the treatment of enuresis only when behavioral approaches have failed. Imipramine was first described to be useful in the treatment of enuresis in 1960. Since then, several well-designed studies have shown its efficacy in the treatment of enuresis when compared with placebo (Greenberg & Stephans, 1977; Gualtieri, 1977). Despite the fact that imipramine stops or reduces bed-wetting in many children, enuresis can recur when the medication is discontinued (Shaffer, Costello & Hill, 1968). The mechanism of action of imipramine in the treatment of enuresis remains unclear although its potent muscarinic receptor antagonistic action which interferes with parasympathetic function is thought to contribute to its efficacy. Its antienuretic action is usually unrelated to its antidepressant effects and usually commences within 48 hours after starting a low dose in the order of 0.5–1.5 mg/Kg. The initial dosage in children between the ages of six to 12 is 25 mg, administered about an hour before bedtime. If the desired response is not obtained, the dose can be increased to 50 mg at bedtime. In children over the age of 12 years, the dose can be increased up to 75 mg.

2. *Attention deficit hyperactivity disorder*: Although most studies find stimulants superior to tricyclic antidepressants, imipramine and more recently desipramine, have been shown to be effective treatments for ADHD (Rapoport & Mikkelsen, 1978; Campbell, Green & Deutsch, 1985). Desipramine has become the tricyclic of choice in the treatment of ADHD because it has fewer anticholinergic and sedating effects than imipramine. Desipramine may be used as an alternative to stimulants in those patients who have either a poor response to stimulants or develop intolerable side effects. Desipramine should also be considered in patients who are at high risk for developing tics. Since desipramine has a much longer half-life than stimulants, it can also be useful in patients who develop such severe rebound hyperactivity on stimulants that they are unmanageable at home in the late afternoon or evenings. Since the

FDA has so far not approved the use of desipramine in the treatment of ADHD, there are no recommended dosage guidelines. However, based on published scientific reports, it is recommended that patients start on a low dose of 0.5 mg/Kg or 10-25 mg per day, with gradual titration upward to a dose not to exceed 2.5 mg/Kg. Rapoport reported more side effects and noncompliance with imipramine than with stimulants, although this may not be the case with desipramine.

3. *Panic disorder and agoraphobia*: Imipramine has been found to be effective in the treatment of adult patients with agoraphobia and panic attacks. These encouraging results led to the first open trial of imipramine in children with separation anxiety disorder and school refusal (Rabiner & Klein, 1969), the results were promising. The same research group undertook a double-blind, placebo-controlled study (Gittelman-Klein & Klein, 1971; Gittelman-Klein, 1973, 1980) demonstrating the efficacy of imipramine not only on school attendance but also on other measures of separation anxiety, such as somatic complaints and depressive affect. By contrast, the same investigators were unable to replicate the efficacy of imipramine (Klein, Koplewicz & Kanner, 1992) in a recently published study in a smaller but similar clinical population. They concluded that imipramine should not be precluded from consideration in the management of separation anxiety disorder, but that a good drug effect cannot be expected with regularity.

4. *Depression*: The treatment of depression with the tricyclic antidepressants began in the early 1960's, long before there was any nosological consensus about what constitutes depression in children (Lucas & Pasley, 1969). With the advent of diagnostic criteria, first by Weinberg et al (1973) followed by the publication of the DSM-III in 1980, several studies appeared in which tricyclic antidepressants were used for the treatment of childhood depression. These early studies, which demonstrated promising results, were open trials (Weinberg et al., 1973; Puig-Antich et al., 1978; Preskorn et al., 1982). More rigorous and better-controlled research designs have not confirmed significant therapeutic effects of antidepressants in child or adolescent depression. This result contravenes a wealth of clinical experience and may be attributable to certain methodologic limitations of the studies. These include: poorly defined patient groups, co-morbidity, small sample size, questionable assessment instruments, short duration of treatment and follow-up, as well as fixed dosages and unmonitored plasma levels

(Kramer & Feguine, 1981; Petti & Law, 1982; Kashani, Shekim & Reid, 1984; Puig-Antich, Perel & Lupafkin, 1987). A recent study (Geller et al., 1992) examined 50 prepubertal children in a double-blind, placebo-controlled design and found a poor rate of response in both treatment and control groups. The patients however had a chronic, unremitting course of depressive illness before the study, with a high percentage of positive family histories of depressive disorder, alcoholism, and suicidality, and a high rate of co-morbidity. Adult study samples with a high degree of co-morbidity and severity have also been reported to be resistant to treatment with tricyclics (Hamilton, 1979; Keller et al., 1990; Liebowitz et al., 1990).

The apparent lack of significant efficacy of antidepressants in the treatment of major depressive disorder of children and adolescents observed in recent well-controlled studies raises some interesting issues. It is presumed that children and adolescents are suffering from the same type of disorder as occurs in adults that has reportedly been demonstrated to be responsive to antidepressants. This assumption has genetic under-pinnings and is based in part on phenomenological similarities between adult- and childhood-onset depression, and in part on the fact that the children and adolescents often have parents with medication-responsive depression. However, these assumptions may be inadequate: early age of onset may signal a more severe form of affective illness, and treatment refractiveness may be related to severity. Alternatively, the immature brain may not be synaptically capable of responding to antidepressant action in a way that reverses an episode of depression in the child or adolescent. This may necessitate the exploration of novel or combined treatment strategies.

Monoamine Oxidase Inhibitors

The use of monoamine oxidase inhibitors (MAOI's) for the treatment of depressive disorders in children and adolescents is limited, as are scientific studies examining their efficacy. Resistance to the use of this group of antidepressants stems primarily from the required dietary restrictions which are difficult to enforce in children and adolescents, especially in outpatient treatment. The two most commonly used drugs are phenelzine (Nardil) and tranylcypromine (Parnate). Only one study examined the efficacy of MAOI's in adolescents (Ryan et al., 1988). This was an open study of 23 adolescents in whom MAOI's were prescribed either alone or in combination with a tricyclic antidepressant. Forty-eight percent of the patients were rated as having both a good clinical response and dietary compliance. Thirteen percent reportedly had a good clinical response but poor dietary compliance. Two patients developed severe hypertension after ingesting food containing tyramine, and required medical treatment. Given this risk along with the availability of a number of tricyclic antidepressants, serotonin selective re-uptake inhibitors (SSRI), and alternative treatments (lithium and anticonvulsants), MAOI'S should be prescribed with particular caution. However, MAOI's have certainly been shown to be beneficial, especially in adult patients with a refractory depression. If one is compelled to use this group of medications, it is advisable to select the patients very carefully, restricting use to patients who are reliable, compliant, and not indulging in substance abuse or impulsive behaviors.

Fluoxetine

Since fluoxetine (Prozac) was introduced in the United States as the first SSRI antidepressant, it has received wide publicity, ranging from its description as a "cure all" and "miracle drug" to an alleged cause of severe aggression and suicidal behavior in patients. Fluoxetine is a potent and highly selective serotonin re-uptake inhibitor. It was introduced for the treatment of depression and obsessive compulsive disorder in adults. To date, fluoxetine has not been approved for use in children and adolescents. Its side effect profile makes it a very attractive choice for the treatment of depression in adults. Unlike the tricyclic antidepressants and the MAOI's, it has minimal cardiac, anticholinergic, and antihistaminic side effects. The most common side effects experienced are nausea, headaches, insomnia and nervousness. Despite a single report of increased suicidality (Teicher, Glod & Cole, 1990), the majority of data do not suggest a cause-and-effect relationship between the use of fluoxetine and suicidality (Fava & Rosenbaum, 1991). Evidence suggests that the rate of suicidality in fluoxetine-treated patients is no higher than in patients treated with other antidepressants. It appears rather to be an effect of the underlying vulnerability of patients with severe depression to suicidal ideation and behavior.

Two studies to date have evaluated the use of fluoxetine in children and adolescents. In one open trial, 14 children, aged five to 15 years, who met DSM-III-R criteria for major depressive disorder, were treated with fluoxetine after treatment failure with a tricyclic antidepressant. The patients had either had a poor antidepressant response or had developed cardiac side effects (Joshi et al., 1989). The majority of the children showed improvement within the first two weeks of initiation of treatment. The second study, the only placebo-controlled study of fluoxetine, evaluated efficacy in 31 adolescents, aged 13 to 18 years (Simeon et al., 1990). Significant clinical improvement occurred in both groups after a few weeks, but the authors could not conclude that fluoxetine was superior to placebo. King et al. (1991), reported the occurrence of hyperactive and self-destructive behaviors in six adolescents with obsessive compulsive disorder who had been treated with fluoxetine.

It is possible that some patients are receiving too much fluoxetine, resulting in a serotonergic overload causing disinhibition, hyperactivity, and impulsiveness, with consequent poor judgment and self-destructive behaviors. These complications result from a rapidly rising blood level caused by the long half life of fluoxetine. This outcome is particularly likely when doctors and patients become impatient in waiting six to eight weeks for a clinical response, and increase the dose too rapidly. In our experience, children and adolescents do better on lower dosages (i.e., 10 mg every other day). Increasing dosage slowly avoids some of the above unwanted effects, while maintaining clinical improvement.

Fluoxetine is now available in liquid form, making it easier to administer smaller dosages. It remains a promising antidepressant for the treatment of major depressive disorders in children and adolescents. It is especially preferred by teenage girls who wish to avoid the weight gain they may experience with tricyclic antidepressants. Caution needs to be exercised when one switches a patient from fluoxetine to a tricyclic antidepressant. Fluoxetine acts synergistically with tricyclics and can cause alarmingly high blood levels. Because of fluoxetine's long half-life, this can happen even after two weeks off fluoxetine, if the tricyclic dose is increased too quickly.

Two newer serotenergic antidepressants are now available for the treatment of depression in adults. Both of these, fluvoxamine and sertraline, have a shorter half-life than fluoxetine. Fluvoxamine has fewer noradrenergic effects and can be administered at bedtime, since it does not disrupt sleep. The half-life of fluvoxamine is 14 to 15 hours in healthy adults, and is 17 to 22 hours in adult inpatients after multiple dosing. There are no current reports of the use of these two drugs in youngsters, though controlled studies are underway examining the efficacy of fluvoxamine in youngsters with obsessive compulsive disorder.

Clomipramine

Clomipramine (Anafranil) is a tricyclic antidepressant which has been well studied for the treatment of obsessive-compulsive disorder (OCD).

Rapoport and Mikkelson (1980, 1989) have carried out several well-designed studies establishing the efficacy of clomipramine in the treatment of OCD in children and adolescents. The usual recommended starting dose is 25 mg/day, gradually increasing in increments of 25 mg/day up to 3 mg/Kg/day or 200 mg/day in divided doses. The side-effect profile of clomipramine is similar to the other tricyclic antidepressants, thus mandating the same pretreatment evaluation, especially cardiovascular status.

LITHIUM

Lithium has been used in children for a variety of conditions ranging from the treatment of bipolar disorders (Youngerman & Canino, 1978) to the management of aggression (Dostal & Zvosky, 1970; Delong, 1978; Lena 1980; Jefferson et al., 1983), self-mutilatory behaviors in autistic children (Campbell, Cohen & Small, 1982), organic mood disorders, especially those secondary to closed head trauma (Joshi, Capozzoli & Coyle, 1985), and hyperactivity (Greenhill et al., 1973; DeLong & Aldershof, 1987). In addition, lithium has been shown to have a favorable antidepressant effect when used as an adjunct to tricyclic antidepressants for the treatment of refractory major affective disorder (Strober, 1989).

Lithium is a monovalent cation from the alkali metal group. It is rapidly absorbed in the stomach and small intestine and is eliminated primarily by renal excretion. Pharmacokinetic studies have shown that the half-life is shorter and the renal clearance is usually greater in children than in adults on the basis of body mass (Vitiello et al., 1988). Lithium has a tendency to concentrate in a few tissues, notably the thyroid gland and the renal medulla. Excretion of lithium depends on the glomerular filtration rate (GFR) and proximal reabsorption. Prior to initiating treatment with lithium, a thorough medical evaluation is mandatory, including an assessment of renal function, thyroid status, and serum electrolytes. There is currently disagreement over the necessity to carry out a quantitative assessment of the GFR by collecting 24-hour urine for creatinine clearance. This poses a practical problem, especially in younger children or seriously ill adolescents who are unable to cooperate fully with this procedure and in those children who have night-time enuresis. The use of calculated creatinine clearance based on a single urine sample has been suggested by Cockcroft and Gault (1976).

Lithium is available as lithium carbonate and lithium citrate. Lithobid, a coated form of lithium carbonate, is somewhat better tolerated and causes fewer initial gastrointestinal side effects. Lithium citrate is available in the liquid form and is therefore useful in younger patients who require smaller or fractional dosages and in others for whom noncompliance by "cheeking" medications may be an issue. The dosage regimen and scheduling in children over five years of age is similar to that of adults (Campbell, Perry & Green, 1984). Dosage requirements are determined by serum lithium levels and vary from one patient to another. Our practice with very young children is to start at a dose of about 150 mgs administered twice daily and gradually titrating it to a therapeutic range from 0.7 m.eq/l to 1.2 m.eq/l. Serum levels should be drawn approximately 12 hours after the last lithium dose. In hospitalized patients, this is effectively done in the mornings. However, in outpatients, it may be more practical to obtain an afternoon or evening serum level, thus avoiding loss of school time that may result from a morning blood drawing. Initially, serum levels are drawn about twice a week; as the patient stabilizes, the frequency of serum levels can decrease. Our practice is to obtain serum levels every two to three months in those patients who are stable and not experiencing side effects.

When treatment is initiated, lithium may cause gastrointestinal symptoms such as nausea, diarrhea, and abdominal cramps. These tend to subside after stable serum levels are attained and can sometimes be alleviated by the prescription of lithobid. The side effects associated with maintenance treatment with lithium are hand tremors, which can be embarrassing or disabling to school-aged children, polyuria (possibly from nephrogenic diabetes insipidus), and hypothyroidism. These side effects must be addressed with the patient because their presence can result in discouragement and noncompliance. The polyuria is accompanied by polydipsia and can sometimes precipitate the reemergence of enuresis. Symptoms of toxicity usually appear at serum levels above 1.5 m.eq/l. With rapidly rising lithium levels, hand tremors can reappear along with gastrointestinal symptoms. More severe toxicity is signaled by cardiac arrhythmias along with impairments in consciousness with lethargy, delirium, and stupor. Lithium toxicity is a serious but largely preventable complication if the patients are monitored closely and effectively.

Children and adolescents treated with lithium must be monitored in several specific ways. Nonsteroidal anti-inflammatory agents, which are commonly used in youngsters, can interfere with renal excretion and can cause elevation in serum lithium, resulting in toxicity (Jefferson et al., 1983). Dehydration, caused by excessive sweating or febrile illness without fluid replacement, will elevate serum lithium levels. There has been concern about the effect of lithium on bone growth, since lithium is known to be deposited in the bone. At the present time, there is no evidence to support any growth impairment secondary to long-term lithium use (Birch, 1980). Facial acne may be exacerbated by lithium; this can undermine compliance, especially in adolescents. The acne can usually be effectively treated with antibiotics, such as tetracyclines, with no known untoward effects (Jefferson et al., 1983).

Lithium is becoming an important pharmacological agent in the treatment not only of bipolar disorder but also of aggression in children and adolescents. In many instances, it is replacing the use of neuroleptics for the management of aggressive and disruptive behaviors, avoiding cognitive dulling and the more serious long-term side effect, tardive dyskinesia, associated with neuroleptic treatment, especially in the mentally retarded.

NEUROLEPTICS

Neuroleptics, also known as "antipsychotic drugs" and "major tranquilizers," have been clinically available for over 30 years. In children and adolescents, they have been used to treat a number of psychiatric disorders, behavior problems, and symptoms. As in adults, they are most widely used specifically for the treatment of psychosis and severe agitation. In lower dosages, they have been used in the treatment of Tourette's disorder, attention-deficit disorder with hyperactivity, and for the control of behavioral dysfunction in patients with mental retardation and pervasive developmental disorders. Neuroleptics are dopamine receptor antagonists. Postsynaptic receptor blockade in the mesolimbic system of the brain is thought to result in the desired therapeutic effect in psychosis, whereas similar blockade in the nigrostriatal dopamine pathway produces the unwanted extrapyramidal effects. Over 20 different neuroleptics are commercially available. The most commonly used ones fall into three broad groups. These are the: (1) Phenothiazines (Chlorpromazine, Thioridazine, Loxapine, Trifluoperazine and Fluphenazine); (2) Thioxanthenes (Thiothixene and Chlorprothixene); and (3) Butyrophenones (Haloperidol and Droperidol).

Among the variety of neuroleptics available, haloperidol has been relatively well studied by several investigators in the management of childhood disorders. In most of these studies, haloperidol proved to be significantly superior to placebo and was usually better than psychotropic medications from other classes, such as psychostimulants and lithium (Serrano & Forbes, 1973; Faretra, Dooher & Dowling, 1970). Low doses of high potency neuroleptics (0.5 to 4.0 mg/day) have been shown to be effective in reducing social withdrawal and stereotypic behaviors in autistic children (Campbell, Anderson & Small, 1982). Similarly, Joshi et al., (1988) demonstrated in an open study, that children with pervasive developmental disorder who received an average dose of 0.04 mg/Kg per day of haloperidol or fluphenazine exhibited significant reductions in hyperactivity and aggressive symptoms, and significant improvement in peer relations. Although serum levels of neuroleptics were not measured in this study, serum levels obtained in a comparable age group of patients with Tourette's disorder, who received similar dosages of haloperidol, found levels to be quite low—at least ten times lower than those typically associated with therapeutic response in adults suffering from schizophrenia (Singer et al., 1982). The untoward side effects were minimal and limited to transient extrapyramidal symptoms, which did not require maintenance treatment with anticholinergic drugs.

Current evidence does not suggest any clear superiority of a particular neuroleptic, once corrected for potency, in the management of psychotic symptoms. The incisive neuroleptics, such as haloperidol and fluphenazine (Prolixin), are generally less sedating and thus interfere less with school performance. Review of the literature suggests that in most instances neuroleptics are generally well tolerated by youngsters without serious ill effects (Faretra et al., 1970; Waizer et al., 1972; Pool et al., 1976; Realmuto et al., 1984). Informed consent is recommended before starting any patient on a neuroleptic, especially in light of the potential for long-term deleterious side effects, such as tardive dyskinesia.

Adverse effects secondary to neuroleptic treatment can be described as early and late. The earlier side effects, which are reversible, include sedation, dystonic reactions, restlessness, akathesia, Parkinsonian symptoms, and postural hypotension. Most of these side effects are subjectively uncomfortable and in the case of a dystonic reaction frightening to the patient. The extrapyramidal side effects can often be reversed by the administration of anticholinergic drugs, such as diphenhydramine (Benadryl) 25 mg. orally or intramuscularly or benztropine (Cogentin) 0.5 to 2 mg. given daily.

Withdrawal dyskinesia, choreaform movements which occur upon discontinuation of neuroleptics, are more frequent in children than in adults. Withdrawal dyskinesia subsides over a period of days to weeks and can be difficult to distinguish from tardive dyskinesia. Although tardive dyskinesia occurs more frequently in the elderly, it can develop in adolescents and young adults as a consequence of long-term and/or high-dose neuroleptic treatment (Gualtieri, 1984). Though there is belief that neuroleptics lower the seizure threshold, there are no systematic studies that demonstrate this. Our clinical experience has been that neuroleptics can safely be used in patients with a seizure disorder, when monitored appropriately. Of particular importance to adolescents are the embarrassing side effects, such as worsening of acne, weight gain, easy sunburning, and, in male patients, sexual dysfunction.

"Neuroleptic Malignant Syndrome"

Neuroleptic malignant syndrome (NMS) is a potentially life-threatening disorder that affects up to 1 percent of patients receiving neuroleptics. The precise cause of NMS remains unclear. While it shares many symptomatic features with malignant hyperthermia, a heritable abnormality of muscular function (Caroff, 1980), there is evidence that individuals with malignant hyperthermia are not vulnerable to neuroleptic-induced NMS; biopsies from patients suffering from NMS have not revealed the metabolic abnormalities of intramuscular calcium disposition as seen in malignant hyperthermia (Tollefson, 1982). The proximate cause of the syndrome appears to be insufficient stimulation of CNS dopamine receptors, since a syndrome identical to NMS occurs in patients with Parkinson's disease who have their dopamine receptor agonists abruptly discontinued (Sechi, Tandi & Mutani, 1984; Bowers et al., 1988). More recent prevalence studies in adult inpatient settings suggest that the risk of NMS ranges from 0.1 to 1.0 percent of all patients receiving neuroleptics (Pope, Keck & McElroy, 1986; Freidman, Davis & Wagner, 1988). The principal clinical features of NMS include striking rigidity, hyperthermia, diaphoresis, rhabdomyolysis, and delirium. Recent studies suggest that an underlying affective disorder may render individuals more vulnerable to developing NMS (Pope, 1986).

While as little as a decade ago children and even adolescents were not thought to suffer from severe affective disorder, more recent studies suggest that affective disorder may be the most common serious psychiatric disorder of late childhood and adolescents, considerably surpassing schizophrenia in its prevalence (Joshi et al., 1990). Furthermore, neuroleptics, the drug of choice in the management of psychosis, may be introduced early in the treatment of affective disorder with psychosis. Supporting this association between affective disorder and NMS vulnerability, two cases of NMS have been described in adolescents who received neuroleptics. Both patients were seriously ill, needing treatment in the intensive care unit. One adolescent was treated with both bromocriptine and dantrolene, and the other with bromocriptine alone (Joshi et al., 1991). Bromocriptine is a dopamine D-2 receptor agonist and is effective in reversing the acute extrapyramidal symptoms of profound rigidity and its secondary consequences, including hyperthermia and rhabdomyolysis. Dantrolene acts by enhancing intramuscular calcium sequestration. It is commonly used in association with agents that potentiate central dopaminergic neurotransmission, since in itself dantrolene does not reverse the rigidity and psychomotor retardation resulting from central dopamine receptor blockade (Sechi et al., 1984; Bowers et al., 1988). The risk for NMS may be increasing in the pediatric population, since psychotropic medications are assuming a greater role in the management of severe psychiatric disturbances in this age group. Pediatricians should be aware of possible NMS in patients, who present with fever of unknown origin, striking extrapyramidal symptoms, and a recent history of psychopharmacologic intervention.

"Rapid Neuroleptization"

Neuroleptics are frequently used to control aggression and agitation on child and adolescent inpatient settings. This is usually most effectively attained with "rapid neuroleptization." Historically, patients on adult and child psychiatry units have been physically restrained when they exhibit dangerous and out-of-control behaviors. Dubin and Feld (1989) described psychotropic medications as more effective, and also more "humane" than physical restraint for the management of aggressive behaviors. Haloperidol has been used with success for rapid neuroleptization for psychiatric emergencies in the United States (Donlon, Hopkin & Tupin, 1979 and Clinton et al., 1987). However, more recently, droperidol (Inapsine) has been receiving much attention for the management of acute psychiatric emergencies involving agitation, violent and threatening behavior, and severe psychosis. Droperidol, like haloperidol, is a butyrophenone, but with a more rapid onset of action (three to 10 minutes), short duration of effect (two to four hours), and significant tranquilizing and sedating effects when administered intramuscularly. Droperidol's side-effect profile, especially the incidence of extrapyramidal symptoms, appears more favorable than other neuroleptics in its class (PDR, 1991; Ayd, 1980). In a double-blind trial, Resnick and Burton (1984) demonstrated marked efficacy and probable superiority of droperidol over haloperidol in managing acute agitation in adults.

There is little literature evaluating the safety and effectiveness of any medication in the management of acute agitation in children and adolescents (Popper, 1990; Vitiello et al., 1987). Droperidol has been routinely used by the authors over eight years on the child and adolescent inpatient services to acutely manage agitated and disorganized patients who have not responded to redirection, time outs, or placement in the seclusion room and have presented as a danger to themselves and others. Walkup et al. (1991) examined the use of droperidol in 17 adolescents in an inpatient setting. The dosage schedule was established according to body weight: 0.25 cc (< 50 lbs.), 0.50 cc (51–75 lbs.), 0.75 cc (76–125 lbs.), and 1 cc (> 125 lbs.). The results showed that droperidol can be safely administered to children and adolescents with negligible untoward side effects, resulting in rapid deescalation of aggression and agitation and return to normal activity after an average of 105 minutes. The effective use of droperidol for the management of severe agitation and aggression has eliminated the necessity for physical restraint. It is important to emphasize that this intervention is used in the setting of intensive behavioral management and family involvement.

ANTICONVULSANTS

The most common anticonvulsant used in the treatment of psychiatric disorders in youngsters is carbamazepine (Tegretol). In the pediatric population, carbamazepine has been used mainly for controlling aggressive behaviors and for the treatment of patients with bipolar disorder. Carbamazepine is an iminodibenzyl derivative with a tricyclic structure similar to imipramine and chlorpromazine. Double-blind, placebo-controlled studies in adults have shown antimanic effects in neurologically normal bipolar patients (Ballenger & Post, 1980). It has also been shown to be prophylactic in mania and depression in lithium-resistant patients, especially those with rapidly cycling bipolar disorder (Post et al., 1983; Potter, 1983). In youngsters, carbamazepine has been reported to be effective in the treatment of explosive behaviors associated with temporal lobe epilepsy as well as in episodic dyscontrol (Tunks & Dermer, 1977).

Other studies of various types including case reports have shown carbamazepine to decrease impulsivity, agitation, aggression, and affective lability to varying degrees (Remschmidt, 1976; Yatham & McHale, 1988; Kafantaris et al., 1992). In adolescents, the dose ranges from approximately 400 to 800 mgs/day, with plasma levels of 6 to 12 ug/mL. Laboratory workup before treatment with carbamazepine should include complete blood count, including differential and platelet count, electrolytes, liver function tests, and an EKG. The most common side effects are an allergic skin rash, initial lethargy and drowsiness, dysarthria, and ataxia. Most can be eliminated by lowering of the dosage. Other ill effects that have been reported and need to be closely monitored are elevated liver function tests, leucopenia, thrombocytopenia, and agranulocytosis (Sillanpaa, 1981). Carbamazepine can be used synergistically with lithium, neuroleptics, and tricyclic antidepressants. Combination with MAOI's requires great caution because of a substantial rise in the plasma concentration of carbamazepine, causing potentially serious toxicity (Rudorfer & Potter, 1987).

CLONIDINE

Clonidine (Catapress) is well known as an antihypertensive drug which was first used in 1979 for the treatment of Tourette's syndrome (Cohen et al., 1980). It is an alpha-2 adrenergic receptor agonist and acts by decreasing noradrenergic functioning. The results of several open and double-blind trials suggest that clonidine is effective in the reduction of tics in patients with Tourette's syndrome (McKeith, Williams & Nicol, 1981; Borison et al., 1983; Leckman et al., 1991). In a double-blind, cross-over design, Hunt, Minderaa and Cohen, (1985) developed evidence that clonidine was efficacious in the treatment of ADHD. For both disorders, clonidine is started at a low dose of 0.05 mg/day and slowly titrated over several days and weeks to achieve the desired behavioral effect. Dosages of over 0.3 mg/day usually result in sedation and hence inattention in the classroom. Clonidine has a slower onset of action than stimulants; therefore, improvement in restlessness, attention span, impulsiveness, or diminution in tics may not be immediately evident. Hypotension with subjective dizziness can sometimes occur, especially if the dose is increased rapidly. Baseline EKG is desirable because of the potential increase in the PR interval.

OTHER MEDICATIONS

Bupropion

Bupropion (Wellbutrin) is a newer antidepressant which has been shown to be superior to placebo in randomized, double-blind, placebo-controlled trials in adults. Bupropion acts by blocking the synaptic re-uptake of dopamine and does not have any appreciable effect on the re-uptake of N E or 5-HT. Bupropion is an attractive alternative to the tricyclic antidepressants in those patients who are unable to tolerate the side effects of the tricyclics antidepressants. It has negligible anticholinergic and cardiovascular side effects. The side effects that have been reported are insomnia, restlessness, and diaphoresis. Seizures can occur if the dosage recommendations are exceeded. There are no reports evaluating the use of bupropion in youngsters. However, the authors have successfully employed bupropion in the inpatient treatment of major depressive disorder in adolescents. The dosage schedule was three divided doses, each dose not exceeding 300 mg. Further studies are needed to establish the efficacy of bupropion in the treatment of depression in youngsters.

Buspirone

Buspirone (Buspar), has been shown to be an effective anxiolytic agent with possible antidepressant effect in adults. It is considered an effective and relatively safe alternative to the benzodiazepines in the treatment of anxiety disorders (Riblet et al., 1982; Goldberg, 1984; Kastenholz & Crimson, 1984; Skolnick, Paul & Weissman, 1984; Taylor et al., 1985; Gardner & Kutcher, 1990). Although there are no double-blind placebo-controlled studies to date in children and adolescents, there is a case report of a 13-year-old boy with overanxious disorder of childhood who responded to treatment with 10 mg/day of buspirone with no ill effects (Kranzler, 1988). Kutcher and MacKenzie (1988, 1990) described their experience with buspirone in youngsters with overanxious disorder of childhood. The dose of buspirone ranged from 15 to 30 mg/day in divided dosages, with significant improvement on the Hamilton Anxiety Scale. The side-effect profile is reported to be relatively benign with a wide margin of safety and low abuse potential. Some of the more commonly reported side effects reported are insomnia, dizziness, head-aches, and gastrointestinal complaints (Newton et al., 1982).

Clozaril

Clozaril is an atypical neuroleptic that has been shown to be effective in a significant portion of chronic, treatment-resistant schizophrenics. The drug does not cause acute extrapyramidal side effects nor tardive dyskinesia. A striking feature of the drug is its ability not only to reduce positive symptoms of schizophrenia but also to abate negative symptoms. Unfor-tunately, clozaril bears the serious, potential fatal risk of inducing aplastic anemia in up to 4 percent of treated patients. As a consequence, patients must be closely monitored with weekly white cell counts. Because of the toxicity, there is little report of its use in children and adolescents. There is only one report in the literature, describing the effective use of clozaril in the treatment of three adolescents with schizophrenia, who had failed treatment with more conventional neuroleptics (Birmaher et al., 1992). However, a number of new atypical neuroleptics without such toxicity are in clinical trials in the United States and could prove useful in psychotic disorders in children and adolescents.

Beta Blockers

The most commonly used beta adrenergic blocking agent in the treatment and management of psychiatric symptoms is propanalol. There have been several reports in the literature of its effectiveness in the management of rage outbursts and aggressive and violent behaviors in youngsters (Rogeness et al., 1987; Yudofsky, Williams & Gorman, 1981; Williams et al., 1982). In a report of 16 youngsters treated with propanalol, the dose range was 80 to 280 mg/day in divided dosage (Kuperman & Stewart, 1987). However, there are no well-controlled studies demonstrating its efficacy and safety. Propanalol acts on both the central nervous system and peripheral sympathetic system and is contraindicated in patients with asthma, diabetes mellitus, bradycardia, and hypotension. It is important to do an EKG and monitor the cardiac status by frequent measurement of the pulse rate and blood pressure.

CONCLUSION

Over the past decade, the use of psychotropic medications in the treatment of severe psychiatric disturbances in children and adolescents has advanced from a treatment shunned by many clinicians and utilized in a rational fashion by a few to an increasingly rigorous and rational approach. The recent difficulties in demonstrating the efficacy of antidepressants in the treatment of child and adolescent major depressive disorders justifiably raise important questions about the facile assumption that knowledge gained in adult-controlled studies can simply be extended to youth. In fact, the Federal Drug Administration (FDA) is considering the possibility of requiring pharmaceutical houses to carry out well-controlled studies of the efficacy of new psychotropic medications on children if it appears that the drug could be used in this age group. This development would certainly go far in advancing our knowledge of the rational use of psychotropic drugs in child and adolescent psychiatry.

The focus on specific indications and dosing parameters does not imply that psychotropic drugs are the most salient feature of treatment. Recent research has emphasized the importance of psychologic, behavioral, and education interventions in combination with appropriate psychotropic medication. As our understanding of psychotropic drug treatment in child and adolescent psychiatry advances, the real challenge will be to establish through controlled studies, the forms and sequence of these ancillary interventions.

REFERENCES

Ayd, F. (1980). Parenteral droperidol for acutely disturbed psychotic and non-psychotic individuals. *Int Drug Ther*, *15*, 13-16.

Ballenger, J. C., Post, R. M. (1980). Carbamazepine in manic-depressive illness: A new treatment. *Am J Psychiatry*, *137*, 782-790.

Bender, L. (1942). Schizophrenia in childhood. *Nerv Child*, *1*, 138-140.

Biederman, J., Baldessarini, R. J., Wright, V., Knee, D., Harmatz, J. S., Goldbatt, A. (1989). A double-blind placebo controlled study of desipramine in the treatment of ADD: Il. Saerum drug levels and cardiovascular findings. *J Am Acad Child Adolesc Psychiatry*, *28*, 903-911.

Birch, N. J. (1980). Bone side-effects of lithium. In F. N. Johnson (Ed.), *Handbook of lithium* (pp. 365-371). Baltimore: University Park Press.

Birmaher, B., Baker, R., Kapur, S., Quintana, H., & Ganguli, R. (1992). Clozapine for the treatment of adolescents with schizophrenia. *J Am Acad Child Adolesc Psychiatry*, *31*, 1:160-164.

Borison, R. L., Ang, L., Hamilton, W. J., Diamond, B. I., & David, J. M. (1983). Treatment approaches in Gilles de la Tourette syndrome. *Brain Res Bull*, *11*, 205-208.

Bowers, M. B., & Swigar, M. E. (1988). Psychotic patients who become worse on neuroleptics. *J Clin Psychopharmacol*, *8*, 6:417-421.

Bradley, W. (1937). The behavior of children receiving benzedrine. *Am J Psychiatry*, *94*, 577-585.

Brown, G., Hunt, R. G., Ebert, M., Bunney, W. E. Jr., & Kopin I. J. (1979). Plasma levels of d-amphetamine in hyperactive children: Serial behavior and motor response. *Psychopharma*, *62*, 133-140.

Campbell, M., Anderson, L. T., Small, A. M., et al. (1982). The effects of haloperidol on learning and behavior in autistic children. *J Autism Dev Disord*, *12*, 167-174.

Campbell, M., Cohen, I. L., & Small, A. M. (1982). Drugs in aggressive behavior. *J Amer Acad Child Psychiat*, *21*, 107-117.

Campbell, M., Perry, R., & Green W. H. (1984). Use of lithium in children and adolescents. *Psychosomatics*, *25*, 95-106.

Campbell, M., Green, W. H., & Deutsch, S. I. (1985). *Child and adolescent psychopharmacology*. Beverly Hills, CA: Sage.

Cantwell, D., Carlson, G.A. (1978). Stimulants. In Werry J.S. (ed.) *Pediatric Psychopharmacology: The use of behaviour modifying drugs in children*, pp. 171-207. New York: Brunner/Mazel.

Caroff, S. N. (1980). The neuroleptic malignant syndrome. *J Clin Psychiatry*, 41:79-83.

Clinton, J.E., Sterner, S., Steimachers, Z., et al. (1987). Haloperidol for sedation of disruptive emergency patients. *Am J Emerg Med*, 16:319-322.

Cockcroft, D.W., Gault, M.H. (1976). Prediction of creatinine clearance from serum creatinine. *Nephron*, 16:31-41.

Cohen, D.J., Detlor, J., Young, J.G., Shaywitz, B.A. (1980). Clonidine ameliorates Gilles de la Tourette syndrome. *Arch Gen Psychiatry*, 37:1350-1354.

Delong, G.R. (1978). Lithium carbonate treatment of select behaviour disorders in children suggesting manic-depressive illness. *J Ped*, 93, 689-694.

Delong, G.R., Aldershof, A.L. (1987). Long-term experience with lithium treatment in childhood: Correlation with clinical diagnosis. *J Am Acad Child Adolesc Psychiatry*, 26:389-394.

Donlon, P.T., Hopkin J., Tupin, J.P. (1979). Overview: Efficacy and safety of the rapid neuroleptization method with injectable haloperidol. *Am J Psychiatr*, 136:273-278.

Dostal, T., Zvolsky, P. (1970). Antiaggressive effect of lithium salts in severely mentally retarded adolescents. *Int Pharmacopsychiat*, 5, 203-207.

Dubin, W.R., Feld, J.A. (1989). Rapid tranquilization of the violent patient. *Am J Emerg Med*, 7:313-320.

Faretra, G., Dooher, L., Dowling, J. (1970). Comparison of haloperidol and fluphenazine in disturbed children. *Am J Psychiatry*, 126:1670-1673.

Fava, M., Rosenbaum, J.F. (1991). Suicidality and fluoxetine: Is there a relationship? *J Clin Psychiatry*, 52:108-111.

Freidman, J.H., Davis, R., Wagner, R. (1988). Brief Report: Neuroleptic malignant syndrome. The result of a 6-month prospective study of incidence in a state psychiatric hospital. *Clin Neuropharmacology*, 2(40):373-377.

Gardner, D., Kutcher, S. (1990). Buspirone-a novel anziolytic. *Family Practice Newsletter*. Sunnybrook Health Sciences Center, 9:1-4.

Geller, B., Cooper, T. B., Graham, D., Felner, H. H., Marsteller, F. A., & Wells, J. (1992). Pharmacokinetically designed double-blind placebo-counselled study of norletplyline in 6-12 year olds with major depressive disorder. *Journal of the American Academy of Child and Adolescent Psychiatry*, *31*, 34-44.

Gualtieri, C.T., Barnhill, J., McGimsey, J., et al. (1980). Tardive dyskinesia and other movement disorders in children treated with psychotropic drugs. *J Am Acad Child Psychiatry*, 19:491-510.

Gittelman-Klein, D.F. (1973). School phobia: diagnostic considerations in the light of imipramine effects. *J Nerv Ment Dis*, 156:199-215.

Gittelman-Klein, D.F. (1980). Separation anxiety in school refusal and its treatment with drugs. In: *Out of school*. Eds., L Hersov & I Berg. New York: Wiley, pp. 321-341.

Gittelman-Klein, R., and Klein, D.F (1971). Controlled imipramine treatment of school phobia. *Arch Gen Psychiatry*, 25:204-207.

Goldberg, H. (1984). Buspirone hydrochloride: A unique new anxiolytic agent. *Pharmacotherapy*, 4:315-324.

Greenberg, L.M., Stephans, J.H. (1977). Use of drugs in special syndromes. In: *Psychopharmacology of childhood and adolescence*, J.M. Weiner, Editor, p. 179, New York: Basic Books.

Greenberg, L. (1985). Attention deficit disorder. In: Kelley V (Ed.), *Practice of Pediatrics, Vol. VI.* Philadelphia, PA: Harper & Row.

Greenhill, L.L., Rieder, R.O., Wender, P.H., Bushsbaum, M., Zahn, T.P. (1973). Lithium carbonate in the treatment of hyperactive children. *Arch Gen Psychiatry*, 28:636-640.

Greenhill, L.L., Puig-Antich, J., Novacenko, H., et al. (1984). Prolactin growth hormone & growth responses in boys with attention deficit disorder and hyperactivity treated with methylphenidate. *J Am Acad Child Adolesc Psychiatry*, 23:58-67.

Greenhill, L.L. (1992). Pharmacologic treatment of attention deficit disorder. *Pediatric Psychopharmacology: Psychiatric Clinics of North America*, 15:1.

Gualtieri, C.T. (1977). Imipramine and children: A review and some speculations about the mechanism of drug action. *Dis Nerv System*, 38:368-375.

Gualtieri, C. T., Quade, D., Hicks, R. E., et al. (1984). Tardirie dyskinesia and other clinical consequences of neuroleptic treatment in children and adolescents. *American Journal of Psychiatry.*, 141, 20-23.

Hamill, P.V.V., Drizd, T.A, Johnson, C.L., Reed, R.B., Roche, A.F. (1976). NCHS growth charts. Monthly vital statistics reports, 25 (suppl 3), *Health Examination Survey Data*, National Center for Health Statistics Publication (HRA) 76:1120, 1-22.

Hamilton, M. (1979). Mania and depression: classification, description, and course. In: *Psychopharmacology of affective disorders*, Eds. E.S. Paykel & A. Coppen. New York: Oxford University Press, pp 4-5.

Hunt, R.D., Minderaa, R.B., Cohen, D.J. (1985). Clonidine benefits children with attention deficit disorder and hyperactivity: Report of a double-blind placebo-crossover therapeutic trial. *J Am Acad Child Psychiatry*, 24:617-629.

Jefferson, J.W., Greist, J.H., Ackerman, D.L., et al. (1983). *Lithium encyclopedia for clinical practice.* Washington: American Psychiatric Press.

Joshi, P.T., Capozzoli, J.A., Coyle, J.T. (1985). Effective management with lithium of a persistent, post-traumatic hypomania in a 10-year-old child. *J Develop and Behavior Pediatr* 6:6, 352-354.

Joshi, P.T., Capozzoli, J.A., Coyle, J.T. (1988). Low-dose neuroleptic therapy for children with childhood onset pervasive developmental disorder. *Am J Psychiatry*, 145:335–338.

Joshi, P.T., Walkup, J.T., Capozzoli, J.A., DeTrinis, R.B., Coyle, J.T. (1989). *The use of fluoxetine in the treatment of major depressive disorder in children and adolescents.* Paper presented at the 36th annual meeting of the American Academy of Child and Adolescent Psychiatry, New York, October.

Joshi, P.T., Capozzoli, J.A., Coyle, J.T. (1990). The Johns Hopkins Depression Scale: Normative data and validation in child psychiatry patient, *Am Acad Child Adolesc Psychiatry*, 29, 2:283-288.

Joshi, P.T., Capozzoli, J.A., Coyle, J.T. (1991). Neuroleptic Malignant Syndrome: A life threatening complication of neuroleptic treatment in adolescents with affective disorder, *Pediatrics*, 87:2.

Kafantaris, V., Campbell, M., Pardonn-Gayol, M.V., et al. (1992). Carbamazepine in hospitalized aggressive conduct disordered children: A pilot study. *Psychopharmacol Bull* (In Press).

Kashani, J., Shekim, W.O., Reid, J.C. (1984). Amitriptyline in children with Manic Depressive Disorder: A double-blind crossover pilot study. *J Am Acad Child Psychiatry*, 23:348-351.

Kastenholz, K., Crimson, M. (1984). Buspirone, a novel benzodiazepine anxiolytic. *Drug Reviews*, 3:600-607.

Keller, M.B., Lavori, P.W., Endicott, J., Coryell, W., Klerman, G.L. (1990). Diagnostic and course of illness variables pertinent to refractory depression. In: *APA Annual Review of Psychiatry*, Eds. A. Tasman, C. Kaufman & S. Goldfinger. Washington, DC: American Psychiatric Press, pp. 10-32.

King, R.A., Riddle, M.A., Chappell, P.B., et al. (1991). Emergence of self-destructive phenomenon in children and adolescents during fluoxetine treatment. *J Am Acad Child Adolesc Psychiatry*, 30:179-186.

Klein, R.G., Landa, B., Mattes, J.A., Kleins, D.F. (1988). Methylphenidate and growth in hyperactive children: A controlled withdrawal study. *Arch Gen Psychiatry*, 45:1127-1130.

Klein, R.G., Koplewicz, H.S., Kanner, A. (1992). Imipramine treatment of children with separation anxiety disorder. *J Am Acad Child Adolesc Psychiatry*, 31:1.

Kovacs, M., Feinberg, T.L., Crouse-Novak, M.A., Paulaukas, S.L., Finkelstein, R. (1984). Depressive disorders in childhood, I: A longitudinal prospective study of characteristics and recovery. *Arch Gen Psychiatry*, 41:229-237.

Kovacs, M., Pollock, M., Finkelstein, R. (1984b). Depressive disorders in childhood, II: a longitudinal study of the risk for a subsequent major depression. *Arch Gen Psychiatry*, 41:643-649.

Kovacs, M., Paulauskas, S., Gatsonis, C. & Richards, C. (1988). Depressive disorders in childhood, III: A longitudinal study of co-morbidity with and risk for conduct disorders. *J Affective Disord*, 15:205-217.

Kovacs, M., Gatsonis, C., Paulauskas, S.L. & Richards, C. (1989). Depressive disorders in childhood, IV: A longitudinal study of co-morbidity with and risk for anxiety disorders. *Arch Gen Psychiatry*, 46:776-782.

Kramer, A.D., Feiguine, R.J. (1981). Clinical effects of amitriptyline in adolescent depression: A pilot study. *J Am Acad Child Psychiatry*, 20:636-644.

Kranzler, H. (1988). Use of buspirone in an adolescent with overanxious disorder. *J Am Acad Child Adolesc Psychiatry*, 27:789-790.

Kuperman, S., Stewart, M.A. (1987). Use of propranolol to decrease aggressive outbursts in younger patients. *Psychosomatics*, 28:315-319.

Kupietz, S.S., Winsberg, B.G., Sverd, J. (1982). Learning ability and methylphenidate (Ritalin(R)) plasma concentration in hyperactive children. *J Am Acad Child Psychiatry*, 21:27-30.

Kutcher, S., Mackenzie, S. (1988). Successful clonazepam treatment of adolescents with panic disorder. *J Clin Psychopharmacol*, 8:299-301.

Kutcher, S. (1990). *High potency benzodiazepines in child and adolescent anxiety disorders*. American College of Neuropsychopharmacology 29th Annual Meeting, Puerto Rico, December.

Leckman, J.F., Hardin, M.T., Riddle, M.A., et al. (1991). Clonidine treatment of Tourette's syndrome. *Arch Gen Psychiatry*, 48:324-328.

Lena, B. (1980). Lithium treatment of children and adolescents. In Johnson FN (ed): *Handbook of lithium therapy*. Lancaster, MAP Press, 405-413.

Liebowitz, M.R., Hollander, E., Schneier, F., et al. (1990). Anxiety and depression: Discrete diagnostic entities? *J Clin Psychopharmacol*, 10:61S-

66S.

Lucas, A., Pasley, F. (1969). Psychoactive drugs in the treatment of emotionally disturbed children: Haloperidol and Diazepam. *Compr Psychiatry*, 10:376-386.

McKeith, I.G., Williams, A., Nicol, A.R. (1981). Clonidine in Tourette's syndrome. *Lancet* 1:270-271.

Newton, R., Casten, G., Alous, D., et al. (1982). The side effect profile of buspirone in comparison to active control and placebo. *J Clin Psychiatry*, 43:100-102.

Physicians' Desk Reference. 45th. ed. (1991). Oradell, NJ (Data). Medical Economic.

Petti, T.A., Law, W. III (1982). Imipramine treatment of Depressed children: A Double-blind pilot study. *J Clin Psychopharmacol*, 2:107-110.

Pool, D., Bloom, W., Mielke, D.H., Roniger, J.J., Gallant, D.M. (1976). A controlled evaluation of loxitane in seventy-five adolescent schizophrenic patients. *Current Therapeutic Research Clinical and Experimental*, 19:99-104.

Pope, H.G., Keck, P.E., McElroy, S.L. (1986). Frequency and presentation of neuroleptic malignant syndrome in a large psychiatric hospital. *Am J Psychiatry*, 143:1227-1233.

Popper, C. (1990). PRN medication and chemical restraint. *AACAP Newsletter*, Summer: 7-8.

Post, R.M., Uhde, T.W., Ballenger, J.C., et al. (1983). Prophylactic efficacy of carbamazepine in manic-depressive illness. *Am J Psychiatry*, 140:1602-1604.

Potter, H.W. (1983). Schizophrenia in children. *Am J Psychiatry*, 12:1253.

Preskorn, S.H., Weller, E.B., Weller, R.A., et al. (1982). Depression in children: Relationship between plasma imipramine levels to response. *J Clin Psychiatry*, 43:450-453.

Puig-Antich, J., Blau, S., Marx, N., Greenhill, L.L., Chambers, W. (1978). Prepubertal major depressive disorder, a pilot study. *J Amer Acad Child Psychiat*, 17, 695-707.

Puig-Antich, J., Perel, J.M., Lupatkin, W. (1987). Imipramine in prepubertal major depressive disorders. *Arch Gen Psychiatry*, 44:81-89.

Puig-Antich, J., Ryan, N.D., Rabinovich, H. (1985). Affective disorders in childhood and adolescence. In: *Diagnosis and psychopharmacology of childhood and adolescent disorders*, ed. J. M. Wiener, New York: Wiley, pp. 151-177.

Rabiner, C.J., Klein, D.F. (1969). Imipramine treatment of school phobia. *Compr. Psychiatry*, 10:387-390.

Rapoport, J.L. (ed.) (1989). *Obsessive compulsive disorder in children and adolescents*. Washington, American Psychiatric Press.

Rapoport, J.L., Mikkelson, E. (1980). Clinical controlled trial of clorimipramine in adolescents with obsessive compulsive disorder. *Psychopharmol Bull*, 16:61-63.

Rapoport, J., Mikkelson, E.J. (1978). Antidepressants. In: *Pediatric Psychopharmacology*, edited by J.S. Werry, pp. 208-233. New York: Brunner/Mazel.

Realmuto, G.M., Erickson, W.D., Yellin, A.M., et al. (1984). Clinical comparison of thiothixene and thiorizadine in schizophrenic adolescents.

Am J Psychiatry, 141:1195-1202.

Remschmidt, H. (1976). The psychotropic effect of carbamazepine in nonepileptic patients. In Birkmayer, W. (ed.), *Epiuleptic Seizures Behaviour Pain*. Hans Huber, Berne.

Resnick, M., Burton, B. (1984). Droperidol vs. Haloperidol in the initial management of acutely agitated patients. *J Clin Psychiatry*, 45:298-299.

Riblet, L., Taylor, D., Eison, M., et al. (1982). Pharmacology and neuro-chemistry of buspirone. *J Clin Psychiatry*, 43:11-16.

Rogeness, G.A., Javors, M.A., Maas, J.W., et al. (1987). Plasma dopamine-B-hydroxylase, HVA, MHPG, and conduct disorders in emotionally disturbed boys. *Biol Psychiatry*, 22:1155-1158.

Rudorfer, M.V., Potter, W.Z. (1987). Pharmacokinetics of antidepressants. In: Meltzer HY, ed. *Psychopharmacology: The third generation of progress*. New York: Raven Press, 1353-1363.

Ryan, N.D., Puig-Antich, J., Rabinovich, H., et al. (1988). MAOIs in adolescent major depression unresponsive to tricyclic antidepressants. *J Am Acad Child Adolesc Psychiatry*, 27:755-758.

Safer, D.J., Allen, R.D., Barr, E. (1972). Depression of growth in hyperactive children on stimulant drugs. *N Engl J Med*, 287:217.

Saraf, K.R., Klein, D.F., Gittelman-Klein, R., Gootman, N., Greenhill, P. (1978). EKG effects of imipramine treatment in children. *J Am Acad Child Psychiatry*, 17:60-69.

Schroeder, J.S., Mullin, A.V., Elliot, G.R., Steiner, H., Nichols, M., Gordon, A., Paulos, M. (1989). Cardiovascular effects of desipramine in children. *J Am Acad Child Adolesc Psychiatry*, 28:376-379.

Sechi, G.P., Tanda, F., Mutani, R. (1984). Fatal hyperpyrexia after withdrawal of levodopa. *Neurology*, 34:249-251.

Serrano, A.C., Forbes, O.L. (1973). Haloperidol for psychiatric disorders in children. *Dis Nerv Syst*, 34:226-231.

Shaffer, D., Costello, A.J., Hill, J.D. (1968). Control of enuresis with imipramine. *Arch Dis Child*, 43,665-671.

Sillanpaa, M. (1981). Carbamazepine: Pharmacology and clinical uses. *Acta Neurol Scand*, 64:1-202.

Simeon, J.G., Dinicola, V.F., Ferguson, B.H., et al. (1990). Adolescent depression: A placebo controlled fluoxetine treatment study and follow-up. Progress in *Neuropsychopharmacology and Biological Psychiatry*, 14:791-795.

Singer, H.S., Tune, L.E., Butler, L.T., Zaczeck, R., Coyle, J.T. (1982). Clinical symptomatology, cerebrospinal fluid neurotransmitter metabolites, and serum haloperidol levels in Tourette's syndrome. In: *Gilles de la Tourette Syndrome, Advances in Neurology, Vol 35*, eds. AJ Friedhoff & TN Chase. New York: Raven, 177-183.

Skolnick, P., Paul, S., Weissman, B.A. (1984). Preclinical pharmacology of buspirone hydrochloride. *Pharmacotherapy*, 4:308-314.

Strober, M. (1989). *Effects of imipramine, lithium, and fluoxetine in the treatment of adolescent major depression*. Washington (DC), National Institutes of Mental Health, New Clinical Drug Evaluation Unit (NCDEU) Annual Meeting (Abstract).

Taylor, D., Eison, M., Riblet, L., et al. (1985). Pharmacology and clinical effects of buspirone. *Pharmacol Biochem Behav*, 23:687-694.

Teicher, M.H., Glod, C., Cole, J.O. (1990). Emergence of intense suicidal preoccupation during fluoxetine treatment. *Am J Psychiatry*, 147:207-210.

Tollefson, G. (1982). A Case of neuroleptic malignant syndrome: In vitro muscle comparison with malignant hyperthermia. *J Clin Psychopharmacol*, 2:266-270.

Tunks, E.R., Dermer, S.W. (1977). Carbamazepine in the dyscontrol syndrome associated with limbic system dysfunction. *J Nerv Ment Dis*, 164:56-63.

Vitiello, B., Behar, D., Malone, R., et al. (1988). Pharmacokinetics of lithium carbonate in children. *J Clin Psychopharmacol*, 8:355-359.

Waizer, J., Polizos, P., Hoffman, S., Engelhardt, D., Margolis, R. (1972). A single blind evaluation of thiothixene with outpatient schizophrenic children. *J Autism Child Schiz*, 2:378-386.

Walkup, J.T., Pizzo, M., DeTrinis, R., Capozzoli, J.A., Joshi, P.T. (1991). *Droperidol in the acute management of agitated children and adolescents*. Paper presented at the 38th Annual Meeting of the American Academy of Child & Adolescent Meeting, San Francisco.

Weinberg, W., Rutman, J., Sullivan, L., Penick, E.C., Dietz, S.G. (1973). Depression in children referred to an educational diagnostic center: Diagnosis and treatment. *J Pediatric*, 83:1065-1072.

Weiner, J.M., Jaffe, S. (1977). History of drug therapy in childhood and adolescent psychiatric disorders. In: Weiner, J.M. (ed.), *Psychopharmacology in childhood and adolescence*. New York: Basic Books, 9-40.

Williams, D.T., Mehl, R., Yudofsky, S., et al. (1982). The effect of propranolol on uncontrolled rage outbursts in children and adolescents with organic brain dysfunction. *J Am Acad Child Psychiatry*, 21:139-135.

Yatham, L.N., McHale, P.A. (1988). Carbamazepine in the treatment of aggression: A case report and review of the literature. *Acta Psychiatr Scand*, 78:188-190.

Youngerman, J., Canino, I.A. (1978). Lithium carbonate use in children and adolescents. *Arch Gen Psychiatry*, 35:216.

Yudofsky, S., Williams, D., Gorman, J. (1981). Propranolol in the treatment of rage and violent behavior in patients with chronic brain syndrome. *Am J Psychiatry*, 138:218-220.

Chapter 8

OCCUPATIONAL THERAPY, ART THERAPY, THERAPEUTIC RECREATION, AND VOCATIONAL SERVICES FOR INPATIENT ADOLESCENTS

Janice J. Jaskulski, Erika Grant, Gregory Kearny, and Vera Roth

OCCUPATIONAL THERAPY

The Concept of Purposeful Activity

A basic premise in the profession of occupational therapy is that humans are motivated to develop and function through what we refer to as "occupation," or via the utilization of purposeful activity. In a healthy state, an individual will occupy his time with activities that support personal or social interests, skills and abilities, and/or occupational roles. Since the early 1900's, psychiatrists have recognized the need for maintaining a healthy balance between the "big four"—work, play, sleep, and rest—and an individual's various life roles (Meyer, 1922). Meyer and others (Reilly, 1962; Llorens & Rubin, 1962; Mosey, 1970; Gazda, 1973; Mumford, 1974) support the theory that one achieves this healthy balance by means of actual doing and practice, even when dysfunction exists. The therapist's fundamental role, therefore, is to provide the patient with the structure and opportunities for functional performance to occur.

Even today, the utilization of purposeful activity underlies many of the major theoretical approaches practiced by occupational therapists who specialize in psychiatry (Clark, 1979; Allen, 1985; Keilhofner, 1985; Allen & Allen, 1987). While not as simplified as in the early 1900's, the concept of a balance in work, play, and self-maintenance still serves as the basis for the development of more formalized theories. In current theories, the concept of "work" involves both educational and prevocational activities, as well as vocational roles. "Play" encompasses any and all personal interests in the areas of socialization, recreation, and self-exploration. "Self-maintenance" predominantly refers to rest, fitness, and self-care activities. The generic terms of "daily living skills" or "activities of daily living" are sometimes utilized to encompass the activities necessary to permit healthy functioning in various daily roles. For example, an adolescent may find himself in the role of student, son, sibling, employee, or friend concurrently. Each role requires a varied set of skills and abilities to function adequately or acceptably in a given situation.

Activity Analysis and Adaptation

When practicing the concept of purposeful activity as defined here, the occupational therapist utilizes the ability to analyze activities and to provide adaptations when necessary to promote successful functioning. Chosen activities are always planned and goal-directed, developmentally appropriate, meaningful and motivating to the patient, and individualized in nature. Cultural differences and environmental factors are likewise considered. Adaptations may be made to the activity itself by breaking a task down into component parts to simplify it or by changing its developmental sequence, adapting the tools or equipment utilized and the physical or cognitive skills required, by applying specific physical techniques such as sensory stimulation and muscle facilitation, or by teaching compensatory methods. Knowledge of the patient's premorbid and current functional level, psychiatric history and life roles, existing strengths and weaknesses, and the ability to analyze and adapt activity provide the basis for treatment planning in occupational therapy.

In psychiatry, as in any setting, the provision of occupational therapy services always relates to one or more of the following guidelines (Lansing & Carlsen, 1977):

1. The *promotion or maintenance* of skills and abilities that are necessary for the performance of desired or required "occupational" activities.

2. The *prevention* of abnormal or inadequate development, deterioration or loss of those skills necessary to engage in prevocational, recreational, educational, or self-maintenance activities.
3. The *remediation* of dysfunction that impacts on performance of daily occupational activities.
4. The *facilitation* of the adaptive skills necessary to influence the quality of life and a healthy status.
5. The *collaboration* and cooperation with significant others in planning and achieving individualized goals.

Assessment Techniques

A common form of assessment utilized in adolescent psychiatry is the structured interview process. One such example often employed by the occupational therapist is the Adolescent Role Assessment (Black, 1976), a semistructured interview leading to discussion of the adolescent's level of functioning in various life roles. In addition, functional levels are also assessed in the areas of self-maintenance, daily living skills, and prevocational tasks via clinical observation and/or standardized evaluation (Cromwell, 1960).

Because of the importance of self-maintenance to healthy functioning in other occupational roles, assessment may focus on daily living tasks, such as money management or budgeting, laundry or cooking skills, or time management and organizational skills. While most healthy adolescents foster a preoccupation with personal appearance and self-identity, the dysfunctional adolescent may demonstrate deficiencies or lack of interest in other self-care activities, such as grooming and hygiene.

Interest checklists or surveys may be administered to elicit areas of personal preference as well as to identify strengths and weaknesses in past performance (Matsutsuyu, 1969). Task-oriented assessment is conducted to evaluate the readiness skills and performance components, i.e., cognitive, perceptual, motor, social, and emotional skills necessary for successful prevocational functioning.

Evaluation of sensory integrative, perceptual and/or motor performance is utilized when an adolescent demonstrates or has a history of poor performance secondary to a physical, developmental, or learning disability. Assessment of these areas will assist in identifying those factors that may impact on the adolescent's overall performance. Developmental histories, screenings, and psychoeducational evaluation may indicate the need for further assessment of these areas as well.

General socialization skills, self-concept, and interactional style of the adolescent is typically assessed by the occupational therapist via self-report and direct clinical observation.

Treatment Planning and Programming

Occupational therapy in practice differs from other therapies in that it is activity-based rather than verbally oriented, may be individualized or provided through group treatment depending on the acuity of illness and the patient's functional level, and is focused on the here-and-now approach. Because the treatment session is seen by the therapist as a microcosm of the manner in which the adolescent typically functions, problems and issues are dealt with as they occur rather than in retrospect. While the activity and/or other existing issues may elicit the behavior itself, the therapist's use of self therapeutically promotes an environment for healthy problem-solving as it relates to interpersonal and work-related issues.

Among the modalities available to occupational therapists working in a psychiatric setting are crafts and games, gross and fine motor activities, insight-oriented awareness groups, behavior modification techniques, and skill-building groups. Typically seen in the adolescent psychiatric setting are occupational therapy groups based upon the "task group" and "project group" concepts (Fidler, 1969; Mosey, 1970). Task group is a parallel-level activity group in which the therapist individualizes and adapts the chosen tasks to meet or promote the patient's skill level and attainment of patient-therapist identified treatment goals. Crafts are a traditional modality utilized in this type of group, as the materials, tools, and equipment can be adapted quickly and easily while offering a sense of personal satisfaction (Kremer Nelson & Duncombe, 1984; Hardison & Llorens, 1988; Boyer et al., 1989).

Project group is a developmentally higher-level group promoting interpersonal skill-building, group cooperation and team-building, leadership, and compromising skills (Fahl, 1970). For the adolescent, peer acceptance and the development of self-identity are of utmost importance to the social and emotional functioning of the patient.

In both types of groups, the adolescent must learn to operate within the rules of the group, recognize acceptable norms, reject or confront inappropriate social behavior, accept and respond to feedback, recognize consequences of actions and adapt behavior accordingly.

Other treatment groups typically led by an occupational therapist in the adolescent psychiatric setting are:

1. Daily living skills group to promote independence in self-maintenance;
2. Socialization group to promote appropriate social behavior, peer interactional skills, and insight into existing styles of interaction;
3. Assertiveness training group to teach and practice assertive methods of communication and to develop insight into passive or aggressive tendencies;
4. Relaxation group to teach progressive relaxation techniques and other forms of self-control, i.e., guided imagery, stop-think-act approaches, etc.
5. Stress management or coping skills group to promote insight into and identification of positive/negative coping mechanisms and to practice alternative forms of coping and problem-solving.

Interdisciplinary Interaction

Occupational therapy treatment may occur with other disciplines on the treatment team as follows:

1. With recreation therapy in a socialization group setting or to promote sensorimotor functioning in a physical activity group;
2. With nursing and the family to promote the use of the adolescent's strengths and realistic options for leisure planning after discharge;
3. With social work to develop assertiveness skills in order to role play parent-child communications;
4. With art therapy to assist in identifying areas of underlying conflict or difficulties in self-expression;
5. With speech therapy to promote the pragmatic use of language in the adolescent's various life roles or functional situations; or
6. With the vocational counselor to assess and promote realistic prevocational skills and interests.

Many treatment settings employ the concept of activity teams which work within the therapeutic milieu to develop and maintain the overall activities program. The members of the team, including the occupational therapist, may act as consultants to nursing staff regarding weekend and evening programming, appropriate and therapeutically oriented leisure activities, and specific unit-based activities such as holiday events, group meal planning, a unit-based store or newspaper, bake sale or other fund-raising events, patient government groups, etc.

In summary, the occupational therapist on the team provides valuable information related to the patient's overall functional level, skills, and abilities to perform adequately in their chosen life roles.

ART THERAPY

The expressive therapies (art and dance/movement therapy) differ from the other forms of activity therapy because they are forms of psychotherapy. They facilitate the emergence of psychodynamic issues and feelings and provide a format for working through such issues.

This section will provide an overview of how art therapy is used with the inpatient adolescent population at Sheppard Pratt Hospital and then will illustrate with a case study.

Art therapy operates on the premise that when people make art, they project their feelings, conflicts, and drives into their artwork which can occur on a conscious or an unconscious level. Art therapy, therefore, can provide diagnostic information and elicit psychodynamic issues, often in one picture. Art therapy is also useful as a treatment modality, particularly with adolescents who are dealing with issues of separation/individuation and have difficulty with authority figures which produces verbal resistance. Art therapy offers an opportunity to sidestep verbal defenses and elicit material, directly or metaphorically. Art therapy treatment can be either group or individual.

Ideally, an adolescent art therapy group should meet weekly and be limited to six to eight patients. Group time is spent half in making art work and half in processing the pictures. The processing period is a form of group psychotherapy in which patients talk about how the pictures express their feelings and other treatment-related issues. It is understood by the group members that the art therapist bring the pictures to weekly multidisciplinary treatment team meetings to provide useful information about current underlying issues that are not being verbally articulated by the patient. Adolescents often enjoy the relaxed atmosphere of art therapy and find they develop feelings of mastery and positive self-esteem from producing artwork and exploring their issues creatively.

Case Study

Paul, a 16-year-old male, was hospitalized on the adolescent inpatient service from age 14 to 16. His history included severe learning disabilities and a long series of behavior problems both at school and at home, culminating in matricide when he was 12. After two years in Detention

Centers and other juvenile facilities, Paul was referred for long-term intensive inpatient hospitalization. He was neatly groomed and usually wore black T-shirts, jeans, and combat boots. He began to shave his head shortly after his arrival. Paul was a guarded, hostile boy who appeared tough, unfriendly, and uncaring. He was observed to push others away through rudeness and deliberate attempts to appear strange.

Paul was referred to individual art therapy with the initial goals of providing him with a less direct or threatening modality through which to work on feelings and grief issues. Paul was seen in individual art therapy for over a year, then transferred to group art therapy for another year to help him work on issues related to peers.

Paul was verbally resistant in art therapy for over a year. He hated art therapy and initially refused to attend sessions. Early art sessions were brief as Paul drew quickly and made minimal comments about his work. When attempts were made to explore the content of his work, he became sarcastic and rude.

Although Paul was verbally silent, his pictures immediately told another story. It became apparent that although he presented himself as tough and intimidating, he suffered from severe anxiety, low self-esteem, and feelings of vulnerability. His drawings conveyed a poignant sense of helplessness and fear. On a sheet of 12" x 18" paper, a one-inch figure would appear at the very bottom of the page, standing on 1/4" of ground (environmental instability), looking very vulnerable. For about a year, Paul drew in pencil; avoidance of color to art therapists is understood as an avoidance of feelings. During this time, he verbalized the belief that there should be no laws, consequences, or responsibility for behavior.

The human figure drawing is generally thought to be an unconscious portrayal of the artist, and the figures that Paul drew vividly conveyed his sense of rage, helplessness, and self-loathing. Six months into treatment, Paul was asked to draw an animal made from parts of other animals. What Paul drew he described as "a human head with eagle ears (to hear attackers), a scorpion's tail (to sting), a snake's body (for flexibility), and crayfish claws (huge, for protection)." The creature had a look of trapped desperation and shame on its face. Paul had portrayed himself as poisonous, dangerous, unapproachable, monstrous, and alone. When asked to draw a self-symbol, he drew a razor, facing outward, clearly a threat. He denied that this was an expression of dangerousness, saying merely that it meant he was clean.

During the first year of treatment, Paul's artwork reflected two themes: grief over loss of mother and loss of home, and violence. Among the grief works were pictures of abandoned fields and farms, fields that were to be paved over (loss of home), leafless trees (depression), and hidden animals that were under stones or in tree trunks, usually waiting for a "safe" time to emerge. These animals were understood by Paul's primary therapist, a psychologist, and the art therapist to represent Paul's feelings which would emerge later when he felt safe. Work which expressed grief for mother included a clay coffin (to keep valuables in) and a clay bear-paw print (he'd seen a mother bear with cubs). The contents of these pictures were not interpreted to him, nor were sustained attempts made to connect the artwork to his life. These were metaphorical expressions; he remained unable to work verbally on these issues in art therapy.

Paul's pictures of violence and dangerousness included pictures of scorpions, battle scenes, murderers (an attempt to contextualize himself and his crime), and stories of violent animals. One such picture portrayed a rattlesnake that killed a rabbit that teased him, and another picture depicted a ballgame in which a crowd jeered at a ballplayer. These two pictures provided an understanding of his violence as a response to a perceived threat and Paul was able to articulate, "You don't kill someone because you're angry, you kill someone because you're afraid."

After a year and a half of treatment, Paul began to speak directly about his antiauthority beliefs and his inability to fit in with peers. About this time, he joined the art therapy group, both to enable him to receive feedback from peers and to provide some anonymity in which to explore feelings. Figure 8.1 was produced at the end of his individual art therapy treatment and is both an example of the vulnerability expressed by his figures and of this shift towards a more direct expression of feelings. Paul described it as "a guy that worries too much." The teeth suggest rage and the hidden hands suggest guilt.

In the art therapy group, Paul began to work in vivid colors and began to express feelings more directly. Figure 8.2 is a drawing of him, about fears. Paul described it as his fear that his aging dog would die before he could see him again. Not only does this picture address feelings of vulnerability, but it is also a statement of emotional attachment.

Themes that emerged in Paul's group work were responsibility, choices, and his concern that he would never regain his freedom. This was in direct contradiction to his early insistence that he would be heading home soon. He talked about the temptation he felt to break rules and be violent and the pressure of knowing that the consequences would be severe. His pictures were increasingly in color, the figures were larger in relation to the page, better composed, and less angry looking. Conversationally, Paul was more open and less guarded, and began to ask questions of others and give feedback.

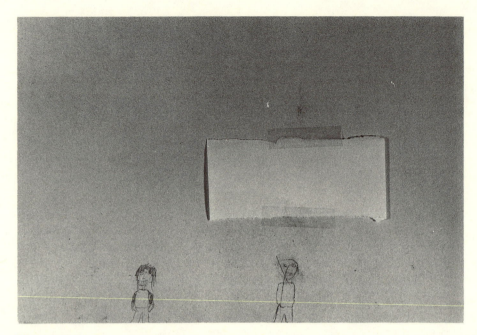

Figure 8.1

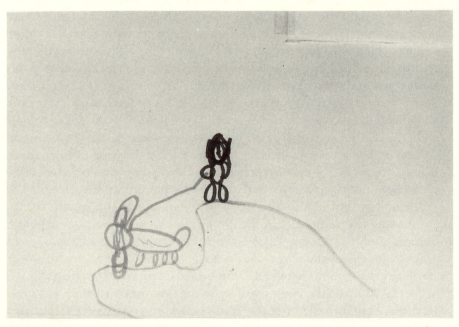

Figure 8.2

Figure 8.3 is a picture drawn late in treatment, when the discharge plan was set to send Paul to a residential treatment center. When asked to draw scenes from his life, he was able to reflect on his changing attitude and level of responsibility. He reported that at age 12, in jail, he'd had no feelings; at age 14, he got in more trouble and wanted the world to leave him alone; at age 15 he was "getting there" (note the increasingly human appearance of the frightened looking figure); and at age 16, "more stable, starting to develop how I want," adding that when he was younger, he had been extremely self-critical. The figure in the picture finally stands on two feet and has fully formed hands, though it looks worried and lacks self-confidence.

The final frame is of an olympic gold medal and represents Paul's hopes for a positive future. It differs markedly from earlier goals which involved his rejection of society and more violence. Around the time this picture was drawn, Paul began to verbalize questions about the personal life and tastes of the art therapist and was able to move from seeing her as an authority figure to seeing her as a real person.

Much of Paul's progress in art therapy was intertwined with his progress in individual therapy. The psychologist and art therapist found it helpful to share information in team meetings, and the pictures provided clues about ongoing issues that were not being verbalized.

THERAPEUTIC RECREATION

The discipline of therapeutic recreation is based on the recognition that leisure, including recreation and play, is an inherent aspect of the human experience (Peterson & Gunn, 1984).

The National Therapeutic Recreation Society states that the purpose of therapeutic recreation is to facilitate the development, maintenance, and expression of an appropriate leisure life-style for individuals with physical, mental, emotional, or social limitations (Peterson & Gunn, 1984). Toward this end, therapeutic recreation professionals provide services which are developed and implemented to enhance an individual's leisure ability. The Therapeutic Recreation Services Continuum Model includes three specific areas of professional service: therapy, leisure education, and recreation participation (Peterson & Gunn, 1984).

The therapeutic recreation professional is an important member of a multidisciplinary team in an adolescent inpatient setting. O'Morrow (1980) noted that no one person can be expected to be knowledgeable about the "whole person." By bringing together various professionals, the institution can give the individual the advantage of the team's combined knowledge and skills (O'Morrow, 1980).

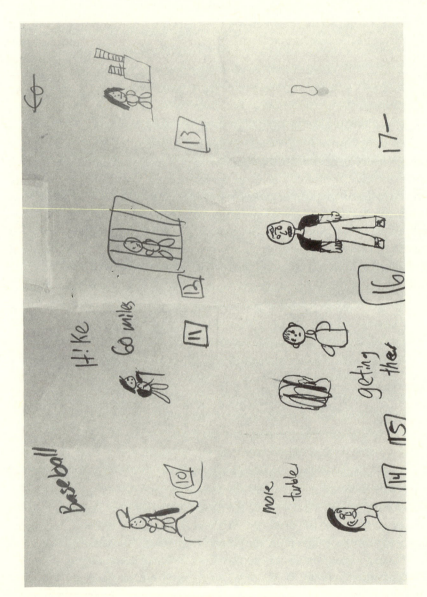

Figure 8.3

In this framework, the therapeutic recreation professional provides an assessment of the patient, develops and implements a program according to individual needs, and provides an evaluation of the patient's progress and problems. A complete assessment is essential for the development of a treatment plan to address the areas that contribute to the patient's inability to function normally out of inpatient setting.

The assessment process of an adolescent in an inpatient setting often includes four areas—the physical, cognitive, social, and emotional domains. Information about these domains is collected in different ways, including an interview with the patient, having the patient complete a self-assessment, and observing the patient in groups and activities. Data from the interview often include the patient's past history, health and social history, and past and present leisure and recreation experiences. The self-assessment provides the therapeutic recreation professional with the patient's perception of his/her strengths or deficits in areas of self-care, social skills, self-esteem, and leisure interests, values, and involvement. Based on observation of the patient in groups and activities, an assessment of the patient's social skills can be made and the patient's investment in, or attitude toward, treatment can be determined.

Groups are frequently used in the treatment of an adolescent in inpatient settings and are developed so that the maximum number of patients can receive maximum benefit and services.

The Therapeutic Recreation Service Continuum Model provides the three categories of service for group development, which include treatment, leisure education, and recreation participation. The purpose of treatment groups is to improve the patient's functional ability. A variety of strategies, interventions, and techniques are used in the process of treatment, which may include gross motor development, anger management, stress management, and relaxation groups.

Leisure education is a broad category of services that focuses on the development and acquisition of various leisure-related skills, attitudes, and knowledge. These services are developed from the Leisure Education Content Model which consists of leisure awareness, social interaction skills, leisure activity skills, and leisure resources. Some groups offered in an inpatient setting with adolescents would include social skills groups, arts and crafts, physical activity groups, values clarification groups, and cooking groups.

Recreation participation is the third component in development of groups. The purpose is to provide opportunities for fun, enjoyment and self-expression within the institution. The types of services offered in this component may consist of hospital-wide activities, such as dances, coffee houses, movies, or special events for specific holidays. Recreation participation allows the patient to experience some normalization while in constant treatment focus of an inpatient setting (Peterson & Gunn, 1984).

A schedule of weekly groups should be available to both staff and patients. This schedule is best developed with input from all who will be affected by the schedule. Any changes in the schedule should be communicated well in advance of their implementation to avoid confusion. It may be helpful for the therapeutic recreator to invite members of the nursing staff to join in groups, to assist or co-lead the groups. Communication is usually enhanced in this manner.

Documentation is also important in communication with a multidisciplinary team. Assessments and weekly progress notes provide important information for the treatment process in psychiatric treatment of adolescents in an inpatient setting.

The multidisciplinary team meetings are key to working effectively in adolescent treatment. The team meetings provide an opportunity for the therapeutic recreator to give information about a patient's progress or problems in the therapeutic recreation groups and to gain information from other disciplines pertinent to the patient's treatment plan.

The therapeutic recreator as a member of the team should also participate in discharge planning to help identify resources that will provide services that the patient may continue to need and/or desire.

VOCATIONAL SERVICES

Vocational services are an important part of aftercare planning for the adolescent patient because they address both short- and long-terms goals in the areas of education and employment.

It is essential for the vocational counselor to help the adolescent's treatment team prioritize the patient's many needs, identity specific services required, consult school records in order to avoid duplication, and contribute to overall planning. Frequently, this patient population requires a great deal of assistance because of their past behavioral and/or emotional problems. Due to the increasingly shorter length of hospital stay, it is important to refer early, to prioritize needs, and to make a quick assessment in order to assist with aftercare planning. Recommendations for follow up and continuity within the school system and community agencies are essential.

Often, referrals are for vocational assessment/testing, counseling, or group services. Because of the broad scope of such requests and the wide range of topics and services available, it is important that the treatment team members be informed about what services are available and the time frame needed to provide them. Specific rather than general requests are more efficiently met. Such services available are vocational interests and aptitude testing, career information, assistance with decision-making, training, and education information planning, GED information and screening, volunteer work information and planning, job-seeking skills, and resources. Most of these areas and topics can be addressed either in group sessions or in individual counseling. The group format is more informational in content while individual sessions allow for more intensive assessment, planning, and implementation.

Testing can be administered in either individual or group settings and seems to be best determined based on the individual's needs and tolerance. The size of the group is also important, and smaller, homogeneous groups appear to be most effective. Consideration of the counselor's caseload is also important. When one is providing information in a group, it is useful for students to have the opportunity to share their experience and to ask questions. This can be a valuable method for peers to learn or to hear from one another rather than from the group leader.

Groups are best operated on a module system by covering specific topics through a rotation of sessions and then repeating them. The frequency of repetition should be synchronized with the average length of stay. It is also helpful to keep each session related to one topic in order to allow for smoother entering and exiting of members. Naming the group sessions can help to create a positive attitude toward the subjects covered and to clarify the content offered. These titles include: Vocational Issues, Work Readiness, Career Planning, or Job-Seeking Skills. Module topics should include interest and value identification skills, job hunting, applications, and interviewing. Follow-up resources are important for all topics. This type of group can be useful for adolescents 13 to 14 years old and older.

Orientation to work or to prevocational skills group is helpful for younger adolescents or to lower functioning adolescents of any age. This can provide them with basic work terminology and expectations, and help them develop basic work habits and skills. A combination of an educational and experiential model is recommended.

Periodically, resistance by an adolescent to testing, individual counseling, or group services can be expected. This resistance appears related to other issues in his life, but he may not be able to articulate this. Vocational planning can stir up issues related to growing up, achieving independence, facing responsibility, and dealing with one's own strengths and weaknesses. There are several ways to handle this resistance. Treatment team input is vital when selecting your approach. In some cases, allowing the individual some control as to the timing or frequency of participation or type of service offered may be useful. Delaying services may be an option if time permits. This can be helpful if the adolescent is not ready to face the issues inherent in vocational counseling. Sometimes, having the adolescent meet with the counselor first or observe a group session may facilitate the individual's involvement and participation. This typically is a treatment team issue and decision.

Testing

Before beginning the testing of the adolescent, it is important to assess if the individual is emotionally and medically stable. To avoid duplication and test-retest factors, a record review of any school or psychological reports is recommended. When selecting testing instruments, it is important to consider the individual's reading level and cognitive functioning. The increasingly shorter length of stay may necessitate a quick assessment of interests, aptitudes, values and skills, and determines the time frame for work with the patient and the time required for administration, scoring, and interpretation of results. These factors also contribute to the choice of assessment tools. An additional outpatient evaluation may be necessary and may require a referral to the home school system or to the Division of Rehabilitation Services (formerly Division of Vocational Rehabilitations) for a more "comprehensive" vocational evaluation where work samples and situational assessments are available.

Many types of tests are available to the adolescent. There are interest tests and surveys, achievement tests, general and specific aptitude tests, personality tests and commercial work samples. Some tests are designed for specific populations and for types of employment or training. When sufficient time is available, administering work samples or placing an individual in a work setting will allow for a "hands-on" opportunity for both the adolescent and the counselor to assess capabilities. This is particularly helpful for those adolescents who typically do poorly in testing or in academic settings.

Following the assessment period, documentation and formulating recommendations based on all information obtained are crucial. Sharing the results with the team, family, and the individual is also important.

In many cases, the testing process can be anxiety-producing, especially with this population. It seems to trigger issues of choice, control, and performance. Often, testing results can be misinterpreted. Counselors are typically asked, "Are you going to tell me what I can do? or be?" Counselors are frequently cautioned against falling into this trap. It is recommended that any information given to the individual and the family be given in the context in which it was taken. For example, qualifiers, such as "At this point in time, the tests results indicate . . .," "You have the ability to learn these types of jobs . . .," or "You may do well in the field of . . .," or "It may be difficult for you to do . . . at this point in time." Suggesting areas for improvement or concentration can often promote positive energy. Focusing on strengths rather than weaknesses is also recommended.

An inpatient hospitalization is a difficult time for the adolescent. In most cases, the intensity of his or her emotional problems often precludes normal vocational development. The primary focus of treatment is psychotherapeutic and psychoeducational in an attempt to assist the adolescent in establishing more positive coping strategies. This is an important key in preparing the individual for career planning. Typically, this group needs more assistance than the general population throughout the stages of career development.

Throughout the hospital stay, the individual is provided with a variety of services from the treatment team. Communication and prioritization is vital in comprehensive treatment facilities. Resource knowledge in the community for aftercare follow up is becoming increasingly important to facilitate a smooth transition back into the community and school system.

REFERENCES

Allen, C.K. (1985). *Occupational therapy for psychiatric diseases: Measurement and management of cognitive disabilities.* Boston: Little, Brown.

Allen, C.K. & Allen, R.E. (1987). Cognitive disabilities: Measuring the social consequences of mental disorders. *Journal of Clinical Psychiatry, 48* (5), 185-190.

Black, M.M. (1976). Adolescent Role Assessment. *American Journal of Occupational Therapy, 30* (2), 73-79.

Boyer, J., Colman, W., Levy, L., & Manoly, B. (1989). Affective responses to activities: A comparative study. *American Journal of Occupational Therapy, 43,* 81-88.

Clark, P.N. (1979). Human development through occupation: Theoretical frameworks in contemporary occupational therapy practice, Part 1. *American Journal of Occupational Therapy, 33,* 505.

Clark, P.N. (1979). Human development through occupation: A philosophy and conceptual model for practice, Part 2. *American Journal of Occupational Therapy, 33,* 577.

Cromwell, F.S. (1960). *Occupational therapist's manual for basic skills assess-*

ment or primary prevocational evaluation. California: Fair Oaks Printing Co.

Fahl, M.A. (1970). Emotionally disturbed children: Effects of cooperative and competitive activity on peer interaction. *American Journal of Occupational Therapy, 24,* 31.

Fidler, G.S. (1969). The task-oriented group as a context for treatment. *American Journal of Occupational Therapy, 23* (1), 43-48.

Fidler, G.S. & Fidler, J.W. (1978). Doing and becoming: Purposeful action and self-actualization. *American Journal of Occupational Therapy, 32,* 305.

Gazda, G.M. (1973). Group procedures with children: A developmental approach. In M.M. Ohlsen (Ed.), *Counseling children in groups* (pp. 117-145). New York: Holt, Rinehart, and Winston, Inc.

Hardison, J. & Llorens, L.A. (1988). Structured craft group activities for adolescent delinquent girls. *Occupational Therapy in Mental Health, 8,* 101-117.

Harrington, Thomas F. (1982). *Handbook of Career Planning for the Special Needs Students*. Texas: Pro Ed.

Keilhofner, Gary (Ed.), (1985). *A model of human occupation: Theory and application*. Maryland: Williams & Wilkins.

Kremer, E.R.H., Nelson, D.L., & Duncombe, L.W. (1984). Effects of selected activities on affective meaning in psychiatric patients. *American Journal of Occupational Therapy, 38,* 522-528.

Lansing, S.G. & Carlsen, P.N. (1977). Occupational therapy. In Valletutti, P. and Christoplos, F. (Eds.), *Interdisciplinary approaches to human service delivery*. Baltimore: University Park Press.

Llorens, L.A. & Rubin, E.Z. (1962). A directed activity program for disturbed children. *American Journal of Occupational Therapy, 16,* 287-290.

Matsutsuyu, J.S. (1969). The interest check list. *American Journal of Occupational Therapy, 23* (4), 323-328.

Meyer, Adolf (1992). The philosophy of occupation therapy. *Archives of Occupational Therapy, 1,* 1-10.

Mosey, A.C. (1970). The concept and use of developmental groups. *American Journal of Occupational Therapy, 24,* 272-275.

Mumford, M.S. (1974). A comparison of interpersonal skills in verbal and activity groups. *American Journal of Occupational Therapy, 28,* 281-283.

O'Morrow, Gerald S. (1980). *Therapeutic Recreation: A Helping Profession*. Reston, VA: Prentice Hall Co.

Peterson, C.A., Gunn, S.L. (1984). *Therapeutic Recreation Program Design: Principles and Procedures*. Englewood Cliffs, NJ: Prentice-Hall, Inc.

Reilly, M. (1962). 1961 Eleanor Clark Slagle Lecture: Occupational therapy can be one of the great ideas in 20th century medicine. *American Journal of Occupational Therapy, 16* (1).

Chapter 9

SPECIAL EDUCATION IN AN INPATIENT SETTING

Burton H. Lohnes

INTRODUCTION

Education is the primary work of adolescents and, as such, is intertwined in all other aspects of an adolescent's life. A school program must therefore be part of the woven fabric that makes up any successful inpatient treatment program serving adolescents. Philosophically, a school program should be part of the overall clinical treatment program and not viewed as an appendage.

Special Education is defined as ". . . specially designed instruction, at no cost to parents or guardians, to meet the unique needs of a child with a disability. . ." (Individuals with Disabilities Education Act of 1990). Many adolescents hospitalized in psychiatric hospitals are educationally handicapped and in need of special education services as well as having a psychiatric disorder. The mere presence of a psychiatric disorder does not guarantee that an individual would also be found to be educationally handicapped. For many inpatients, education is a strength and their psychopathology has not interfered with the acquisition of knowledge.

In the case of an adolescent I shall call "Mary," there is a clear interplay between the educational process and a psychiatric disorder, but without an observable negative impact on her education. In Mary's case, she did very well at school by everyone's standard but her own. As a high school student, she received excellent grades, made the honor roll, and was involved in extracurricular activities at school and in the community. Mary's standards for herself were unrealistically high. She collected perceived insults, unnoticed by anyone except herself. A grade of "A" was not sufficient in a particular subject, since she did not receive the highest grade in the class. Having a major part in the school play did not measure up, since it was not the lead role. One after another, year after year, Mary collected the perceived insults as if adding a small pebble to her backpack each time, until the weight, in its cumulative form, overwhelmed her. Mary attempted suicide, was admitted to a general hospital in a comatose state, was stabilized, and was eventually admitted to a long-term adolescent inpatient unit.

Mary's case illustrates the difference between a psychiatric disorder, which she clearly has, and an educationally handicapping condition, which she does not manifest. Mary's psychopathology, which almost caused her death, did not exhibit its symptoms in school or impact on her grades or her social skills. In order for an individual to be identified as severely emotionally disturbed, i.e., educationally handicapped, the psychopathology, along with other criteria, must be of a type " . . . which adversely affects educational performance" (Programs for Students with Disabilities, 1991). The criterion which requires that there be an adverse impact on educational performance in order for a student to be identified as severely emotionally disturbed is the standard cited most often when a request that an individual with a psychiatric condition be identified as educationally handicapped is denied. If someone cannot be identified as educationally handicapped, he/she is not entitled to special education services or special education funding while on an inpatient unit.

The issue of whether or not a particular adolescent is eligible for special education services and/or funding, although very important, obscures the main issue at times. The point is that school is the work of adolescents; an educational program must be provided that encourages and facilitates the continuation of a student's normal developmental activities. A secondary school student simply cannot miss a month or more of instruction while he is hospitalized on an inpatient unit. This is especially true for the building block courses, such as the upper-level math and science courses. If a student misses a month or more in these subjects, he is usually lost for the remainder of the school year.

Thus, the overriding question for an educator when a student is admitted to an inpatient unit is: What does this *individual* student need educationally? Is this patient admitted for a short-term stay and thus in need of an itinerant home and hospital teacher to keep up with the subjects in his/her home school? Is the adolescent going to be hospitalized for several months so that the hospital school becomes the school of record and needs to provide and coordinate all the activities leading toward grade advancement and/or graduation? Is the individual a previously identified special education student who comes with an individual education plan that the school must implement? Or is the student coming from a regular high school program and, most likely, returning to the same program? Some adolescents are admitted to the impatient program after they have quit school. School dropouts may attend classes, work towards a General Education Diploma (GED) (Maryland State Department of Education, 1988), or formally re-enroll in school.

Each question has its infinite variations depending upon the history, strengths, and weaknesses of the student. Each student is unique. The answers to these questions, along with the requirements that govern secondary schools in this country and the student's wishes and desires, dictate an individual education plan for each adolescent.

MODELS

Separate, stand-alone educational models are good for the sake of theoretical comparison but do not reflect the current educational practice in the field. Inpatients are not admitted as if punched out by cookie cutters. Students present themselves representing many themes and infinite variations of those themes. Their educational needs are distinctly varied and individualized, not completely fitting smoothly into model X, Y, or Z. In reality, most school programs in psychiatric hospitals are hybrids, offering elements of two or more of the following models due to the different programmatic needs of the population they serve.

Self-Contained Classrooms

Self-contained classrooms at the high school level are normally found where there is a high concentration of low-functioning students. A group of students spend most or all of the school day with the same teacher or teacher and aide. A teacher certified to teach special education is expected to instruct the students in all major subject areas. The students may go to other specialty teachers periodically during the week, such as physical education, art, music, and practical arts, etc., if the program is large enough to warrant their existence. The main focus however is the home base, self-contained classroom.

Advantages
Self-contained classrooms are easy to administer and organize. Communication lines are simplified, with inpatient units needing to deal with only one classroom teacher per patient instead of five to seven teachers.

Behavioral programs are easier to design and monitor with students working with one teacher instead of many. The chances of splitting staff are decreased.

Disadvantages
Students are not taught by subject-certified teachers. Material presented does not have the breadth or depth as compared to classes taught by subject-certified teachers, and this model is not appropriate for students who are on or near grade level.

Departmentalized Classrooms

Departmentalized classrooms at the secondary school level are normally found in most programs, especially where a high percentage of students are operating at or near grade level. Students rotate between classes, as in a normal high school, seeing five to seven different teachers each day. Each teacher instructs the students in the subjects in which they are certified.

Advantages
Departmentalized classrooms offer superior academic instruction by subject-certified teachers. This model replicates the educational reality that most inpatients will return to upon discharge and offers the best chance for students to keep up with their regular school classmates.

Disadvantages
Communication lines are complicated with inpatient units needing to interface with five to seven classroom teachers. Behavioral programs are more difficult to design and administrate. The chance of splitting is markedly increased as more teachers are working with students on a daily basis.

Home and Hospital Instruction

Home and hospital teaching usually occurs when, as an example, a student is hospitalized with a broken leg or psychiatric illness, or is at home recuperating from a similar experience. The local boards of education, according to Public Law 101-476, must provide instruction in institutions and hospitals as part of their continuum of alternative placements. Typically, a local board of education sends one or more teachers to a hospital to instruct an individual student, on a one-on-one basis, for a few hours per week. The minimum number of home and hospital instructional hours per week required by the State of Maryland, for example, is six (Programs for Students with Disabilities, 1991). Unfortunately, the minimum six hours of instruction per week routinely ends up to being maximum number of hours provided.

Advantages

Home and hospital instruction is productive when the length of stay is short and the student is going to return to his regular school placement. The home and hospital teacher(s) involved can coordinate the educational activities presented in the hospital with what is going on in the inpatient's normal school setting. The teachers are usually provided and paid for by the local board of education. The hospital needs only to provide a quiet space, conducive to the educational process, and a contact person to facilitate the communication process.

Disadvantages

The number of instructional hours per week is insufficient to help an inpatient keep up with his regular school program for very long. This is especially true of the higher level courses for which home and hospital teachers are usually not properly trained.

Mainstreamed Placements

Placing adolescents confined to psychiatric hospitals into public school programs is an infrequent occurrence due in part to the need for constant supervision. Students could be, however, mainstreamed for as little as 10 minutes per day initially, gradually working up to a full day. A more common occurrence would involve placing a hospitalized adolescent back into the school he attended before becoming an inpatient. Another option would involve placing a student into a public school during his last weeks of hospitalization as a transition or as a trial before discharge.

Advantages

Mainstreaming an inpatient gives the student a chance to try out newly acquired coping and social skills while still having the backup and support of a hospital setting. A mainstreamed class can also be the same class the inpatient will attend once discharged. This helps the transition while lessening the stigma attached to a stay in a psychiatric hospital.

Disadvantages

Public schools cannot provide the constant close supervision needed by most adolescent inpatients. The communication process can be somewhat cumbersome, especially if a student has many different teachers. The issue of transportation can be highly problematic, depending on the ability of the local school system, hospital, or parent to be a reliable resource.

As can be seen by reviewing the four models presented above, there are advantages and disadvantages to each. In general, there is no right or wrong model. In practice, it is often necessary to use segments of each model in order to meet the varying needs of a school population. Each student's needs must be evaluated individually and programmed on an individual basis, often by using parts of more than one model.

As an example, a bright high school student whose major academic courses could be easily programmed was hospitalized on the adolescent inpatient program. The student was, however, taking an advanced computer course. At that point, the inpatient school had just started offering beginning computer courses. In order to provide for the advanced computer course, the local home and hospital teaching program was contacted, which provided a qualified teacher who came to the school, used the school's equipment, and provided the appropriate instruction to the student. Parts of two models were simply used together in order to provide a program that made sense for that student.

EDUCATIONAL PROGRAM

The educational program at the Sheppard and Enoch Pratt Hospital will be described as it proceeds from day of admission, through hospitalization, to discharge. To keep matters simple, the material presented in this section describes mainly the school program. It is worthwhile to note, however, that the operation of the school program is intimately intertwined with the overall hospital program.

Intake

During the admissions process, records are requested from all the previous schools attended by an adolescent. The records requested include copies of transcripts or all previous report cards, results of standardized tests, immunization history, and any anecdotal information available. Once all the necessary information is gathered, the guidance counselor determines if any additional educational testing is required in order to place the adolescent in the appropriate class sections. If further assessments are necessary, the guidance counselor refers the case to the diagnostic and prescriptive (D&P) teacher. The D&P teacher is responsible for assessing a student's strengths and weaknesses, along with designing an approach to teaching that will be successful with a specific student.

After further reviewing the patient's record in conjunction with the guidance counselor or other members of the education staff, the D&P teacher selects and administers the instruments required to round out the adolescent's educational profile. The D&P teacher remains available throughout the adolescent's stay to assist the classroom teachers in understanding the individual's needs and to help the teachers successfully program for the patient. The D&P teacher is also available to conduct further evaluations as conditions warrant.

Courses

Thirteen classroom teachers provide the high school instructional program offering a wide array of courses. There are two classroom teachers in each of the four major subjects—English, history, social studies, math and science—with one classroom teacher each in art, basic education, business education, computers, industrial arts, and physical education. Courses in the four major subjects are offered at three different levels. The majority of the 73 class periods offered each day in the high school are taught at grade level and may have up to 10 students per class. For students who are two or three years behind in reading, a series of courses, the Skills Level, with up to eight patients per section is offered. For high school students who are reading at the elementary level, a series of Basic courses with a maximum of six per class is offered. Depending upon the strengths and weakness of a given student, classes from various levels are combined to create a schedule. The patients interact with five to seven different subject-certified classroom teachers per day, much the same as in regular school experiences.

Classes run for 40 minutes each, totaling seven periods per day. Four marking periods of approximately 45 days each combine to total the normal 180-day school year. Many adolescents who are hospitalized in psychiatric units have a history of missing segments of their formal education for various reasons. They often lag behind their peers in their credit standing and need to make up course work in order to graduate on time. A 35-day summer session is included in the program in an attempt to offer an opportunity for lagging students to catch up to their classmates. In order to have enough time in class to be able to grant original credit for the courses, classes are 55 minutes in length during the abbreviated summer session.

Adolescents who are nearing their discharge date may be mainstreamed into their local public school or another that is located in the community adjacent to the hospital. Courses are offered to support those students who are working towards a GED diploma. Students who have previously graduated from high school may sharpen their skills by taking classes from our course offerings. Adults from the adult section of the hospital also have the opportunity to take courses in the school depending on their particular interests and/or needs.

Support Services

A full-time librarian and an assistant are available daily for the high school students. Local public library services are utilized when necessary to supplement the library collection. The services of two D&P teachers and the guidance counselor are available. The guidance counselor works intensively with the seniors, as they prepare for college or the world of work, and is the focal person of the work-study program for adolescents on campus. Speech and language diagnostic services as well as ongoing speech/language therapy are available for the adolescent population.

The resource room, with a staff of three, is the focal point of the behavioral intervention services provided within the high school program. The resource staff provides academic help to students who need extra attention, monitor study halls, and maintain the highly structured environment needed to get most of the adolescents through a typical school day. It is the center where many of the minute-to-minute decisions are made. Most of the communications that occur during the school day between the high school and the inpatient units are funneled through the resource room. Material that cannot wait until the more formal written communication is passed on at the end of the school day is expeditiously transmitted as needed.

After the normal school day, extracurricular sports activities take place within the framework of a statewide athletic association. Students travel through the state during the year, participating in league games and activities. While some institutions participate in league play as part of their recreational program, we have found it advantageous to include it as part of the normal school routine. The school spirit that the team activities generate has proven to be a positive influence.

Discharge

As soon as an adolescent is admitted to the hospital, the planning process for school placement after discharge is begun. This is particularly important as the average length of stay has decreased sharply in recent years. The benefits of hospitalization would be potentially diminished if an adolescent were discharged to a good living arrangement only to sit at home during the day for lack of an appropriate school placement.

The special education identification, funding, and placement process is cumbersome and time-consuming. This is especially true if placement is being sought in a residential treatment center and a local board of education is being asked to fund the entire bill, not just the school portion. If a particular student has never been identified as needing special education services, it can take many months to complete the screening, assessment, identification, and placement process. Nothing is lost and much is to be gained by starting the process as early as possible. Parents can always stop the process whenever they like if plans change or if the avenue of exploration does not prove to be fruitful.

POTENTIAL PITFALLS

All programs that rely on eight-hour shift work, such as an inpatient unit, have created an environment that has a number of built-in problems. Communication between shifts, between school and inpatient units, and the timing of team meetings/staffings are critical issues that must be addressed and solved if a program is to be successful. If only there were 26 hours in a day and the extra two hours were added at normal inpatient nursing shift change time, 2 p.m. to 4 p.m., the timing and communication issues would be mostly resolved.

Communication

Successful communication is the lifeblood of all inpatient programs. There are two concepts that must be indelibly inscribed in each individual who works with an inpatient population from the day he or she is first employed; they are *communication* and *consistent, predictable environment*. The two concepts actually feed into each other, with excellent communication being a prerequisite for a consistent, predictable environment that enhances the chances of excellent communication patterns being developed.

Overcommunication, however wasteful and inefficient the management engineers may deem the practice, is far preferable to poor communication or no communication at all. A high-pressure environment, such as an inpatient unit, only intensifies the problems created when players are left out of the communication loop. Adolescents usually force us to be good communicators, as they are normally adept at "splitting." Good communication becomes a necessary survival skill and must be a way of life for everyone involved in inpatient care and school in order for a program to succeed.

Collaborative Meetings

Team meetings, staff meetings, and case conferences need to take place when all or most of the staff can be present to enhance and ensure good communication. Problems arise when specific segments of the staff need to attend a meeting at the same time that they are programmatically responsible for the patients. For example, teachers may be needed for a meeting, but the meeting is scheduled during the school day when they are in the classrooms; or meetings might be scheduled for later in the afternoon at a time when the evening inpatient shift is responsible for supervision and programming.

Meetings scheduled when day and evening shifts overlap enable representatives from both groups to attend meetings. This time tends to coincide with the end of the school day when teachers are also available. If enough staff are available to cover a classroom or group activity, a teacher or group care worker would be available for meetings. The amount of time a group care worker or teacher is missing from his or her primary assignment in a given week is always a concern that must be kept in mind.

Competing Activities

Most schools that are part of adolescent inpatient programs enroll a relatively small number of students. Many offer only one section of various subjects, such as Algebra I, Sociology, or Biology, thus dictating when a student must attend class. Seniors are a special group that cannot miss a substantial amount of school without putting their graduation at risk. At the same time school is in session, there are various groups, therapies, and evaluations that need to be scheduled and are competing for the same prime-time slots. The problem is more pronounced on short-term units where a number of evaluations must be completed in a compressed time frame. Everyone would like to work 8:30 a.m. to 4:30 p.m., Monday through Friday, but this is not possible. We are also responsible for and must program for these adolescents on a 24-hour-per-day basis, seven days a week.

Academically, a student cannot miss more than one class period in a given subject per week and still expect to pass the course. The rule of thumb within our adolescent programs is that a student may be taken out of a given course only one class period per week. In this manner, students can make up the work missed, hopefully, without falling behind their class. Many courses are offered in multiple sections enabling the guidance counselor to offer some flexibility in scheduling.

Parental Concerns

Almost all parents have been through school to one extent or another. They have lived through their children's educational experience and have opinions about what should be done educationally for their hospitalized offspring. For some parents, school presents an arena where one can concentrate energies and concerns while denying the reason their adolescent was hospitalized. It becomes a smoke screen, in most instances, an effort to hide from the truth. In some cases, parents refuse to allow contact with the previous school in an attempt to keep the hospitalization a secret. Adolescents are not hospitalized because they need the specific educational services associated with a particular inpatient unit. However, an excellent school program may influence parents to admit their adolescent to one hospital over another facility with a mediocre school program.

The closer a school program in a psychiatric hospital replicates the academic offerings of a public school, the more accepting parents tend to be of the program. The same Carnegie Units that are required by a given state govern public schools and nonpublic schools alike, serving educationally handicapped students.

Integration of Programs

A school calls the education plan for an adolescent an Individual Education Plan (IEP), while on the inpatient unit, it is called an Individual Treatment Plan (ITP). Laws and regulations govern hospitals and schools somewhat differently regarding formats and wording. Both plans contain different names, different emphases, but hopefully the same goals and objectives, especially the behavioral ones.

It is the communication process between the school and inpatient unit that is critical in aligning the goals and objectives for an individual adolescent. A teacher/advisor system is one method for keeping the channels open. The teacher/advisor transmits the information from the school to the inpatient unit and from the unit to the school. This person attends team meetings in the school and on the inpatient unit, transmitting information in both directions. Other devices used to keep the lines of communication open are point cards and homework sheets. Both devices can be utilized with an individual adolescent as needed. The adolescent carries the card(s) to school each day where each teacher records points earned, comments, and/or nightly homework assignments. The information is transmitted to the inpatient unit each afternoon where the evening staff monitors, comments on, and signs off the homework assignments. The next morning, the information regarding the evening activities is transmitted to the school. The system needs daily monitoring in order to minimize the splitting in which adolescents are so prone to engage.

FUNDING PROCESS

With the passage of Public Law 94-142 (Education of the Handicapped Act of 1975), the process of obtaining public funds to pay for the education of educationally handicapped students attending an accredited special education school while hospitalized on an inpatient psychiatric unit became easier. The thrust of the law was to ensure that each student who was identified as educationally handicapped receive an appropriate educational placement. Special education students identified as Seriously Emotionally Disturbed (SED) who needed to be educated in a separate school program could have their education paid for while they were hospitalized on an impatient psychiatric unit. The regulations adopted by the Federal and State governments to implement PL 94-142 made the process clear but also made it very time-consuming. The step-by-step approach of the implementing regulations follows, starting with a parent's request to screen their child for possible identification as a special education student all the way through placement.

> STEP 1. The parents must request the public school system to screen their child for possible identification as an educationally handicapped or special education student. This should be done in writing, through the U. S. Postal Service, with the parent keeping a copy of the letter. If there is any mistrust at all between the parents and the school system, the letter should be sent with a return receipt requested. The date the public schools receive the letter is very important, since it is the start date of the timeline to which the public schools must adhere in order to be in compliance with the law.
>
> STEP 2. The public school system must convene an Admission, Review and Dismissal (ARD) committee meeting within 30

calendar days of receiving the parents' request in order to screen the student for special education. At the screening ARD committee meeting, the members of the committee consider all the records available to them, including all records or private assessments provided by the parents. If the screening committee concludes that there is a possibility that the student in question may meet the criteria to be identified as educationally handicapped, they will identify what public school assessments must be conducted to help the committee decide the issue. The parents must give the school system their written permission so that the evaluations can proceed.

STEP 3. The public schools have 45 calendar days to conduct all of their evaluations.

STEP 4. A second ARD committee meeting must be held within 30 calendar days of the completion of the assessments. The committee must decide if the student is educationally handicapped and what type of disability he has. For the most part, students who are inpatients on a psychiatric unit are coded SED, either by itself or in combination with another disability code. It should be noted that there is no mild or moderate emotional disturbance in the Federal Government's coding system, only severe.

STEP 5. The public school system, in conjunction with the parents, has 30 more calendar days in which to write an Individual Educational Plan (IEP) for the student and have it approved by an ARD committee. The IEP must be completed prior to the placement decision. A common but inappropriate practice within the field of special education is to decide on the placement and then write the IEP to fit the placement. The IEP must be written to fit the student, then the placement follows.

STEP 6. The school system has an additional 30 school days to start the student in an appropriate special education program. If there is not an appropriate placement within the public school system, a nonpublic school placement is an option, paid for by public funds.

As one can see, the process can be quite time-consuming, taking up to 177 days. Given the fact that the vast majority of stays in psychiatric hospitals are for substantially shorter amounts of time, the special education funding option to pay for the educational component of an inpatient stay is usually limited to those students already identified as educationally handicapped. The special education identification and funding process can be an important aspect in discharge planning. If a patient is identified as educationally handicapped, a wider array of educational placement options are usually available upon discharge. This may include funding a placement in a residential treatment center for educational reasons.

SUMMARY

Education is the work of adolescents and must be appropriately carried on when a student is a patient in a psychiatric hospital. The educational model used to deliver the service depends on many variables, chief of which is the anticipated length of stay of the student. The key is to be able to individualize the adolescent's program in order to meet his needs. Short-term stays of a week or two dictate a program that keeps the adolescent abreast of his studies in his home school. A stay of two or three months or more indicates the hospital's school must take responsibility for the direction and planning of an individual's program.

The interrelationship between an inpatient unit and the school program is critical to a student's success. Excellent ongoing communication between the inpatient unit and the school is the key factor in assuring success. Given adolescents' ability to split adults, a clear, dependable communication system is essential for any psychiatric hospital. The consistent predictable environment that is so important to our charges is our responsibility to engineer, maintain, and improve.

REFERENCES

Education of Individuals with Disabilities Act, 20 U.S.C. § 1401 (1990).

Education of the Handicapped Act, 20 U.S.C. § 1401 (1975).

Maryland State Department of Education. (1988) *The Maryland High School Diploma by Examination* (Maryland School Bulletin, Vol. 36–3). Baltimore, MD: Author.

Programs for Students with Disabilities, Code of Maryland Regulations § 13A .05 .01 (October, 1991).

PART III

Special Treatment Considerations

Chapter 10

TREATMENT OF EATING DISORDERS

Elizabeth Williams, David Roth, and Fereidoon Taghizadeh

Adolescents' preoccupation with their bodies has been long recognized and robustly documented. Successive generations will be remembered for their experimentation with drugs and alcohol, signature hairstyling, distinctive forms of dress, the introduction of jewelry into men's ears, and surgically engendered cosmetic changes. It is in this vein, that future psychiatric texts will probably describe the last quarter of the 20th century as the "golden years of diet." The general public's appreciation, recognition, and understanding of dietary abuses and associated disorders have increased markedly over the past decade alone. As recently as the 1970's, few families had ever heard of the terms anorexia nervosa and bulimia nervosa. Now, these eating disorders are the substance of made-for-television movies, feature articles in popular magazines, and both public and private school prevention programs.

The scientific community has responded in kind. Over the last 10 years, we have witnessed an explosion in the number of published articles and chapters on eating disorder topics. Investigators are refining our diagnostic system, identifying significant risk factors, assessing the efficacy of various treatment interventions, and recommending specific prevention protocols. This chapter will be divided into two sections. First, we will briefly review pertinent diagnostic, etiologic, and treatment issues. Next, a detailed, clinically oriented description of the Sheppard Pratt inpatient adolescent eating disorders program will be provided.

Currently accepted psychiatric nosology (DSM-III-R, American Psychiatric Association, 1987) allows for the diagnosis of two primary, syndromal-level eating disorders: anorexia nervosa and bulimia nervosa.

As will become more evident, the clinical features of these disorders are quite different. The classic anorexic starves, whereas the classic bulimic is prone to large-scale binges. Nonetheless, a rather fundamental dynamic unites both disorders, in that eating-disordered individuals harbor a disdain of fatness, which is accompanied by an overvaluation of thinness. The eating disorders also share another characteristic, namely, that upwards of 90 percent of all patients with bulimia nervosa and anorexia nervosa are women (Halmi, 1987).

Syndromal-level classification of anorexia nervosa and bulimia nervosa requires the presence of a constellation of weight-related attitudes, appetitive behaviors, and circumscribed bodily states. Essentially, to meet DSM-III-R criteria for anorexia nervosa, one needs to have lost a minimum of 15 percent of premorbid body weight (children who have not yet achieved adult height must weigh at least 15 percent less than predicted weight), manifest extreme body image disparagement or misperception, experience profound fear of weight gain, and have been amenorrheic for three or more consecutive months. Typically, anorexic-level weight loss is achieved through rigorous dietary restriction and extreme exercise. The age of onset of this disorder has been found to range from 10 to 40 (Hsu, 1990). Scrutiny of epidemiological findings reveals a bimodal pattern of onset with anorexia nervosa first appearing around the ages of 13–14 and 17–18 (Halmi, Casper, Eckert, Goldberg & Davis, 1979). Research on prevalence indicates that upwards of 5 percent of young women will develop a subclinical case of anorexia nervosa (Button & Whitehouse, 1981) and approximately 1–2 percent will develop the full syndromal disorder (Crisp, Palmer, Kalucy, 1976; Szmuckler, 1983).

The central feature of bulimia nervosa is recurrent episodes of binge eating. A binge refers to the consumption of more food than an "average" person would eat in a 30-minute to two-hour period of time. To meet diagnostic criteria, one must binge two or more times per week for at least three months. Binges are typically experienced as being uncontrollable. The bulimic engages in compensatory caloric reduction practices, including, but not limited to, vomiting, laxative and/or diuretic abuse, and periods of dietary restraint. The bulimic, much as the anorexic, is concerned with her weight and appearance. The bulimic can present at anorexic, medically optimal, and obese weights. While the age of onset of bulimia nervosa has been reported to range between 10 and 51, most cases begin between the ages of 15 and 30 (Hsu, 1990; Johnson & Connors, 1987). Research indicates that as many as 90 percent of college-age women have binged (Hawkins & Clement, 1980). However, investigators using rigorous diagnostic criteria and methodologically sophisticated assessment batteries report a 2–4 percent prevalence rate for syndromal level bulimia nervosa (Fairburn & Beglin, 1990).

The eating disorders are rarely "free-standing," self-contained clinical entities. Medical problems, characterological disturbance, and other psychiatric syndromes frequently co-exist in the eating-disordered patient. Physical complications typically stem from prolonged malnutrition, dehydration, and purgative abuse (e.g., ipecac, laxatives). Eating-disorder related disturbances are not limited to a single site and have been detected in the gastrointestinal, hormonal, musculoskeletal, dermatological, cardiovascular, and metabolic systems, (Sheinin, 1988). The mortality rate for eating-disordered patients ranges from 5–20 percent (Garfinkel, Garner & Goldbloom, 1987). Co-morbid Axis I and Axis II disorders are quite common in anorexic and bulimic patients, particularly those presenting at a tertiary care facility. Major depression and/or dysthymic disorder has been diagnosed in 24–28 percent of eating-disordered individuals (Mitchell, Specker & deZwann, 1991). Substantial lifetime prevalence rates have also been reported for anxiety disorders (33–91 percent), substance use disorders (9–55 percent), and sexual victimization (20–50 percent) (Fairburn & Cooper, 1984; Laessle, Wittchen, Fichter & Pirke, 1989; Mitchell, Hatsukami, Eckert & Pyle, 1985; Mitchell et al., 1991; Weiss & Ebert, 1983). Improvements in assessment methodology and diagnostic sophistication have resulted in rather interesting characterologic findings. Specifically, Cluster A traits (i.e., paranoid, schizoid, and schizotypal) are relatively uncommon in eating-disordered patients, Cluster B traits (i.e., antisocial, borderline, histrionic, and narcissistic) are overrepresented in bulimic patients, and Cluster C traits (i.e., avoidant, dependent, obsessive-compulsive, and passive-aggressive) are also overrepresented in anorexic patients (Swift & Wonderlich, 1988; Wonderlich & Mitchell, 1991).

As an in-depth examination of theories of causality is well beyond the purview of this chapter, only a review of central etiologic constructs will be presented. Fundamentally, the biopsychosocial pressures and demands of adolescence provide a context for the development of an eating disorder. Thus, it is not a matter of coincidence that anorexia nervosa and bulimia nervosa typically begin during the teenage years. Adolescence is a period of dramatic change physically, sexually, affectively, cognitively, and interpersonally (Hsu, 1990; Strober & Yager, 1985). The negotiation of these changes and the tasks of separation-individuation are not easily accomplished by all adolescents (Freud, 1958). Moreover, a variety of factors adversely impact on the adolescent's capacity to successfully adapt to developmental demands such as low self-esteem, interpersonal anxiety and skill deficits, inadequate tension reduction and affect management skills, maladaptive personality traits, and dysfunctional familial environments (e.g., overprotective or chaotic). The adolescent at risk for developing an eating disorder typically fits the aforementioned profile (Garfinkel et al, 1987; Hsu, 1990).

The eating disorders provide a culturally congruent means of handling common, age-appropriate life stresses. Western culture's glorification of feminine thinness provides a medium through which many of the developmental tasks of adolescence can be approached. Weight loss promises peer acceptance and self-esteem enhancement. In fact, upwards of 70 percent of adolescent girls have seriously dieted (Nylander, 1971; Rosen & Gross, 1987) even though most were not obese. The highly vulnerable adolescent is apt to become overreliant on the constellation of eating disorder behaviors, attitudes, and body states. For instance, bingeing and purging can become a mode of self-regulation, thinness can be equated with specialness, and cachexia can provide an avenue of "retreat" from adolescence, per se (Crisp, 1980; Johnson et al., 1987). Once established, the eating disorders are apt to be reinforced by periodic compliments regarding "dietary achievements," the further diminishment of general functioning brought on by nutritional mismanagement, and the illusory effectiveness of these newly acquired skills.

Advances in our understanding of the pathogenesis of eating disorders have markedly shaped the substance and scope of therapeutic services provided to anorexic and bulimic patients. Gradually diminishing are the internecine struggles between proponents of psychosocial and biological orientations (Minuchin, Rosman & Baker, 1978; Hudson, Pope & Jonas, 1983). Instead, there is a growing recognition of the multifactorial nature of eating disorder pathology and the importance of multimodal, interdisciplinary treatment regimens (Hodes, Eisler & Dare, 1991; Hsu, 1990). Unfortunately, because of the difficulties inherent in conducting treatment-outcome field studies, there is a remarkable dearth of easily interpretable research regarding the efficacy of adolescent, inpatient eating disorder programs (Steinhausen, Rauss-Mason & Seidel, 1991). However, there is a growing consensus regarding acceptable criteria for hospitalization, cardinal treatment goals, and fundamental aspects of treatment.

There are four primary treatment goals for the hospitalized patient. These include: (1) the remediation of symptomatic behavior (e.g., weight restoration, normalization of diet, discontinuation of bingeing and purging); (2) further identification/correction of pathogenic factors; (3)

alleviation of co-morbid psychiatric problems; and (4) restoration of physical health. The optimal achievement of these goals requires the services of an interdisciplinary team. Members of the team must address psychological, medical, pharmacological, familial, interpersonal, nutritional, and rehabilitative issues. There is considerable debate about the necessity of a highly stringent behavioral program within the treatment milieu to manage the eating disordered behaviors (Eckert, Goldberg, Halmi, Casper & Davis, 1979). Nonetheless, there is agreement about the need for formal monitoring and supervision of weight and weight-related activities (Touyz, Beaumont & Glaun, 1984). Without question, follow-up outpatient treatment is needed to sustain and promote additional clinical gains.

THE SHEPPARD AND ENOCH PRATT PROGRAM

Our eating disorders program is part of a general adolescent psychiatric inpatient unit, where six of the unit's 24 beds are allocated for the treatment of eating disorders. This integration ensures that treatment addresses not only the eating disorder, but also the broad range of developmental needs unique to adolescents and any other concomitant psychiatric problems which are so often present in individuals with eating disorders. In order for the patient to internalize important educational, behavioral, and psychological benefits from the program, we encourage a hospitalization of at least one month.

Admission Criteria

Criteria for admitting a patient to the adolescent eating disorders program include a diagnosis of a full or subclinical syndrome of anorexia nervosa or bulimia nervosa. Presently, reasons accepted for hospitalization rather than outpatient treatment include severe medical risk, (e.g., marked and/or rapid weight loss, significant electrolyte imbalance, etc.); the presence of multiple, disabling co-morbid psychiatric syndromes; or a suicidal crisis. Also, a brief hospitalization may be indicated for a moderately to severely impaired bulimic who has had a refractory response to a reasonable trial (e.g., six months) of intensive outpatient treatment.

We do not accept patients who are in need of acute medical care until after they are medically stabilized. Eating disordered patients who have a primary psychiatric condition that impairs their cognitive ability to benefit from the entire eating disorder program (such as active psychosis or the very severe dissociation present in some cases of multiple personality disorder) are often accepted into a limited segment of the program, such as being included only in the nutritional rehabilitation protocol.

Preadmission Interview

During preadmission interviews, the parents and the patient meet with the chief of the service, who obtains the clinical history, explains the program fully, discusses the importance of the parents' support of the program's policies (such as eating all prescribed food, despite discomfort), receives informed consent, and arranges for a tour of the unit.

Treatment Program

There are four components to the adolescent eating disorder program: assessment, nutritional rehabilitation, psychotherapy, and discharge planning.

Component #1: Assessment

Thorough, multidisciplinary assessment is essential for appropriate treatment. Assessment is ongoing, with weekly team meetings to share and incorporate new information. The following information is gathered and shared by the treatment team within the first week of hospitalization.

Medical. Patients receive a comprehensive physical examination by a pediatrician upon or just prior to admission. Patients are weighed regularly, with frequency of weighings decreasing, as described below, as the patient progresses through the nutritional rehabilitation protocol.

Patients do not see their weights for the first two weeks, after which a clinical decision whether to tell the patient her weight is made by the staff with the patient. The relationship between physiological status and eating disorder behavior is shared with the patient and family throughout the hospitalization through discussion with staff, readings, and in therapy groups.

Nutritional. Detailed, dietary histories, eating disorder behavior patterns (e.g., binge, purge, restrict, etc.) and weight attitudes of the patient and the family are obtained. Importantly, both patients and families act as informants. The relationship between menstrual status, eating disordered behaviors and body weight is also assessed. Standardized questionnaires assessing eating disorder symptoms and attitudes, such as the Eating

Disorders Inventory (Garner, Olmstead & Polivy, 1983), are used to supplement this subjective data base. Patients are also observed during meals, providing behavioral information on attitudes and feelings about food.

Psychiatric and Developmental: Thorough developmental, psychiatric, and family psychiatric histories are obtained. Areas of particular importance that are assessed in this population include the presence of an affective disorder, sexual abuse, sexual attitudes and behaviors, obsessional characteristics, borderline personality characteristics, social phobias, and deficits in leisure skills. Also, an attempt is made to assess the extent to which parental prescriptions about eating and dieting are etiologic or reactive.

Component #2: Nutritional Rehabilitation
Nutritional rehabilitation for eating disordered patients involves physiological, educational, and behavioral elements. A three-stage graduated protocol is used, whereby patients are moved from high to low levels of external support and structure. The indicators for readiness to decrease external support include: eating all prescribed food, not bingeing, not purging, exercising only when scheduled, and, for anorectics, appropriate weight gain. Setbacks (such as, restricting food intake) are viewed as indicating a need for an increased level of staff support. Patients progress through these levels of support at different rates, with some patients requiring only one to two weeks per stage, most requiring two to four weeks per stage, and a few requiring even a longer time period, per stage. Unfortunately, it is increasingly common that insurance limitations necessitate a decision to progress someone more quickly through the protocol than would be indicated by symptom severity.

An individualized dietary exchange plan emphasizing adolescent nutritional needs is constructed for each patient to guide her until she can internally judge appetite and normal amounts of food. The exchange plan helps patients revise their beliefs about food. Instead of viewing food as an enemy, they learn to conceive of it as an essential fuel made up of one or more of the nutritional components of carbohydrates—meat, milk, fat, vegetables, and fruits. Calories are largely de-emphasized.

With underweight patients, the exchange plan aims for the achievement of two–three pounds per week weight gain until a minimally healthy weight level is achieved so that menses could either begin or resume. A six-pound goal weight range is established by using the age-adjusted Metropolitan Life Insurance "normal" weight as an approximate upper limit for females and males. The Frisch & MacArthur (1974) table provides menstrual threshold weights and is used as a lower limit for females. Intake for anorectic patients is typically begun at 1200–1500 calories, due to physical discomfort and medical risk associated with refeeding. Calories are increased every three days, in 300 calorie increments, with daily levels peaking between 2500 and 4500 calories.

With normal weight or obese bulimics, the exchange plan is designed to help patients maintain their weight. Obese bulimics are discouraged from attempting to lose weight until recovered from the bulimia, as dieting predisposes one to bingeing. For weight maintenance, caloric needs are initially estimated to be 15 calories per pound of body weight adjusted up or down over the course of treatment if the patient appears to be gaining or losing weight. The nutritionist schedules weekly meetings with the patients throughout the hospitalization to revise the exchange plan and help the patient become increasingly self-sufficient in its use. Unscheduled meetings with the dietician are discouraged as such visits almost always represent a dysfunctional mode of coping with food and weight-related anxiety. Instead, staff point out to the patient the exaggerated phobias underlying this behavior in order to reassure the patient. Maladaptive food phobias are also addressed by exposure of the patient to the full gamut of cafeteria foods. In fact, with the exception of premorbid vegetarianism, patients are expected to consume all but three specific disliked foods, such as hotdogs, brussel sprouts, etc.

The Nutritional Rehabilitation Stage One: Support Phase. In this stage, patients are observed 24-hours a day for prevention of purging and bingeing. This also ensures that *all* their prescribed food, is eaten so that they receive the message, "Food is medicine." Thus, all therapies are conducted on the hall, and patients must be escorted to the bathroom. Patients are weighed daily during this stage, exercise is not allowed, and some patients may be placed on bedrest if their medical condition warrants it. Patients are given 30 minutes to complete their meals, which are preselected by the dietician. If patients fail to consume the entire meal or purge the meal, they are required to consume a nutritional supplement, such as Ensure, equivalent of the meal. Refusal to drink the Ensure first results in a 30-minute time out; if necessary, the patient is then given the nutritional supplement through nasogastric tube feeding. In this way, patients are given the clear message that the staff will not allow them to starve. This procedure begins after a 24-hour orientation period, so that the patients clearly understand these measures. Tube feeding rarely occurs, apparently because patients clearly understand and wish to avoid the consequences of not eating.

It is imperative that staff clearly communicate that the powerful external control they are imposing on patients' basic bodily functions is supportive in purpose and intent. Patients understandably see protocol-driven staff control as punitive. Moreover, control struggles are usually central for these patients, as most of them have experienced excessive pressures to conform their needs to please other people. The basic message is that the patient's unique decisions, actions, and opinions are indeed to be honored *except* where they threaten the patient's health. Unnecessary struggles can also be avoided if the patients are prepared for the discomfort associated with refeeding, such as bloating, slowed gastric motility, edema, and constipation after cessation of laxatives. Patients need to be reassured that these discomforts will pass and are not signs of complete discontrol. Finally, it is critical in this stage to remember that very serious, even fatal complications, such as acute gastric dilatation or massive peripheral edema, can sometimes occur in refeeding, particularly if the refeeding is too fast.

Nutritional Rehabilitation Stage Two: Stabilization Phase. Patients enter this stage when they have demonstrated three consecutive days of refraining from eating disorder symptoms. Also anorexics must no longer be dangerously underweight, as indicated by being at least three pounds above 70% of their goal weight range.

During this phase, patients are allowed to attend therapies off the hall and, if appropriate, the school on the hospital campus. Patients are weighed three times a week during this stage. They continue to be observed for one hour post meals and during bathroom visitations. As they demonstrate continued ability to refrain from bingeing and purging, to feed themselves healthily by eating all prescribed food, and, for anorexics, to gain weight appropriately, postprandial observation is gradually eliminated.

Setbacks, which include not eating all prescribed food, bingeing, purging, and, for anorexics, weight loss, are met with 24-hour hall restriction and observation after all meals. After this contingency has been enforced, patients resume their previous position in the protocol. The message conveyed is that setbacks mean that patients need to give themselves increased support to get back on track, but *not* that their progress is undone.

During this phase, supervised meals are begun in the cafeteria and patients are encouraged to begin choosing their own meals. Patients and staff together decide how to make these changes, for example, deciding which meals to start eating in the cafeteria at first, how quickly to phase in off-hall meals, etc. This process gives patients practice requesting external support to help cope with eating-related anxiety.

Moderate exercise can be initiated in this phase if weight is in the minimally healthy range. Exercise must be supervised and psychologically healthy, meaning a decreased emphasis on solitary activities oriented towards appearance, such as solo calisthenics, and an increased emphasis on activities oriented towards socializing and enjoyment, such as dancing and basketball. The exercise program is developed with the activities therapist, who emphasizes exercising for fun, a sense of well being, and health, *not* for appearance or weight loss.

Nutritional Rehabilitation Stage Three: Maintenance Phase. Patients are moved to this stage when they have demonstrated sufficient internal ability to refrain from purging and bingeing, and to feed themselves healthily. Specifically, they should be eating and self-selecting all meals in the cafeteria. Bulimic patients should be free of bingeing and purging for two days, and anorectics should be in their goal weight range for two days.

Patients are encouraged to eat all meals with peers and check dietary plans with staff two–three times per week. Setbacks are handled in the same way as previously described. Patients are weighed randomly once a week.

Patients are encouraged to identify problem situations involving food and weight that may occur outside the hospital, and to set up programs with staff to help them practice coping with these situations. For example, patients are encouraged to have meals with their families and at restaurants. Another common practice situation involves going shopping for clothes and trying on different outfits.

Component #3: Psychotherapy
The eating disorder is viewed as a way to cope with psychological dilemmas caused by societal pressures for thinness, family dynamics, the demands of adolescence, and individual vulnerabilities. Therefore, the individual and family are assisted in learning other ways to cope with these dilemmas.

Case Management and Individual Therapy. Treatment is coordinated by the patient's attending therapist, who is a psychiatrist or psychologist. This attending therapist also provides individual therapy three times a week in which the patient explores healthier ways to express feelings and needs and obtain a sense of worth and power. Discussions of food and weight are limited by the therapist, but must occur to ensure that the patient feels understood. The patient is also assigned a primary nurse who provides psychoeducational readings and assignments relevant to recovery, such as planning restaurant sign-outs.

Family Therapy and Support Group. During weekly family therapy, families are helped to construct a nonblaming understanding of etiology and to utilize adaptive intrafamilial coping skills. Families receive relevant reading material and have an opportunity to discuss separation-autonomy issues in a support group for families of hospitalized adolescents.

Group Therapy. There are four weekly eating disorders groups. The Eating Disorders Psychoeducational Group addresses issues such as cultural pressures and basic physiological concepts concerning weight and dieting. Also, in this group, patients plan and prepare at least one meal. Tray Group is run by the nutritionist, often over lunch. In this group, patients learn about food exchanges, how to integrate all types of food into their diets, (including "junk" foods), and how to plan menus. Body Image Group is a structured group using experiential methods, (e.g., sculpture, movement, collages), to evoke and explore different aspects of body image. Eating Anxiety Group is an unstructured, psychodynamic group where eating disorder symptoms are related to underlying issues of self-esteem and relationships.

Patients also attend weekly general psychotherapy groups, that is, groups not specific to eating disorders. These heterogeneously composed groups help the eating disorder patients realize that many of their struggles are common to every adolescent. These groups include assertiveness training, relaxation training, recreational skills, and "girl's issues," where female sexuality is one of the issues discussed.

Milieu Therapy. Eating disorder patients are extremely vulnerable to perceived approval from others as a determinant of their self-worth. With this in mind, non-eating disordered patients are discouraged from applauding thinness and dieting. Instead, conversation is directed to the more substantive aspects of interpersonal relationships. Also, efforts are made to move eating disorder patients from a posture of perfectionism and compliance to a position of healthy assertiveness and rebellion.

Medication. Hospitalization provides an opportunity to conduct medication trial(s) with patients who are medically compromised and/or have been noncompliant with outpatient regimens. Antidepressants are used with a large subgroup of patients who evidence significant depressive or obsessional disorders. However, since depressive features may clear with nutritional rehabilitation, it is optimal to defer an antidepressant trial, if possible. A low dose of antianxiety medication may be used before meals for anorexics whose level of anxiety prevents them from participation in the refeeding protocol.

Component #4: Discharge Planning

Sound discharge planning is crucial, as full recovery from a severe eating disorder requires prolonged treatment. First, financial resources must be assessed and allocated wisely. Staff help the patient and their family assess the relative benefits of using the resources on a longer inpatient stay versus more extended treatment in intensive or traditional outpatient programs. Discussions often concern the importance of ensuring that insurance coverage is available, or ensuring that resources are available for another inpatient stay if a crisis occurs.

Patients and families extensively prepare how they will handle food and weight issues. Families are reminded to not monitor food consumption and weight, transferring these functions to the patient and their outpatient therapist. For anorexics, clear weight criteria for rehospitalization are determined. Patients prepare for two weeks of meals after discharge. They brainstorm with staff and other patients about potential high-risk situations, such as being alone or feeling fat, and how to cope with them. Patients routinely assess their wardrobe and discard clothes that don't fit or tend to evoke "fat" feelings.

Case Description

Megan was a 16-year-old girl who was hospitalized at Sheppard Pratt due to anorexia nervosa. She was 5 foot 3 1/2 inches tall and weighed 98 pounds. She manifested depression, suicidal ideation, anxiety, social withdrawal, ritualistic behavior and delusional thinking regarding food, such as fearing that she would absorb calories through her skin if she touched food. Megan had been hospitalized at two other psychiatric facilities during the preceding year; however, after being discharged, she decompensated and her depression became more acute, culminating in suicidal wishes and extreme delusional ideation.

The patient's family history was positive for affective disorders. Megan had a sister 14 months younger than herself. As a child Megan had colic, difficulty adjusting to formula and food, and difficulty soothing herself when distressed. At age three, the patient precipitously regressed and became mute. Throughout her adolescence, Megan regularly avoided competition with peers and had difficulty both experiencing and expressing anger. Megan's pubertal development was profoundly impacted by an experience where she was verbally harassed by older male teenagers. Subsequently, she evidenced deep fears about her evolving sexuality. Megan was socially anxious and would make frantic attempts to be accepted by her peers. Megan's mother felt ill-prepared and overwhelmed by this parenting challenge. At the same time, her father became overinvolved and tried both to "spoon feed" her school work and to shelter her from the stresses of adolescence.

During the summer of her 15th year, Megan attended a two-week church camp. The camp experience represented the worst of Megan's fears: separation from her parents, extensive peer involvement, further sexual pressure, and little protection from these forces. To cope with these same stresses, Megan enlisted her sister into a collaborative diet. Megan continued the diet well after her sister resumed normal eating. Megan quickly achieved an anorexic weight level.

The course of Megan's hospital treatment was long and complicated. Her diagnosis was anorexia nervosa, major depression, and identity disorder. Mellaril and Tofranil were used to help her alleviate symptoms of depression and delusional thinking related to food. Megan also received intensive individual therapy, group therapy, activity therapy, and art therapy and was involved in the unit's psychoeducational program. During family therapy sessions, she was encouraged to directly deal with feelings of guilt and anger, as well as with issues of separation and individuation. Megan's parents were helped to promote the process of family growth by addressing and correcting their own marital problems. During individual therapy, the patient's poor self-image, low self-esteem, fear of fatness, aversion to food, need to please others, inability to deal with anger and, later, sexuality were addressed. Over the course of 12 months' hospitalization, the patient made considerable strides in emotional, social, academic, and physical spheres.

At the time of discharge, it was decided that the patient still needed considerable structure in her life. Accordingly, she was referred to a boarding school. The patient was also followed by a multidisciplinary team and received a comprehensive array of individual, family, group, and medical therapies for the next four years. It is significant to note that Megan successfully graduated from high school and entered college. She remains in recovery, has a number of close friends, frequently asks other people to meet her needs, and has actively been dating.

Future Directions

The inpatient psychiatric treatment of eating disordered adolescent patients is a tremendously complicated process. Therapy requires a multidisciplinary effort with close attention paid to the interaction of genetic, psychosocial, and developmental forces. Insurance companies are shortening the length of stays for eating disorders, thus dramatically affecting the manner in which inpatient treatment is being conducted. Gone are the days when a moderately ill child could be hospitalized as a therapeutic maneuver to create distance within a highly enmeshed family (Andersen, 1985). In fact, an increasing number of insurance carriers are eliminating inpatient coverage for bulimia nervosa. It has been our experience that shortened hospitalizations lead to an overemphasis upon rapid weight restoration and symptomatic remission. We have found that symptomatic improvement quickly unravels when there is insufficient time to address pathogenic influences and learn alternative coping skills. Of course, treatment outcome studies will need to be conducted in order to assess the effects of changing patterns of insurance coverage and hospital lengths of stay. If these trends continue, new models for providing intensive treatment to eating disordered individuals will need to be developed, piloted, and refined if we are to effectively meet the mental health challenges of the 1990s.

REFERENCES

American Psychiatric Association (1987). *Diagnostic and Statistical Manual of Mental Disorders* (Third edition—revised). Washington, D.C.: American Psychiatric Association.

Andersen, A. E. (1985). *Practical comprehensive treatment of anorexia nervosa and bulimia.* Baltimore, MD: Johns Hopkins University Press.

Button, E. J. & Whitehouse, A. (1981). Subclinical anorexia nervosa. *Psychological Medicine, 11,* 509-516.

Crisp, A. H. (1980). *Anorexia Nervosa: Let me be.* London: Plenum Press.

Crisp, A. H., Palmer, R. L. & Kalucy, R. S. (1976). How common is anorexia nervosa? A prevalence study. *British Journal of Psychiatry, 128,* 549-554.

Eckert, E. D., Goldberg, S.C., Halmi. A., Casper, R. C. & Davis, D. M. (1979). Behavior therapy in anorexia nervosa. *British Journal of Psychiatry, 134,* 55-59.

Fairburn, C. & Beglin, S. J. (1990). Studies of epidemiology of bulimia nervosa. *American Journal of Psychiatry, 147,* 401-408.

Fairburn, C. G. & Cooper, P. J. (1984). The clinical features of bulimia nervosa. *British Journal of Psychiatry, 144,* 238-246.

Freud, A. (1958). Adolescence. *Psychoanalytic Study of Children, 13,* 255-278.

Frisch, R. E. & MacArthur, J. (1974). Menstrual cycles: Fatness a determinant of minimum weight for height necessary for their maintenance or onset. *Science, 185,* 949-951.

Garner, D. M., Olmstead, M. P. & Polivy, J. (1983). Development and validation of a multidimensional eating disorder inventory for anorexia nervosa and bulimia. *International Journal of Eating Disorders, 2,* 15-34.

Garfinkel, P. E., Garner, D. M. & Goldbloom, D. S. (1987). Eating disorders: Implications for the 1990's. *Canadian Journal of Psychiatry, 32,* 624-631.

Halmi, K. A. (1987). Anorexia nervosa and bulimia. *Annual Review of Medicine, 38,* 373-380.

Halmi, K. A., Casper, R., Eckert, E., Goldberg, S. C. & Davis, J. M. (1979). Unique features associated with age of onset of anorexia nervosa. *Psychiatry Research, 1,* 209-215.

Hawkins, R. C. & Clement, P. F., (1980). Development & construction validation of a self-report measure of binge eating tendencies. *Addictive Behaviors,* 219-226.

Hodes, M., Eisler, I. & Dare, C. (1991). Family therapy for anorexia nervosa in adolescence: A review. *Journal of The Royal Society of Medicine, 84,* 359-362.

Hsu, G. (1990). *Eating Disorders.* New York: Guilford Press.

Hudson, J. I., Pope, H. G. & Jonas, J. M. (1983). Phenomenological relationship of eating disorders to major affective disorder. *Psychiatry Research, 9,* 345-354.

Johnson, C. & Connors, M. E. (1987). *The etiology and treatment of bulimia nervosa.* New York: Basic Books.

Laessle, R., Wittchen, H., Fichter, M. & Pirke, K. (1989). The significance of subgroups of bulimia and anorexia nervosa: Lifetime frequency of psychiatric disorders. *International Journal of Eating Disorders, 8,* 569-574.

Minuchin, S., Rosman, B. L. & Baker, L. (1978). *Psychosomatic families.* Cambridge, MA: Howard University Press.

Mitchell, J. E., Hatsukami, D., Eckert, E. D. & Pyle, R. L. (1985). Characteristics of 275 patients with bulimia. *American Journal of Psychiatry, 42,* 482-485.

Mitchell, J. E., Specker, S. M. & DeZwann, M. (1991). Co-morbidity and medical complications of bulimia nervosa. *Journal of Clinical Psychiatry, 52,* 13-20.

Nylander, I. (1971). The feeling of being fat and dieting in a school population: Epidemiologic interview investigation. *Acta Sociomedical Scandinavia, 3,* 17-26.

Rosen, A. C. & Gross, J. (1987). Prevalence of weight reducing and weight gaining in adolescent girls and boys. *Health Psychology, 6,* 131-147.

Sheiwin, J. E. (1988). Pathophysiologic and Chemical aspects of medical, endocrine, and nutritional abnormalities and adaptations in eating disorders. In B. J. Blinder, B. F. Chaitin & R. S. Goldstein (Eds.). *The eating disorders: Medical and psychological bases of diagnosis and treatment.* New York, NY: PMA Publishing.

Steinhausen, H., Rauss-Mason, C. and Seidel, R. (1991). Follow-up studies of anorexia nervosa: A review of four decades of outcome research. *Psychological Medicine, 21,* 447-454.

Strober, M. & Yager, J. (1985). A developmental perspective of the treatment of anorexia nervosa in adolescents. In D. M. Garner and P. E. Garfinkel (Eds.), *Handbook of Psychotherapy for Anorexia Nervosa and Bulimia.* New York, NY: Guilford Press.

Swift, W. J. & Wonderlich, S. A. (1988). Personality factors and diagnosis in eating disorders and structures. In D. M. Garner and P. E. Garfinkel (Eds.), *Diagnostic Issues in Anorexia Nervosa and Bulimia Nervosa.* New York, NY: Brunner/Mazel.

Szmuckler, G. I. (1983). Weight and food preoccupations in a population of English School girls. In G. J. Bargman (Ed.), *Understanding Anorexia Nervosa and Bulimia.* Columbus, OH: Ross Laboratories.

Touyz, S. W., Beaumont, P. J. & Glaun, D. (1984). A comparison of lenient and strict operant conditioning in refeeding patients with anorexia nervosa. *British Journal of Psychiatry, 144,* 517-520.

Weiss, S. R. & Ebert, M. H. (1983). Psychological and behavioral characteristics of normal weight bulimics. *Psychosomatic Medicine, 45,* 293-303.

Wonderlich, S. & Mitchell, M. (1991). *The Co-morbidity of Eating Disorders and Personality Disorders.* Washington, DC: American Psychiatric Press.

Chapter 11

INTEGRATING ALCOHOL AND DRUG ABUSE TREATMENT INTO AN ADOLESCENT PSYCHIATRIC HOSPITAL PROGRAM

Steven L. Jaffe

Problems with substance abuse and chemical dependency have become epidemic in our adolescent population. Violent deaths due to accidents, suicide, and homicide make up 80 percent of teenage mortality. Half of these deaths involve alcohol and drugs. A large proportion of hospitalized teenagers have abused alcohol and drugs, and this situation must be assessed and addressed as part of their integrated treatment programs. In this chapter, I will describe the specific components and therapeutic processes involved in a model chemical dependence recovery track of a general inpatient psychiatric treatment program.

Follow-up studies of treated chemically dependent adolescents (Harrison & Hoffman, 1987; Brown, in press) indicate that regular attendance at support groups (after care and Twelve Step groups) is a major factor of how well teenagers are functioning one year after discharge from hospital/residential treatment. This result supports the use of a diagnostic and treatment program that integrates the Twelve Steps with a developmental psychodynamic framework.

If initial evaluations of adolescents raise the issue of significant alcohol or drug abuse, then these teenagers are asked to write a First Step as developed in *The Step Workbook for Adolescent Chemical Dependency* (Jaffe, 1990). Writing specific answers to specific questions presses these teenagers to commit to look at their lives and experiences. Answers in the workbook can be checked to make sure teenagers are answering the questions in detail. The written answers are also presented verbally for discussion and feedback, especially at a First Step Group. Teenagers usually tend to be very resistant to examining their alcohol/drug use and are generally not very motivated to stop using substances. The Workbook First Step becomes a diagnostic process for the teenagers to examine how alcohol and drugs have affected their lives.

The Workbook begins with some screening questions such as:

- Have they cut school and used drugs or alcohol?

- Have they missed school because of drinking? (Halikis, J., 1990)

- Have they been in trouble with the police because of drinking or using?

- Does alcohol or drug abuse exist in any family members?

The questions of the First Step (Part 1) cover the following topics: How have drugs put their own or others lives in danger? Have they been suicidal? Have there been times when they have been hurt or hurt others? Have they done things they said they would never do? Have they broken the law when using or trying to get money to use? The effects of drugs on the loss of trust by their family as well as physical effects, like blackouts and flashbacks, are covered. Specific questions also examine how alcohol/drugs have been used to run away from painful feelings, how drugs interfered with getting things done and future plans. These issues are then related to the concepts of the First Step.

Only after careful examination of these issues can the teenagers decide if their lives are a mess because of drugs and consider whether they are addicts. Addicts are unable to use alcohol or drugs in moderation; once beginning drug use, they must continue even though their lives are increasingly chaotic; and they no longer care about school, job, family or friends.

Step One—The First Step of AA states, *"We admitted we were powerless over alcohol—that our lives had become unmanageable."* However, most teenagers flee from the word "powerless," for no self-respecting teenagers are interested in admitting that they don't have power. Our approach has been to emphasize that addicts are powerless if they use alcohol or drugs. If they do not use alcohol or drugs, then they will have the power to have a life. This places the First Step into a context that emphasizes having power. Acknowledging that they cannot use alcohol and drugs in moderation gives them the power to become responsible persons with a future. The other helpful concept for teenagers working a First Step is that the teenagers may be "on the way to becoming an addict." Here teenagers recognize that if they continue along their alcohol and drug abusing pathway, they will develop all the signs, symptoms and problems of chemical dependency.

There are two positive therapeutic goals that are pursued in the First Step. The first goal involves the development of honesty. Since most abusing and chemically dependent teenagers *lie* to deny and minimize the severity of their alcohol and drug use, honesty must be developed through staff and peer interaction and confrontation. Sometimes, adolescents will need to write and present their First Step a second or third time until they have been honest and thorough.

The second therapeutic goal is overcoming the defense mechanism of disavowal. Disavowal relates to teenagers who acknowledge extensive alcohol/drug use and its severe effects on their lives, but do not experience the painful, connected emotions. For example, teenagers may relate to being beat up or raped while drunk or high, but feel this was "no big deal." This is dealt with in the First Step by having teenagers write, in a very concrete manner, the details of these experiences. The detailed writing is then verbalized since speech facilitates the process of making these objective events become affectively meaningful memories. For example, if each incident of driving while drunk is remembered in detail, it is recalled as a threat to their own life and the lives of others. Each traumatic event must be remembered in detail. As one teenager described, "Until I wrote it down, it never bothered me. I didn't like it at first because I got upset and then the feelings came out. I cried even though I always thought crying was for sissies. I guess that has to happen first before you can start to come clean and stay that way." Realizing the seriousness of the effects of alcohol and drugs on their lives enables teenagers to make the decision that they *need* to stop drinking and using.

The second part of the First Step involves teenagers writing their life history. Some of the areas covered include: memories as a young child, childhood friends, and happy as well as terrible and/or scary times (i.e. physical or sexual abuse). Adolescents are required to describe their family constellation and the quality of these relationships. Serious problems within the family and their own emotional responses are emphasized. Grades, as well as behavior and learning problems in school, are also examined. Another important issue considered is a listing of what they have done that was illegal even if they didn't get caught. Reflecting on their life history helps them to look at what they wished were different but was out of their control. The life history part of the First Step directs teenagers to identify sad and traumatic events in their lives from which getting drunk and "high" became an escape. The importance of exploring one's own thoughts and feelings and of beginning to develop a sense of self is established. The teenagers also learn that many past experiences were not in their control and not their fault. The feelings associated with their life stories need to be expressed when this part of the First Step is presented to a group.

If the First Step reveals that the adolescents are unable to moderate the use of alcohol or drugs resulting in life-threatening and self-destructive behavior, a full chemical dependency program is needed to help achieve abstinence. The continuation and integration of a Twelve Step program into the teenagers' local community is critical for continued abstinence after discharge from the hospital or residential program.

Along with the Twelve Steps, specific other chemical dependency recovery components are needed.

1. **Chemical Dependency Groups.** These include Step study groups where the First Step is presented along with the issues of Steps Two through Five. Other chemical dependency groups will include lectures, discussions, and testimony groups where recovering persons present their "life story." Honesty is the crucial aspect of this step, along with the adolescents' life history.

2. **Contacts and Sponsors.** After the First Step and life history have been presented and approved as being honest and well done, adolescents are given the names of one or two "contacts." Contacts are volunteers to the program who are older, recovering members of the local community and have achieved at least one year of abstinence. Adolescents are to telephone their "contact" every day to begin developing a special relationship. If a positive relationship develops, the contact may visit in the hospital and later take the adolescent to community meetings. Often, the contact becomes a sponsor and is the person to whom the Fifth Step is presented.

   Although chemically dependent teenagers typically are involved in many high-risk behaviors when "high" on alcohol or drugs, contacting a stranger by telephone while sober can cause intense anxiety. Therefore, support and encouragement in learning to initiate and maintain a telephone conversation can be accomplished through role playing.

3. **Community AA/NA Meetings.** It is essential that adolescents continue their recovery program after leaving the hospital in order to maintain abstinence. Therefore, increasing attendance and participation at community meetings should occur as adolescents

make progress in the hospital. The adolescents attend local meetings with staff as a group, individually with their contacts or volunteers, and then each time they leave the hospital or residential program on a home pass. Recovering adolescents must become familiar and comfortable with participation at local AA/NA meetings. Joining a group meeting that is located close to their home better assures that adolescents will emotionally connect with several of the regular members.

4. **Family Groups.** Intense therapeutic work with the adolescents' family is essential for progress. Family turmoil almost universally occurs in response to the adolescents' behavior. "Enabling" attitudes and behavior by the family that positively reinforce the continued use of alcohol or drugs have usually developed. Often, other family members are also chemically dependent and will need treatment. These issues, as well as any premorbid family psychopathology, need to be treated by an intense family program that includes education groups, individual family therapy, and multi-family groups. Attendance at support groups such as Alanon, Naranon, and Adult Children of Alcoholics (ACOA), may also be helpful.

5. **Other.** Other program components include spiritual groups and relapse prevention groups.

After the diagnostic First Step, it is important to try to complete Step Two through Step Five. Methods for "working" these Steps (as described in detail in the Workbook), are as follows:

Step Two—*"Came to believe that a power greater than ourselves could restore us to sanity."*

The first part of the Second Step involves helping teenagers to look at the numerous bad things that have happened in their lives as a result of drinking or drug using (i.e., problems at home, school, etc.). When teenagers keep repeating behaviors that cause hurt to themselves, these behaviors don't make sense. Dwelling on these repetitions helps teenagers to realize that they were not able to moderate use of alcohol or drugs, and this caused irrational, self-destructive behavior to repeat again and again.

The second part of the Second Step is often very difficult for teenagers to process. Here, they are asked to begin to turn to a "Higher Power" to help them with those parts of their life that are beyond their control. Teenagers have the most difficulty with this component because they generally have not dealt with traumatic experiences in their early lives. As young children, the significant adults who raise them are their early "higher powers." Children look and turn to these adults for nurture, love, and guidance. This is often problematic since most chemically dependent teenagers have had severe traumatic events related to their early parental relationships. Frequently these childhood "higher powers" have hurt them through emotional, physical, and/or sexual abuse, or have let them down by neglect or abandonment. The teenagers must deal with the pain and sadness resulting from the disappointment in their childhood "higher powers" and must mourn these losses. This mourning must occur before the teenagers can begin to develop a sense of something positive in the universe that they can turn to for help.

Another part of the Second Step that is helpful to teenagers is for them to examine the belief systems they developed when using alcohol and drugs. These beliefs often involve lying, "My way is the only way," "Take what you want," and "You can live without pain or distress." These beliefs make the adolescents feel strong and in control, but they just don't and won't work. Once they recognize this, the teenagers are then required to look at the belief systems of people who are in good Twelve Step programs. These positive beliefs include honesty, responsibility, caring about oneself, and caring about others. Turning to a positive "Higher Power" and a positive belief system is the needed positive step to sanity.

Step Three— *"Made a decision to turn our will and our life over to the care of God as we understand Him."*
The Third Step involves the development of a decision for the teenagers to *commit* themselves to working the Steps while having a positive spiritual higher power. This Step involves taking the leap and trying a new way. Having teenagers look at what they fear when giving up their old ways is often very helpful at this time. Getting them to admit they don't need to have all the answers and that it is okay to weaken their tough image will help them tolerate the anxiety of trying something new. The teenagers are encouraged to recognize that they turned over their lives to alcohol and drugs and went to any length to get what they wanted. Now they are being asked to turn things over to a positive program. Many teenagers feel that the "God" part is too religious. In such instances it is often helpful to reframe or redefine the "God" part as being a "Good Orderly Direction."

Step Four—*"Made a searching and fearless moral inventory of ourselves."*

In this step, it is helpful to create a questionnaire containing specific questions relating to early aspects of the adolescents' life. Written details concerning their early life, family life, school life, worries, anxieties, fears, self-image, sexuality, actions, and jobs are required. Written response to these past actions, thoughts, and feelings can cause teenagers to become anxious, sad, and angry. However, a successful Fourth Step requires that these painful memories be reexperienced. The adolescents must be helped to understand that through dealing with the painful experiences of the past, they can begin to grow and have a new future.

At the end of this Step, the adolescents must examine the issues still causing any anger, sadness, or guilt. They should also summarize their best and worst experiences in life, which will give some indication of their self-worth. Studies have shown that chemically dependent teenagers have numerous co-morbid problems, such as severe depressions with suicide attempts, learning problems, behavior problems, family instabilities, family use of alcohol and drugs, and the devastating traumas of physical and sexual abuse. These issues are touched upon by answers to the specific questions of the Fourth Step.

Step Five.

The Fifth Step involves sharing, with another person, all the terrible and hurtful experiences of their lives, deeds done unto others, and the feelings of hate, guilt, failure and fear that were identified in the Fourth Step. The person with whom this information is to be shared is usually a recovering member of AA or NA who, due to past personal experience, understands the importance of this step. The person should be someone the adolescents will not meet in their everyday work, home or school environment; perhaps their sponsor within the program. Teenagers also may choose to accomplish the Fifth Step with their therapist. Although the discussion and processing of these issues often takes a number of hours, this important cathartic experience is usually followed by a feeling of great relief and peace.

Follow-up studies (Jaffe, 1992) have shown that returning to relationships with alcohol/drug-using friends is the most prevalent cause of relapse after hospital treatment. Therefore, it is extremely important that teenagers make friendships with nonusing peers who most often will be other recovering teenagers. Also, Twelve Step support groups of AA and

NA are free and available in virtually every city in the United States and many foreign countries.

Working the first Five Steps will help the teenagers to feel better about themselves, to be more honest, and to care about themselves and others in a new way. Teenagers are helped to understand that they must work their First Step everyday, recognizing that they are addicts and can't use in moderation. However, all aspects of the Twelve Step program are extremely important. The teenagers must regularly attend meetings, call their contacts or sponsors often, and continue their psychiatric treatment, including appropriate medication. They need to avoid contact with any old friends who are still using, and new friendships need to be developed with other teenagers who are working good AA/NA programs.

CONCLUSION

Helping teenagers to work the Steps becomes the core of their chemical dependency recovery program and connects them to support groups. The intensive work with the family during the hospitalization should help the family to function in a healthier manner and to be supportive of the teenagers' Twelve Step Program.

This chemical dependency recovery program can be readily integrated into hospital/residential adolescent psychiatric programs. It has the unique advantage of using the structure of the standard Twelve Steps. This program, as modified for adolescent developmental issues, provides an extensive, free group and peer support system in their home community.

REFERENCES

Brown, S. A., Recovery Patterns in Adolescent Substance Abuse. In J. S. Baer, G. A. Marlott and R. J. McMahon (Eds.), *Addictive Behaviors Across the Lifespan: Prevention, Treatment and Policy Issues*. Sage Publications, Beverly Hills, CA, In Press.

Halikas, J. (1990), Substance Abuse in Children and Adolescents. In B. D. Garfinkel, G. A. Carlson and E. B. Weller (Eds.), *Psychiatric Disorders in Children and Adolescents*. Philadelphia: W. B. Saunders Co.

Harrison, P. A. and Hoffman, N. G., CATOR report: "Adolescent Treatment Completers One Year Later," Ramsey Clinic, St. Paul, MN.

Jaffe, S. L. (1992), Pathways to Relapse in Chemically Dependent Adolescents. *Adolescent Counselor*, pp. 42, 43, 55, 1992.

Jaffe, S. L. (1990), *Step Workbook for Adolescent Chemical Dependency Recovery: A Guide to the First Five Steps*, American Academy of Child and Adolescent Psychiatry, APA Press, Inc., Washington, D.C.

Chapter 12

SECLUSION, ECT, AND HYDROTHERAPY

Paramjit T. Joshi, Harinder S. Ghuman, and Erika E. Wilmoth

SECLUSION

Seclusion and restraint of psychiatric patients has been the subject of debate and controversy for over a century since Pinel first advocated the humane treatment of psychiatric patients (Pinel, 1862). In recent years, because of the perception on the part of some that seclusion and restraint may restrict the rights of patients, legal statutes have stipulated the constraints on their use (American Psychiatric Association, 1984). Several reports on the prevalence and impact of the use of seclusion and physical restraints in adult settings (Mattson & Sacks, 1978; Phillips & Nasar, 1983; Soloff & Turner, 1981) have indicated that seclusion is used primarily to reduce danger to others or to self in patients who are severely aggressive or suicidal, or patients who are quite agitated (Gutheil, 1978; Plutchik et al., 1978).

The issue of seclusion and restraint with children and adolescents is much more complex (Garrison, 1984), and the literature is sparse regarding this topic. Redl and Wineman (1952) articulated the clinical rationale for restraining youngsters who were out of control, but only a few other studies appear in the literature in which the developmental perspective is incorporated into the discussion of the use of seclusion and restraint in children and adolescents (Treischman,Whittaker & Bendtro, 1969; Gair, 1984; Cotton, 1989). Plutchik et al. (1978) found that adolescent patients were much more likely than adults to be secluded, and ethnic differences were not a factor. They further reported that the professional staff, as compared to the paraprofessional staff, such as a psychiatric aide, felt regretful that the patient crisis was not resolved in a different way and in fact experienced some guilt and misgivings about the necessity for secluding the patient. The nonsecluded adolescents in this study stated that they felt safe when the staff secluded a peer who was out of control and felt that the secluded patient "got what he deserved." Patients who had experienced seclusion, reported being angry with the staff and worried about future episodes.

The use of the quiet room on an inpatient setting was examined by Joshi, Capozzoli, and Coyle (1988), who indicated that the frequency and time spent in the quiet room decreased significantly over time during hospitalization and that the majority of the episodes involved self-seclusion. Furthermore, in the majority of the episodes, the patients calmed down quickly and in half of the episodes they were able to explain the reason for the quiet room usage. Joshi suggested that the quiet room may be a useful, therapeutic management tool that enhances self-control in children who have serious psychiatric disturbances. In examining the predictability of the use of seclusion on a psychiatric unit, Millstein and Cotton (1990) showed that children who were secluded were more likely to have a history of physical abuse and assaultive behaviors, and have neurological and cognitive impairments. They concluded that seclusion may meet specific needs of children who are unable to respond to environmental controls and found a relationship between the use of seclusion and specific coping strategies, as determined by the Zeitlin coping inventory (Zeitlin, 1985).

Environmental stimuli can trigger destructive behaviors and occasionally aggressive outbursts in children with attentional problems, oppositional behaviors, or psychotic symptoms. Accordingly, reduction in the stimuli through removal of the patient from the environment can often assist children in gaining self-control. Thus, removal of the child to a quiet room would be seen as a final step in a behavioral strategy to reduce stimuli and assist the child in gaining mastery over his behavior, and not simply as an adverse event to extinguish disruptive behaviors.

It is common for parents or guardians to set limits on children. This is usually accomplished through a variety of methods such as having a child go to his room to calm down and/or be "grounded" for a period of time. These normal child-rearing practices are not dissimilar to what occurs on a psychiatric inpatient service. The responsible adults on the inpatient service take over the day-to-day care of the patient, which includes among other things the setting of limits on undesirable behaviors. Therefore, seclusion or restraint can be viewed as a natural extension of the normal child rearing practices of adults.

Inpatient psychiatric facilities for children and adolescents are expected to be capable of addressing serious and problematic behaviors of their patients. Prominent among these are suicidal and self-injurious behavior, assaultive behavior, destruction of property, and disruptiveness on the unit. Generally, such behaviors are of complex and multifactorial etiologies but are closely entwined with the underlying psychopathology that led to hospitalization.

The psychiatric evaluation of children and adolescents is complex, labor-intensive, and time consuming, involving the child, the family, the school, and other agencies and institutions. It is during this early period in the child's hospitalization that behavioral approaches, along with empathic support and structure, are essential in minimizing disruptive and destructive behaviors.

In this context, the use of the quiet room can be seen as part of a greater continuum to reduce sensory stimuli, diffuse aggravating circumstances that cause disruption and aggression, and, hopefully, encourage behavioral control on the part of the patient. Nevertheless, such behavioral approaches must be given constant scrutiny to ensure that the treatment goals are positive and not in any way punitive. One way to minimize the adverse effects of the use of the quiet room, is described by Joshi et al. (1988). The parents and the patient are given a tour of the inpatient unit by a staff member who explains the behavioral program on the unit. This orientation hopefully minimizes some of the anxiety that is naturally associated with hospitalization and also gives the parent/guardian and the patient an opportunity to have concerns addressed before they decide to accept admission to the inpatient program. Our experience has shown that those patients who are admitted directly from the emergency room, or for some reason do not get this opportunity to tour the unit, have more serious concerns about the use of the quiet room, once admitted. This often interferes with treatment. Such patients and their parents often show significant anger when the quiet room is used, feeling that the patient is being confined and punished. On occasion, this very issue results in the parent requesting discharge of the patient before completion of treatment.

Inpatient units have guidelines as part of their policy and procedures for the use of the quiet room. One of the distinctions made between the quiet room and the seclusion room is that if the door is left open, it is the quiet room, and if the door is locked, it is a seclusion room. Closing the door of the quiet room and thus turning it into a seclusion room is not a frequent occurrence on child inpatient units, but may be more frequent on an adolescent unit. Factors that may influence the effect of such interventions often depend on the particular child's developmental and psychopathological status. Therefore, it is extremely important to take into account the patient's cognitive, physical, and emotional limitations when making such a restrictive intervention.

The following guidelines may be considered for the use of the quiet room or seclusion, depending on legal statutes:

1. The use of seclusion should be considered clinically justifiable only to prevent a patient from injuring himself or others, to prevent serious disruption of the therapeutic environment, and/or to reduce external stimuli that significantly increase the risk of injury or serious disruption.
2. Before writing an order authorizing the use of seclusion, a physician must conduct a clinical assessment of the patient and this assessment must be documented in the medical record with the rationale for the use of seclusion, that should address the inadequacy of less restrictive intervention techniques.
3. The use of seclusion requires a written order by a physician which specifies both the rationale and the time limit for seclusion.
4. In an emergency, seclusion may be initiated by a member of the nursing staff. Such emergency seclusion requires an order signed by the nurse and documentation in the medical record of the rationale that addresses the inadequacy of a less restrictive intervention technique. Such an emergency seclusion should not exceed one hour without further authorization from a physician, who should conduct a clinical assessment of the patient.
5. Orders for seclusion should not be written on a PRN basis.
6. During the time that the patient is in the seclusion room, the patient should be observed through a monitor screen at all times to ensure that he or she does not become self-injurious. If the patient does become self-injurious, such as head-banging or throwing himself against the wall, it is advisable to give a PRN medication to calm the patient.

Our experience with droperidol (Inapsine) in the latency-aged children and adolescents which has been described in Chapter 7 has been a positive one, allowing us to avoid the use of physical restraints. The usual practice is to have a patient in the quiet room for a specified period of time or until the termination of the undesirable behavior.

As an alternative to the use of the quiet room or seclusion, very young children can be redirected in their activity or held in a chair for a few minutes until they can attain control of their disruptive behaviors. Developmentally, the young child has a very poor sense of the cause-and-effect relationship and also of time, making placement in the quiet room or seclusion counterproductive. In such instances, the use of a timer can often be helpful.

Behavioral constraint with self-injurious, aggressive, or disruptive behaviors is a reality of the management of severely psychiatrically disturbed children and adolescents in an inpatient setting. Behavior programs of progressive but temporary isolation from the group, involving time-outs and use of the quiet room, can be an effective nonpunitive means of managing these problems in the majority of children and adolescents. Nevertheless, much more objective information needs to be developed with regard to the least restrictive, most effective, and least aversive ways of addressing these problem behaviors in psychiatrically disturbed youngsters.

ELECTROCONVULSIVE TREATMENT

Since its introduction in 1938, electroconvulsive treatment (ECT) has been found to be an effective treatment for selected psychiatric disorders in adults (Cerletti & Bini, 1938). Though it has been well researched in adults for the treatment of severe depressive illness and acute forms of schizophrenia (APA task force report: 14, 1978), there are no controlled studies of the use of ECT in children and adolescents. The modern clinical use of ECT was addressed in a NIMH-sponsored conference in 1985, but its use in children and adolescents was never discussed (Rose, 1985). Despite reports of increased rates of prevalence of mood disorders, an earlier age of onset, and an increase in the rate of suicide attempts in youngsters (Klerman, 1986), there exist only a handful of articles, primarily case reports, describing the use of ECT in children and adolescents.

The use of ECT in children and adolescents was first reported by Bender (1947). She described the use of ECT with 98 prepubertal children, diagnosed with childhood schizophrenia, over a five-year period. The children received up to a maximum of 20 treatments each with minimal complications, resulting in improvement in their primary psychiatric disturbances. Bender reported that the children were less withdrawn, less anxious, and better able to respond to individual and group psychotherapy.

Clardy and Rumpf (1954) criticized Bender's original report by questioning both the diagnosis and outcome of the 98 children. They followed up on Bender's original cases and found that the patients had only a temporary positive response to ECT, 35 of the children were still in mental hospitals, and 13 were in schools for the mentally defective. They concluded that one ought to exercise caution in using ECT with children, especially the "very young," since there was no clear understanding of the long-term effects of this form of treatment on the developing brain of the young. They urged that ECT should be reserved as a last resort for severely ill patients in whom all other measures had failed.

In 1973, Bender reported on a follow-up study of 87 of her original cases and justified the use of electroconvulsive treatment in her study population. She concluded that ECT can improve the clinical and behavioral adjustment of schizophrenic children and bring about remission. Black, Wilcox and Stewart (1985) reported on an 11-year-old boy with major depression who had a positive response to ECT. Although he relapsed frequently in subsequent years, the authors proposed that ECT was a valid treatment for children with depression, mania, or acute schizophreniform psychoses, who were refractory to pharmacotherapy. Several other case reports in the literature describe a positive response to ECT in children with depression or manic depressive illness (Heuyer, Dauphin & Lebovici, 1947; Gallineck, 1952; Campbell, 1952; Gillis, 1955; Warneke, 1975; Carr et al., 1983; Mansheim, 1983; Berman and Wolpert, 1987; Bertagnoli & Borchardt, 1990) and early onset bipolar illness (Hassanyeh & Davison, 1980).

Another report on one child and three adolescents found that only one of the four patients responded favorably and three patients had seizures lasting more than four minutes. The authors hypothesized that children and adolescents are prone to having prolonged seizures and are more refractory to ECT treatment (Guttmacher & Cretella, 1988). In another study (Hift, Hift & Spiel, 1960) of 14 patients, nine of the 12 patients between the ages of 12 and 14 years, who were diagnosed to have childhood schizophrenia and had significant affective symptoms showed significant improvement in their affective symptomatology after ECT treatment. However, two other patients, both aged seven, did not respond. Despite noting memory and cognitive impairments soon after treatment, none of these reports suggest long-term cognitive side effects or complications secondary to ECT treatment. Some of the authors reported post-ECT anxiety, whereby patients worried and resisted receiving future treatments (Bender, 1947; Campbell, 1952; Clardy & Rumpf, 1954).

The issue of consent for the use of ECT in children and adolescents has generated considerable discussion within the professional community.

With the adolescent patient, it is prudent and advisable to obtain written consent from both the adolescent and the parents. With a child, the issue is far more complex. Regulations differ in different states around the country. For example, some states require two child and adolescent psychiatrists to render second independent opinions about the need for ECT in a patient under the age of 18 years. Legal consultation and/or a hearing may be necessary when the patient and the family refuse ECT treatment.

Historically, there has been a bias against the use of ECT in psychiatric patients in spite of modern techniques free of the frightening practices of the past. In the absence of well-controlled, rigorous scientific studies of the use of ECT with children and adolescents that examine its efficacy and potential cognitive side effects, especially in the school-aged child, it is hard to justify the use of ECT in the young. With the advent of newer and more sophisticated pharmacotherapies, perhaps the need for the use of ECT in children and adolescents will not be a pressing one.

HYDROTHERAPY

"The history of hydrotherapy forms the most interesting chapter of the history of medicine, it illustrates how prejudice may hinder progress and how enlightened physiology and pathology have tended to reinstate values but neglected remedy. What remedies have survived since the day of Hypocrites and Galen? The application of diet and the use of water are really the only remedies which have withstood the test of time" (Baruch, 1903).

Cold wet-sheet pack is a form of hydrotherapy. In the 18th and 19th centuries, hydrotherapy was used for various physical ailments and for some mental conditions. In the early 1900's, Baruch described the usefulness of sheet packs in the treatment of various mental conditions, including melancholia, acute maniacal attacks, general paresis, insomnia, and agitated delirium. Black (1936) reviewed the use of cold wet-sheet packs in 800 cases and advocated their use for "acute excitement." The use of cold wet-sheet packs declined after 1940 as a result of a number of factors, including the introduction of psychotropic medications, a change in the social climate, the increased amount of staff time required to implement the procedure, and the lack of experienced staff.

Kilgalen (1972) recommended packs for patients who could not tolerate medication, or for those waiting for medication to become effective. She emphasized that packs facilitated verbal communication and the development of close relationships between patient and the staff with very low risk to the patient since the sheet packs provided total immobilization and induced passive relaxation, acceptance, and sleep, whereas other forms of restraints may predispose the patient to struggle and cause resentment, hypothermia, and exhaustion. Singh (1986) reported the use of packs in the treatment of a severely disturbed self-destructive adolescent and described how packs were helpful in controlling the patient's self-destructive behavior. He also commented on conducting individual sessions while the patient was in packs and how this facilitated and accelerated the formation of a trusting therapeutic relationship. Ross et al., (1988) conducted a retrospective review of 46 psychiatric patients hospitalized at their facility who received packs during their treatment and they reported on the results of a national survey on the use of cold wet-sheet packs, concluding that packs had a useful effect in 83 percent of the cases. A number of patients were able to become in touch with regressed feelings or previously repressed memories and were able to talk about them while placed in packs.

Indications

Cold wet-sheet packs are used in the following ways:

1. On a PRN basis when a patient is extremely agitated, violent, or self-destructive, and not responding to the structure of the treatment program and medication. Patients may require packs once or several times during their hospital stay.
2. On a scheduled basis when a patient is chronically and extremely agitated, violent, and/or self-destructive, and not responding to various hospital interventions, including medications. In these cases, packs can be used on a scheduled basis up to twice a day until the patient is more in control of his/her behavior.
3. During individual and group therapies to better enable the patient to participate in these therapies without fearing loss of control.

If packs are used on a planned basis, it is important to schedule around the time when the patient experiences the most difficulty. Like any other treatment, packs prove more beneficial if the patient is invested in using them as a method of controlling their dangerous and/or life-threatening behavior. However, patients who are either too embarrassed of getting exposed or upset with the idea of packs may not benefit. Best results may be achieved under the following three conditions: (1) the patient is cooperative with the procedure; (2) the staff involved are experienced and skilled in implementing the procedure; and (3) the pack is applied and utilized under the appropriate conditions. For example, if the patient requires a pack due to overstimulation, it should be administered in the quiet room; if a pack is used for a patient to maintain control in order to participate in group therapy or community meeting, it should be instituted just prior to the therapy and the patient brought to the area where the therapy/meeting is to take place.

The Procedure

The adolescent patient and family need to receive a full explanation of the clinical rationale for packs, of the procedure itself, and of the expected results. After consent and documentation are received, a physician's order is required to start the procedure. Unless the packs are scheduled routinely, all equipment should be assembled and made ready prior to initiating the pack to avoid delay and confusion. Often, when the patient is well into a series of scheduled packs, he may initiate or be asked to participate in setting up the pack with staff support. The pack table is prepared with a blanket and two sheets that have been wrung out after having been immersed in cold water. Special care should be taken to eliminate as many wrinkles as possible by "snapping" the sheets and not smoothing them. Smoothing them will decrease coolness. Sheets are folded to the height and width of the patient. The patient is asked to remove all clothing (except underpants) and put on a hospital gown. When able, the patient should go to the toilet before the procedure. When numerous packs are used, lanolin-based cream should be applied to bony prominences. These preparations will increase the patient's comfort level and decrease the possibility of skin breakdown.

The patient is then helped onto the pack table and placed directly on the folded sheets in a supine position. A series of wrappings and turning of the patient from side to side is then begun involving the arms, legs and trunk. The wrapping is done quickly with the first sheet, followed by the second and finally by the blanket. While the wrapping is taking place, the hospital gown is carefully removed, with care taken not to expose the patient. This is particularly important with a co-ed pack team. A minimum of five staff members are required, two on either side and one supporting the patient's head. The patient is kept in proper body alignment to decrease the possibility of injury and discomfort. To provide maximum safety and hypothermic effect, the procedure should be instituted quickly and securely.

After the series of wrapping is completed, a large pillow is placed under the patient's knees to ensure proper blood flow and a small pillow under the head for comfort. Loose linen and blankets should be tucked away from the patient's face and neck to decrease annoyance. Straps and/or belts are applied to secure the patient to the pack table and decrease the possibility of falling. Straps must be placed over the patient to provide security and restriction without the possibility of discomfort or injury. The number of straps is dependent upon how active the patient is or becomes; a minimum of three is recommended. An additional blanket is then placed over the patient to assist in retaining body heat. Additional blankets may be requested by the patient and applied without fear of interfering with the desired effect.

Once wrapped in this mummy-like fashion, the patient becomes totally dependent upon the staff for his safety and having his needs met. It is absolutely critical that a staff member remain in attendance throughout the entire procedure to closely monitor the patient's pulse, respiration, and skin color. Additionally, staff must help decrease the patient's level of fear and anxiety by providing support, comfort, and encouragement to enhance the sedating effect. Throughout the procedure, staff should offer liquids, readjust pillows or straps, and provide explanation regarding the treatment. Chewing gum or eating foods or candy in the supine pack position must be avoided as this may cause the patient to choke. If necessary, medications in pill form may be administered with extreme caution to enhance the sedating or calming effect.

Patients respond differently while in the pack. Some become quite active and talkative, while others prefer to remain still and nonverbal. Initially, most patients are frightened and anxious about being in such a restrictive and dependent state. Explanations regarding the procedure and frequent reassurances that they are safe and will not be left unattended are very useful in assisting them to feel more secure and relaxed. Bright overhead lighting and sunlight can be quite annoying or uncomfortable to the patient. If dimming of the lights or drawing of the curtains is not possible, it is advisable to reposition the patient on the pack table for maximum comfort level.

It is imperative that staff anticipate the patient's needs and respond accordingly, since patients often do not request assistance or verbalize discomfort. The amount of time prior to a patient's warming up varies. Generally, the more active or agitated a patient had been prior to the pack, the quicker he/she will warm up. While in a pack, the patient may become so warm that his face begins to feel uncomfortably flushed and warm. A cool wash cloth is helpful.

The procedure lasts for up to two hours. When the treatment is discontinued, the patient is carefully unwrapped and assisted into a dry gown. The patient is then helped into a sitting position with the legs dangling over the pack table for several minutes until the sensation of weakness and dizziness is gone. Supporting the patient on either side as he/she descends is important to avoid an unsteady fall. If possible, the patient should be encouraged to bathe or shower and return to wearing street clothes. Rejoining the milieu is dependent upon the patient's emotional status and personal preference.

How the Cold Wet-Sheet Pack Works

Ross et al. (1988) conceptualized sheet packs as a complex treatment modality with biological, psychological, and social components. Bailey (1920) wrote that wet-sheet packs appear to cause an initial contraction of subcutaneous vessels followed by a marked dilatation, which creates a feeling of warmth and relaxation. Packs also produce motor confinement similar to the swaddling of infants (Lipton, Steinschneider & Richard, 1965).

Psychologically, the use of packs demands close human contact, thereby offering the potential for development of a positive, caring, and trusting relationship between the patient and the staff member.

Singh (1986) emphasized that packs provide gratification of the patient's dependency needs, increase external control over his/her dangerous impulses, and reassure the patient and others in the environment by controlling dangerous behavior. They also provide for an increased sense of involvement, hope, and ability to receive attention without indulging in self-defeating patterns of acting-out behaviors. Ross et al. (1988) reported that many patients, especially seriously ill borderline patients threatened with psychotic decompensation, were able to express intense and conflicted affects while they were in a pack. Ross et al. also noted that the cold wet-sheet pack treatment allowed very disturbed patients to be part of the therapeutic milieu.

Case Report

Helen, a 16-year-old female, was transferred from another hospital due to severe self-mutilating behavior, including self-cutting, self-burning, and head banging. The patient's self-destructive behavior started around age eight years with attempts to damage her eyes by staring at the sun. This was her third psychiatric hospitalization. Helen had been in outpatient treatment intermittently for three years and received various medications, including Carbamazepine, Imipramine, Lithium, and Phenelzine, all in therapeutic levels, and moderate doses of Thioridazine, Perphenazine, and Haloperidol. Prior to this admission, she had taken an overdose and tried to drive over a cliff.

During the current hospitalization, Helen continued to be defensive but superficially cooperative. One night, she was found by staff under the table in her hospital room with cuts from head to toe and burn marks on her breasts and groin area; severe cuts to both wrists required suturing. Following this incident, cold wet-sheet packs were instituted. The patient received 120 packs total with 45 individual therapy sessions while she was in pack. Packs enabled the patient to control her self-destructive behavior and assisted her in developing trusting and meaningful relationships with the staff and her therapist. She was gradually able to control herself without packs and eventually was discharged to an outpatient status after 14 months of hospitalization.

CONCLUSION

The use of seclusion, ECT, and hydrotherapy in the treatment of adolescents remains controversial. These procedures have been considered restricting and inhumane by some mental health professionals, as well as by some segments of our society. Perhaps there is less rationale for the use of these procedures when one considers advances in modern pharmacotherapy.

There remains, however, a role for use of seclusion, ECT, and hydrotherapy when other interventions have failed or have been only partially successful. Due to controversies surrounding these techniques, it is imperative to involve the adolescent and the family in the decision-making process. These procedures require care, precision, and an experienced staff to gain the optimal results.

REFERENCES

American Psychiatric Association (1984). Seclusion and restraint, *Task Force Report No. 22.*

American Psychiatric Association (1978). ECT, *Task Force Report No. 14.*

Bailey, H. (1920). *Nursing mental disease.* New York: MacMillan.

Baruch, S. (1903). *The principles and practice of hydrotherapy: A guide to appreciation of water in diseases for students and practitioner of medicine.* New York: William Wood.

Bender, L. (1947). One hundred cases of childhood schizophrenia treated with electric shock. *Tran. Am. Neurol. Soc., 72,* 165-169.

Bender, L. (1973). The life course of children with schizophrenia. *Am. J. Psychiatry, 130,* 783-786.

Berman, E. & Wolpert, E. (1987). Intractable manic-depressive psychosis with rapid cycling in an 18-year-old woman successfully treated with ECT. *J. Nerv. Ment. Dis, 4*, 236-239.

Bertangoli, M. W., Burchardt, C. M. (1990). A review of ECT for children and adolescents. *Journal of the American Academy of Child and Adolescent Psychiatry, 29*, 302-307.

Black, D.W., Wilcox, J.A., Stewart, M. (1985). The use of ECT in children: Case report. *J. Clin. Psychiatry, 46*, 98-99.

Black, N.D. (1936). The value and application of hydrotherapy in a mental hospital. *Psychiatric Quarterly, 10*, 344-44.

Campbell, J. D. (1952). Manic depressive psychosis in children: Report of 18 cases. *Journal review of Meme-Dis., 16*, 424-439.

Carr, V., Dorrington, C, Schader, G. & Wale, J. (1983). The use of ECT in childhood bipolar disorder. *Br. J. Psychiat., 143*, 411-415.

Cerletti, V., Bini, L. (1938). L'elletroshock. *Arch. Gen. Neurol. Psichiat. Psichoanal, 19*, 266-268.

Clardy, E.R., Rumpf, E.M. (1954). The effect of electric shock treatment on children having schizophrenic manifestations. *Psychiatr. Q., 28*, 616-623.

Cotton, N. (1989). The developmental-clinical rationale for the use of seclusion in the psychiatric treatment of children. *Am. J. Orthopsychiatry, 59*, 442-450.

Gair, D.S. (1984). Guidelines for children and adolescents. In K. Tardiff (Ed.), *The psychiatric uses of seclusion and restraint* (pp.69-85). Washington, D.C.: American Psychiatric Press, Inc.

Gallineck, A. (1952). Controversial indications for electroconvulsive therapy. *Am. J. Psychiatry, 10*, 361-366.

Garrison, W.T. (1984). Aggressive behavior, seclusion, and physical restraint in an inpatient child population. *Am. Acad. Child Psychiat., 23*, 4:448-452.

Gillis, A. (1955). A case of schizophrenia in childhood. *J. Nerv. Ment. Dis., 121*, 471–472.

Gutheil, T.G. (1978). Observations on the theoretical basis for seclusion of the psychiatric inpatient. *Am. J. Psychiat., 135*, 325-328.

Guttmacher, L.B. & Cretella, H. (1988). Electroconvulsive therapy in one child and three adolescents. *J. Clin. Psychiatry, 49*, 20-23.

Hassanyeh, F., Davison, K. (1980). Bipolar affective disorder with onset before age 16 years. Report of 10 cases. *Br. J. Psychiatry, 137*, 530-539.

Heuyer, G., Dauphin, M., Lebovici, S. (1947). La practique de l'electrochoc chez l'enfant. *Z Kinder Jugendpsychiatr, 14*, 60-64.

Hift, E., Hift, S. & Spiel, W. (1960). Ergebnisse der schockbehandlungen bei kindlischen schizophrenien. *Schweiz. Arch. Neurol. Psychiatr., 86*, 256-272.

Joshi P.T., Capozzoli J.A.,and Coyle J.T. (1988). Use of a quiet room on an inpatient unit. *J Am Acad Child Adolesc Psychiatry, 27*, 642-644.

Kilgalen, R.K. (1972). Hydrotherapy, Is it all washed up? *Journal of Psychiatric Nursing, 10*, 3-6.

Klerman, J. L. (1986). *Suicide and depression among adolescing and young adults.* Washington, D.C.: American Psychiatric Press.

Lipton, E.L., Steinschneider, A., Richard, M.B. (1965). Swaddling, a child care practice: historical, cultural and experimental observations. *Pediatric* (Supplement), *35*, 519-567.

Mansheim, P. (1983). ECT in the treatment of a depressed adolescent with meningomyelocele hydrocephalus and seizures. *J. Clin. Psychiatry, 44*(10), 385-386.

Mattson, M.R. & Sacks, M.H. (1978). Seclusion: Uses and complications. *Am. J. Psychiat., 135,* 1210-1213.

Millstein, K.H. & Cotton, N.S. (1990). Predictors of the use of seclusion on an inpatient child psychiatric unit. *Am. J. Child. Adol. Psychiatry, 29,* 2:256-264.

Phillips, P. and Nasar, S.J. (1983). Seclusion to restraint and prediction of violence. *Am. J. Psychiat., 140,* 229-232.

Pinel, P. A. (1862). *Treatise on Insanity.* New York: Hafner Press

Plutchik, R., Karasu, T.B., Conte, H.R., Seigel, B. & Jerrett, I. (1978). Toward a rationale for the seclusion process. *J. Neuro. Ment. Dis., 166,* 571-579.

Redl, F. & Wineman, D. (1952). *Controls from within.* New York: Free Press, 1952.

Rose, R.M. (1985). Electroconvulsive therapy: Consensus conference. *JAMA, 254,* 2103-2108.

Ross, D.R., Lewin, R., Gold, K., Ghuman, H.S., Rosenblum, B., Salzberg, S., Brooks, A.M. (1988). The psychiatric use of cold wet sheet packs. *Am. J. Psychiat., 145:*2, 242-245.

Roth, E.A. (1982). Children's self-images: Before, during, and after psychiatric hospitalization. *Am. J. Art Therapy, 21,* 125-131.

Singh, H. (1986). Treating a severely self-destructive adolescent with cold wet sheet packs. *Hospital and Community Psychiatry, 37:*3, 287-288.

Soloff, P.H. & Turner, S.M. (1981). Patterns of seclusion: A prospective study. *J. Nerv. Ment. Dis., 169,* 37-44.

Treischman, A., Whittaker, J. & Bendtro, L. (1969). *The other 23 hours.* Chicago: Aldine Publishing Company.

Wadeson, H. & Carpenter, W.T., Jr. (1976). Impact of the seclusion room experience. *J. Nerv. Ment. Dis., 163*(5), 318-328.

Warneke, L. (1975). A case of manic-depressive illness in childhood. *Can. Psychiatr. Assoc. J., 20,* 195-200.

Zeitlin, S. (1980). Assessing coping behavior. *Am. J. Orthopsychiatry, 50*(1), 139-144.

Zeitlin, S. (1985). Coping inventory: A measure of adaptive behavior. Vensenville, IL: Scholastic Testing Service.

Chapter 13

DEVELOPMENTAL CONSIDERATIONS IN THE INPATIENT TREATMENT OF ADOLESCENTS

Thomas R. Pentz

THE DEVELOPMENTAL TREATMENT MODEL

The adolescent inpatient treatment program is based upon a developmental model that views the adolescent both as a developing individual and as a product of his or her developmental past (Rinsley, 1983; Berlin, Critchley & Rossman, 1984). Development is conceived of as continuous, a progressive series of tasks to be mastered by the individual over the course of the life span. It is viewed as proceeding along a variety of interrelated developmental lines (Freud, 1946) with mastery of successive tasks dependent upon successful mastery of antecedent tasks, unfolding potentials of the individual, and provision of a context of opportunities for growth together with interpersonal encouragement, enrichment, and support.

The treatment approach on the adolescent inpatient unit is integrally bound to and molded by this conceptual view of human development. The adolescent is viewed in the context of his or her developmental experience. As such, the treatment program is specifically designed to address adolescent developmental needs, while at the same time assessing and remediating developmental deficits and lags. In addition, the treatment methodology is sensitively geared to the developmental levels and resources presented by adolescents within the treatment population.

The developmental model generates a number of guiding principles for assessment and treatment. The progressive nature of development establishes the basis for our theoretical understanding of psychopathology as representing an exaggeration or distortion of normal development or as a reflection of deficits in the mastery of earlier developmental tasks. The goal of treatment is to remediate such deficits through a developmentally corrective experience and to retrack the adolescent on a normal developmental course.

Adolescents who present for psychiatric inpatient treatment invariably display deficits and lags along various developmental lines which have, in turn, impacted adversely upon mastery of adolescent developmental tasks. Disruptions along the developmental lines of object relations are reflected symptomatically in unstable, insecure relationships and an impaired capacity for establishment of trust. Rinsley (1983) describes these youngsters as presenting "weak ego," and ego-skill deficits, including reliance upon primitive defense mechanisms, failure to sublimate or to interpose thought between impulse and action, poor frustration tolerance, and limited social skills with affective and behavioral concomitants of anxiety, depression, and impulsivity.

The inpatient treatment program is designed not only to remediate developmental deficits, but also to address adolescent developmental needs. The goal of treatment is to return the adolescent to a normal developmental course. The assessment process views adolescent psychopathology within a developmental framework and identifies progress along various developmental lines. The object relations line is viewed as crucial as it has been established that successful treatment outcomes are associated with the establishment of stable relationships between the child and the people who treat him (Gossett, Lewis & Barnhart, 1983). Supportive attachment relationships provide a context for other treatment interventions. The hospital treatment program functions as a corrective emotional experience and as a learning lab for confronting maladaptive behavior patterns while promoting development of adaptive ones.

The components of an effective inpatient treatment program for adolescents have been discussed elsewhere in this volume. This chapter will focus on how treatment programs adopting a developmental model establish treatment strategies that correlate with the developmental needs, capacities, and resources presented by the adolescents being treated. While adolescent inpatients present significant disruptions in the developmental process, they have achieved adolescence. Therefore, the normal developmental features of adolescence must be recognized and addressed in the treatment approach. Miller (1983) has emphasized that "the provision of good psychological treatment and general emotional care depends on the ability of an environment to meet the nonspecific developmental needs of the adolescent within it." The goal of treatment is to restore progressive development. The treatment program must be oriented to adolescent developmental realities, recognize developmental deficits and needs, and adopt strategies adjusted to developmental capabilities.

Adolescence as a Development Stage

Adolescence encompasses the general age range from 12 to 19+ years but is best defined in terms of maturational variables and developmental progress rather than by chronological age. It represents a stage of transition from childhood to adulthood and is marked by significant change physiologically, psychologically, cognitively, and socially. Adolescence is ushered in by the physiological changes of puberty and incorporates the psychological reactions to this physiological process. It has been defined by Blos (1962) as the "process of adaption to puberty." It is a biopsychosocial process that encompasses the developmental ego tasks of resolution of childhood dependencies and achievement of adult autonomy, consolidation of identity including sexual identity and capacity for intimacy, integration of ego skills including internalization of self-regulation and soothing, and establishment of separation from the family together with the development of a peer support system (Hartman, 1958; Erikson, 1968; Josselson, 1980).

The rate of progress through adolescence varies between individuals and by gender, with females entering puberty up to two years in advance of males. The nature in which any given child experiences and negotiates adolescence will depend upon earlier life experiences and the nature of prior ego development. While adolescence has been historically represented as a period of turbulence, research has demonstrated that most adolescents traverse the adolescent period without presenting significant disruptive emotional turmoil (Offer, 1969; Offer, Marcus & Offer, 1970).

Adolescence is divided into three distinct substages, each representing different tasks, stressors, conflicts, and capabilities. These substages are early adolescence (12–15 years), middle adolescence (15–18 years), and late adolescence (19 years up). This chapter will focus upon a description of the early and middle substages of adolescence and implications for treatment planning and implementation.

EARLY ADOLESCENCE

Early adolescence is ushered in by the endocrinological triggering of puberty with its attendant physiologically based changes, including rapid physical growth and resurgence of sexual and aggressive drives. Rapid physical changes in size and shape create a sense of unfamiliarity and clumsiness with the body as the adolescent seeks to adjust to a changing body image. There is a psychological experience of helplessness and loss of control that accompanies the significant biological changes faced by the pubertal child. The establishment of a sense of control over one's body and one's sexual and aggressive feelings and impulses represents a significant developmental challenge. The defensive structure of the young adolescent remains rigid, and the child is prone to feeling affectively overwhelmed.

Early adolescents are very much action-oriented. Feelings of anxiety and tension associated with significant physical and psychological change are expressed and ventilated through motoric activity. Feelings are often expressed through action in view of limitations in cognitive skills as well as emotional sensitivities which block reflection or introspection. Action may also serve as a means of communication that invites adult intervention, support, and control.

During early adolescence, the adolescent begins to decathect and deidealize the parents as childhood attachment and primary identification figures (Kohut, 1977). This process engenders a significant internal conflict for the adolescent, who must begin to move away from parental supports in the face of an internally generated sense of dyscontrol. The loosening of parental ties creates a hunger and quest for new attachment objects that fuels the adolescents' propulsion into the peer group as a source of acceptance, approval, security and support. Young adolescents also seek to compensate for their developmental sense of loss and dyscontrol by turning to extra-parental adults for support and control. Young adolescents enter relationships with adults cautiously as a product of projection of their lack of self-trust and wariness regarding the regressive pull of dependent relationships. Adults who have been tested and found worthy function as identification models and auxiliary egos who support the adolescent in his/her growth toward mastery, identity, and autonomy.

Cognitive development is marked by progressive growth in thinking skills and performance over the course of adolescence (Elkind, 1974; Flavell, 1963; Piaget & Inhelder, 1958). Most adolescents do not achieve formal operations until middle adolescence (Dulit, 1972). The appearance of formal operational thought allows for more abstract thinking as thought becomes less tied to concrete reality and the consideration and manipulation of possibilities become cognitively available. The thought of the early adolescent remains concrete and often self-centered, with attendant limitations in the capacity for self-observation, empathy, and consideration or appreciation of alternative viewpoints.

EARLY ADOLESCENCE: IMPLICATIONS FOR TREATMENT

The developmental realities presented by younger adolescents pose significant implications for the design and implementation of psychiatric inpatient treatment programs.

Assessment

The assessment process itself assumes substantial significance in terms of defining the progress of the adolescent along the various developmental lines and identifying deficits targeted for remediation. It is also crucial for developing an appreciation of developmentally based cognitive and psychological factors to which treatment methodology must be geared The assessment process is guided by an appreciation of the fact that while a certain amount of emotional upheaval may be developmentally normative for early adolescence, prolonged and intense upheaval represents a reflection of psychopathological process (Baittle & Offer, 1971).

The assessment process must also be guided by an appreciation of the fact that various psychopathologies may assume variant symptomatic presentations over different development levels. Early adolescent developmental tasks seriously challenge the adolescent's sense of mastery and self-esteem and render it difficult for the adolescent to acknowledge or portray dysphoria, self-depreciation, hopelessness, or helplessness. Adolescents tend to be action-oriented and to act out their depression in ways designed to ward off threatening, unpleasant affective experience or to signal an appeal for assistance and support. The "psychological toll of depression" (Weiner, 1980) is reflected in fatigue, somatization, and impaired concentration. Adolescents may seek to ward off depression through restlessness, immersion in activity, or a desperate need for companionship. Action communications signaling a need for help, in view of the adolescent's psychologically and cognitively mediated inability to verbally express emotional pain and a need for support, may include problematic behaviors such as delinquent activity, tantrums, truancy, and runaways. The adolescent's defiant and rebellious acting out often serves to compel adult intervention.

Psychotherapy

Developmentally normative realities of early adolescence exert a significant impact upon psychotherapy. Young adolescents are not normally psychologically minded. Cognitive development retains thinking at a concrete level which legislates against attempts at insight-oriented therapy requiring more advanced analytical and abstract thought processes. In addition, the young adolescent's experience of inner conflict and turmoil makes introspection threatening and painful, and often renders the adolescent not a good candidate for therapeutic self-examination and exploration. The ego strength of the early adolescent remains fragile, based upon a rather primitive defensive structure reliant upon denial, repression, and externalization, yet beset by escalating intensity of drives and feelings. Psychotherapeutic approaches that intrude upon these immature defenses and seek to uncover intense emotional material may serve instead to overstimulate and overwhelm the adolescent in such a way as to disrupt development of a working relationship. It is important to remember that with early adolescents we are facing a normal and developmentally adaptive disconnection between feelings, drives, and thought processes that should be treated differently than a pathological defense, i.e., respected rather than attacked. Psychotherapy with early adolescents is focused upon ego building and strengthening of defenses rather than on self-exposure and stimulation of affect.

As the personality development of the young adolescent is very much in flux, so must the psychotherapist remain flexible in technique. Prolonged silences are contraindicated as they tend to stimulate anxiety and may be interpreted as disinterest or withdrawal by the hypersensitive adolescent. An active and directive approach is indicated with young adolescents, focused upon provision of a supportive relationship, reality clarification, permission to express feelings, supplementation of fragile internal controls, and building of skills for managing feelings and interpersonal experiences. Much of the therapy proceeds in the transference as a corrective working-through experience without seeking any explicit statement or understanding of the psychodynamics involved. Questions and interpretations that fail to respect the adolescent's cognitive limitations and emotional vulnerabilities leave the adolescent feeling invalidated, criticized, or persecuted.

> A 13-year-old boy who alternately experienced murderous impulses toward his estranged father and intense worries regarding the father's physical health and well-being presented for hospitalization with declining academic performance, physi-

cally aggressive behavior toward his younger brother, and suicidal ideation. Psychotherapy focused upon providing appreciation for the intensity of his anger toward father and problem-solving around how to manage the anger without harming others or himself. Sessions focused on developing specific strategies for controlling and channeling angry feelings, including verbalization as well as discovery of physical outlets for the anger. Limits were set on redirections of anger that resulted in harm, physical or emotional, to others and self. In the transference, subtle manifestations of anger were recognized and tolerated. Expressions of anger toward the therapist were generally followed by the child's engaging the therapist in some conciliatory activity or play. This working through was supported without emphasis upon verbal interpretation of the transferential negotiation or of the intense and confusing mixture of anger, hurt, and disappointment generated toward the father.

The young adolescent retains certain childlike ways of perceiving and communicating, and psychotherapy must conform to the child's natural way of relating to others. Young adolescents often "play out" their feelings and conflicts in action and in interaction with the therapist. Psychotherapy with young adolescents often requires a transitional, hybrid model between actual play therapy and insight-oriented verbal work. These adolescents may feel less threatened, for example, when psychotherapy sessions are structured around a shared activity. In the course of psychotherapy, young adolescents deliver action messages that convey feelings and embody internal experiences and conflicts. The therapy promotes a corrective emotional experience by understanding the communication and, in turn, delivering a sensitive, growth-promoting action response rather than a verbal one. Adolescents tune into and interpret the action communications of adults, which must be consistent with verbal communications if they are to earn the adolescent's respect. Therapeutic relationship and counteraction do not, however, require verbal formulation in order to be effective. The action orientation of early adolescence calls for careful attention to and awareness of the therapeutic process.

A 13-year-old boy with a chaotic developmental history replete with disruption, neglect, and abuse presented for hospitalization because of recurrent and uncontrolled aggressive as well as self-abusive behaviors. Many early sessions involved sitting with the child in quiet room. Eventually, when the child was able to join the therapist for walks on grounds, he displayed an acute interest in nature and many sessions involved monitoring the caretaking and growth of a nest of baby birds. While cognitive and developmental limitations precluded verbal exploration and interpretation, this child responded favorably to the implicit, metaphorical, and relational aspects of the psychotherapy.

Another 13-year-old adolescent with a serious history of violence was noted to become threatened, defensive, angry, and resistant when feeling pressured to engage in verbal interchange. He became clearly more relaxed and animated, however, during walks to a nearby pond. He displayed a preoccupation with unclogging water dammed up by debris. After many sessions of shared "unclogging," this child became progressively more verbal regarding his history of violence and was ultimately able to acknowledge with a smile the therapist's interpretation of the analogy between the psychotherapeutic process and his undamming of the stream.

A relationship with the young adolescent must be earned based upon perceived consistency, strength and respect, and provision of assistance with self-control as well as willingness to be active and directive. The adolescent's hunger for extraparental attachments renders him simultaneously needy and cautious. The young adolescent rarely issues verbal requests for assistance and guidance or expresses appreciation for it. Formation of a therapeutic alliance essentially takes much longer than development of the therapeutic relationship. The transference can be highly ambivalent and volatile, reflective of the adolescent's significant dependency conflict. Young adolescents are more likely to act out in the transference and may require firm limit setting. The therapist also needs to be highly attuned to countertransference as young adolescents engage in much testing, provocation, and projective identification. They may seek to manipulate the therapist into a role consistent with their developmental experience of adults. The therapist is disadvantaged, as well, by the lack of opportunity to diffuse the transference through verbal interpretation. Once the adolescent has found the therapist to be trustworthy, then the therapist also becomes an identification model to the adolescent.

Psychotherapy with early adolescents is largely implicit, transferential, relational, and action-oriented, proceeding more so in the doing than in the saying. Young adolescents have a limited capacity for self-observation and are not likely to own their problems at an intellectual or emotional level. The therapist is essentially challenged to formulate a therapeutic response in the context of the action metaphor. Verbal interventions may be most effective when delivered in generalized, displaced, third person analogy or story form. Verbal interchanges may also focus at a concrete level in the here and now on the developmental problem-solving strategies and skills that support the adolescent's sense of mastery.

Milieu

Many of the same principles that guide the psychotherapeutic process with early adolescence can also be applied to inpatient program development and milieu management. The milieu treatment program focuses on ego support and strengthening, object relations, impulse control, affect management, and reality testing (Redl, 1966; Noshpitz, 1983). The disturbed adolescent's vulnerability to anxiety and impulsivity are appreciated and the program is designed to maximize implicit controls through structure and consistency so as to minimize the need for application of reactive controls. The environment is designed to provide structure, consistency, predictability, and clarity of expectations and rules to convey a sense of safety and control and to minimize tension and stress. Thorough staff training and communication are essential for provision of firm, consistent, nonpunitive, sensitive, and at times anticipatory application of limits and controls. Staff training allows for appreciation and understanding of the action messages of adolescents and promotes the ability to formulate a sensitive therapeutic action response. Adolescents tune into the action messages of adults. They respond to respectful controls by feeling safe and cared for. The issue of control is central in the psychological life of the early adolescent, and disturbed adolescents in hospital must achieve a sense that they can and will be controlled before further treatment can occur toward the goal of increased internalization of controls.

The inpatient treatment program for young adolescents is both action-oriented and relationship-based. Relationships with staff members follow principles similar to those discussed in terms of the psychotherapist. Ego building takes place over time based upon corrective emotional experiences and identifications in the context of supportive attachment relationships. The staff responds to losses of control with containment, consistency, and confidence. The program provides opportunities for problem solving, skill development, experience of success, and emotional working through. As in psychotherapy, much of the treatment proceeds through relationships and activities. The life space interview (Redl, 1966) entails patient-staff interactions focused on processing of the here and now in concrete terms, identification of feelings to enhance a sense of affective mastery, definition of problems, formulation of problem-solving strategies, and development of skills for managing feelings and interpersonal experiences. An emphasis on short-term concrete goals serves to enhance the adolescent's sense of mastery.

The staff target ego deficits and function as auxiliary egos as well as role models. There is often an emphasis on action intervention and redirection of energies rather than on verbal processing. Verbal interventions may focus on concrete teaching of self-care, self-soothing, or social skills. Problems are often framed concretely followed by development of concrete strategies for solving problems. Adolescents are guided to identify behavioral helps, reinforcers, and lists and plans for dealing with commonly encountered difficulties. The adolescent's day is highly structured, with the schedule geared toward meeting the developmental needs of young adolescents, i.e., earlier bedtimes, ample opportunity for physical activity, and guidance with nutrition. Individualized daily schedules are also developed to meet the special needs of adolescents. The easily overstimulated adolescent, for example, may have a zoning program that schedules periodic quiet times in the patient's room throughout the day.

Activities

In keeping with the action orientation of early adolescents, the treatment program places a strong emphasis on activities. These activities are specifically structured and designed to promote the fulfillment of therapeutic goals such as enhanced body image and self-awareness, sense of mastery and self-esteem, impulse control and frustration tolerance, and coping and affect management skills.

Therapeutic activities are generally implemented in a group setting in recognition of the young adolescent's developmental attraction to the peer group. Many hospitalized adolescents are lacking in social skills. In addition, they often present disturbances in object relations that interfere with the establishment of healthy peer relations. Activity therapy groups provide a structured opportunity for addressing and remediating deficits in social skills by focusing on active interpersonal problem solving in the here and now. Activities are designed to promote sharing and cooperation.

In recognition of the young adolescent's transitional status between childhood and adolescence, along with his/her proper and continued reliance upon childhood coping mechanisms, the activity therapy group incorporates significant elements of play. Throughout the course of development, play has been instrumental in the establishment of defenses and skills for coping with drives and emotions (Sarnoff, 1976). Hospitalized young adolescents are characteristically lacking in skills for affect management and impulse control, and tend to act out feelings in destructive ways. Physical activities provide a constructive outlet for the adolescent's tensions and anxieties. The development of a capacity to control and manage anger is a central goal of treatment and activities are structured to promote sublimation and redirection of aggressive energies. Conceptually similar to play therapy with children, the activity therapy group allows for indirect expression, working through, and management of feelings by channeling affect into constructive activities (Olds, 1982). In the course of these activities, the adolescent experiences success, which contributes to a sense of mastery and self-esteem.

While promoting growth and mastery of developmental tasks, the playful element of these activities also allows for controlled, structured, constructive regression (Erlich, 1983). The adolescent essentially chooses to participate in childlike activities rather than experiencing the regressive pull of childhood in a helpless fashion. The developmental shift from childhood to adulthood, often conceived and experienced by adolescents in a disruptive all-or-nothing fashion, is rendered less stressful and problematic if adolescents are assisted in experiencing this transition as a more gradual, progressive shifting from child to adult and from dependency to independence.

Activity therapies with younger adolescents focus on nonverbal modes of communication and relationship such as games, arts and crafts, role play, music, and movement. These therapies are designed to build ego skills, social skills, and self-esteem as well as to provide a context for corrective emotional experiences in relation to therapists and peers (Kottman, Strother & Deniger 1987; Schiffer, 1984). In view of the developmental variations between adolescents, flexibility is warranted in terms of available activities for any group session so that activities can be individually geared to the developmental levels and capacities of the group members. The need of younger adolescents for higher levels of external direction and control requires that group size be kept small, i.e., six to eight members for two therapists. Advance planning of activities and availability of multiple activities per session promote the capturing of the group's attention, adjustment to shorter attention spans, and provision of short term gratification and success to bolster a sense of mastery. The therapist adopts an active, directive, facilitative approach providing firmness, clarity, and consistency of limits, as well as concrete guidance with social skills and strategies for problem solving and affect management.

The role of the therapist is focused upon providing a caring relationship and a healthy role model, and teaching adolescents how to handle interpersonal and affective situations, rather than exploring the nature of relationships. At the same time, however, the therapist's interventions are guided by an understanding of the underlying psychodynamics reflected in the actions and interactions of the adolescent. The adolescents are encouraged to communicate verbally, to make feeling statements, and to provide one another with feedback, but therapeutic emphasis remains upon activities rather than upon discussion and processing. A typical intervention might involve the therapist responding to a peer conflict by setting limits to establish control, suggesting techniques by which the adolescents can calm down, concretely framing and defining the conflict with the adolescents, encouraging them to problem solve alternative ways for dealing with the situation, and finally walking them through a healthier interaction.

Group Therapy

The more traditional model of group therapy is also a component of the adolescent treatment program, but again with modifications in methodology and approach to address the developmental vicissitudes of early adolescence. Group therapy takes advantages of the young adolescent's attraction to the peer group as a source of acceptance, validation and support while diffusing the intensity of the transference with the therapist and providing an alternative source of support to compensate for the developmental letting go of adult supports. Group therapy also provides an arena of peer interaction in which to address deficits in object relations and social skills. The capacity of the young adolescent to establish peer relationships is crucial to the continuation of healthy developmental progress (Weiner & Elkind, 1972). The high levels of tension common in young adolescents require that the therapist adopt an active role in establishing limits, rules, and structure that create and convey a sense of control and allow for therapeutic work. Therapeutic work is facilitated when the structure and design of the group implicitly reinforce control in a way that obviates the need for repeated setting of explicit limits.

The group therapy model is based upon a modified amalgam of traditional psychodynamic, cognitive, and behavioral techniques (Halpin & Rosenberg, 1990). Adolescents earn points for attendance, respectful behavior (based on clearly defined rules and expectations), presentation of a topic of concern to the group, and offering of constructive feedback to peers. The therapist assumes an active role in the concrete framing of topics to allow the group to apply problem-solving techniques. Out of respect for the cognitive limitations of young adolescents, there is less emphasis on exploration and more on concrete teaching and guidance with social skills, conflict resolution, and cooperative support. While the limited capacity for abstract thinking also places limits on the capacity for empathy, young adolescents can be assisted in appreciating other points of view by engaging in role-playing activities.

Behavioral techniques represent a significant component of inpatient treatment programming with young adolescents. A generalized point system focuses on self-care, daily responsibilities, and treatment compliance. A system of established consequences imposed for lapses in responsibility is helpful in avoiding persistent power struggles. Younger adolescents respond better to concrete rather than symbolic rewards and privileges. Individualized behavioral programs are also designed and addressed specifically to symptom alleviation.

Knowledge has been shown to render developmental changes less anxiety provoking and more desirable. Young adolescents benefit from a didactic treatment approach, particularly in the area of sex education.

Family involvement in treatment is essential as young adolescents retain a developmentally normative intense and dependent relationship with their parents.

MIDDLE ADOLESCENCE

Middle adolescence extends roughly from the age of 14 or 15 to 18 years. During this time period, physiological and anatomical changes continue to occur, but the adolescent in general has come to feel more comfortable with his or her body, and sexuality and drive energies are experienced with lessened intensity. In addition, ego strength has matured to the extent that the adolescent presents with enhanced frustration tolerance, impulse control, and affect management skills, more flexible defensive style, and the capacity and willingness to recognize and acknowledge subjective distress. Based upon successful achievements and healthy peer relationships, there also develops increased internalization of self-esteem with lessened reliance upon parents for the mirroring of value.

Major developmental tasks of middle adolescence include the internalization of self-esteem and control together with consolidation of separation and individuation from parents and integration of a sense of identity.

The adolescent during mid-adolescence begins to achieve a more real sense of separation and autonomy from parents rather than "playing at" independence. While early adolescence parallels Mahler's practicing subphase (Mahler, Pine & Bergman, 1975), middle adolescence parallels the rapprochement subphase (Josselson, 1980). With an increasingly secure sense of autonomy, the adolescent achieves increased freedom, both functional and psychological, from childhood dependencies. With an increasingly stable sense of separation from parents, the adolescent can feel more comfortable to return to the parents as role models and a source of support. The adolescent continues to expand a support base of extrafamilial relationships, and there is growth toward a capacity for interpersonal intimacy (Erikson, 1963). The "object hunger" (Blos, 1962) associated with the sense of loss of the parents continues to fuel the search for extrafamilial attachment objects. These attachments, in turn, represent identification objects that widen the adolescent's horizons and supplement the elements from which the adolescent will construct and integrate a sense of self. The sense of identity, what Erikson (1963) has called "a conscious sense of individual uniqueness," represents an essential developmental product of the mid-adolescent period.

An essential feature of the middle adolescent period involves cognitive growth toward formal operational thinking (Piaget & Inhelder, 1958). Many adolescents during the mid-adolescent period achieve formal operations, the ability to engage in logical abstract thinking, to consider possibilities not directly experienced, and to reason on pure hypothesis (Elkind, 1974; Flavell, 1963; Keating, 1980, Piaget & Inhelder, 1958). This cognitive growth in turn allows for a significant surge in the development of adaptive ego skills. With the capacity to generate and test hypotheses, the adolescent becomes better able to plan and to problem solve. When formal operations are applied introspectively to the probing of internal states, the adolescent can develop increased self-awareness and understanding as well as consolidation in the sense of identity. Changes in thought add a new dimension to interpersonal experience with an enhanced capacity for empathy. The coping strategies and defensive style of the adolescent also become more flexible and adaptive.

It should be noted that many variables affect the development and implementation of formal operational thought and that not all adolescents, or adults for that matter, achieve formal operations (Neimark, 1975; Keating, 1980). There is a dynamic interactive relationship between the cognitive and other developmental lines. Piaget's concept of "decalage" (Piaget, 1954) is particularly relevant in that the successful application of cognitive abilities may be clearly influenced by the affective charge associated with emotionally laden cognitive material. Whether or not an adolescent will actually engage in introspection or empathy is determined not only by cognitive but also by emotional factors.

MIDDLE ADOLESCENCE: IMPLICATIONS FOR TREATMENT

While maturity brings to the mid-adolescent an increased proclivity toward dealing with experience in an ideational, expressive fashion, these adolescents continue to present a potential for acting out in a maladaptive quest for excitement and stimulation, companionship, attention, self-medication, and pseudoindependence. Older adolescents may be more inclined to display adult-like symptoms of depression, but they also continue to present acting out in the form of drug abuse, sexual promiscuity, and self-destructive behaviors, for example. In dealing with an emotionally disturbed population, it is important to recognize that the developmental stages may be blurred and that progress along various developmental lines may be uneven. The assessment of psychopathology and of developmental levels must be interdependent. Dysphoria and mood swings in mid-adolescence may reflect the normal mourning process that accompanies object relinquishment (Blos, 1983). Assessment of resistance, acting out, and symptom formation needs to be carried out in the context of an appreciation of what is developmentally normative. Another important aspect of assessment is to determine whether, in fact, the adolescent has achieved formal operational thinking. It should also be kept in mind that older adolescents have evolved more sophisticated defenses that can serve to mask and obscure their underlying pathology.

Psychotherapy

The transferential quality and therapeutic focus of treatment relationships are different from younger to older adolescents. The progress of mid-adolescents toward an increasingly secure and stable sense of individuation renders them more accessible to the establishment of supportive relationships with adults. With cognitive growth and enhanced ego strength, the adolescent becomes better able to recognize a need for treatment, to assume more responsibility for treatment, and to establish a working alliance. The therapeutic relationship can assume more a flavor of working together as opposed to working through. From a countertransferential viewpoint, older adolescents tend to be more openly appreciative of adult support and thus more directly gratifying to work with. Nonetheless, the mid-adolescent remains conflicted regarding the impending approach of adulthood and will continue to enact conflicts around dependency in relationships with adults.

The achievement of formal operations affords the abstract thinking required for engagement in more insight-oriented forms of psychotherapy. Such therapies may take advantage of the enhanced capacity for self-observation and analytic thinking to foster development of increased intellectual and affective understanding of behavior in the context of developmental experiences and current realities. The adolescent is encouraged to consider the impact of developmental experience on current behaviors, perceptions, and relationships with accrued insights applied to behavioral control and change.

It is important to recognize, however, that ego skills for modulation of affective experience and impulse control are necessary before cognitive growth can be applied to consideration of affective and interpersonal experience. Self-examination of affective experience requires that the adolescent possess a sense of mastery and control over his affective life. The middle adolescent who has achieved formal operations is rendered a candidate for insight-oriented psychotherapy by an increased capacity for introspection, appreciation for disparate points of view, recognition of the subjective nature of interpersonal perception, awareness of the symbolic meaning and value of life experiences, and ability to recall the affective correlates of earlier life experiences (Looney et al., 1980). The older adolescent may be guided to recognize and compensate for, if not to overcome, their developmentally sensitized and, at times, distorted interpersonal perceptions.

The older adolescent's enhanced capacity for verbal communication and sharing of thoughts and ideas renders the spoken word a more potent therapeutic tool. Whereas with younger adolescents actions are more meaningful, with older adolescents thoughts and words become more powerful. While much therapy with younger adolescents proceeds in the transference with conflicts displaced, projected and worked through, the older adolescent is able to apply ego observation and mastery to those same conflicts. While psychotherapy with older adolescents assumes a more exploratory approach, therapists will still need to be often active as adolescents continue to require and appreciate direction and guidance. Judicious and limited interpretation of the transference remains advisable. In addition, the therapist needs to be sensitive to the adolescent's developmentally appropriate efforts to establish autonomy and to countertransferential stimulation of the therapist's own issues regarding separation (Anthony, 1969).

> A 17-year-old high school senior became progressively more depressed to the point of developing suicidal ideation and paranoid, delusional thinking. Following psychopharmacological interventions addressed to the psychotic

symptomatology and depression, this bright young man became readily engaged in insight-oriented psychotherapy. He was able to uncover significant concerns and conflicts related to separation which dated back to the turbulent divorce of his parents when he was four years of age. He was also able to trace back the symbolic value of the delusional material to a longstanding fear of Satan that had also arisen in the throes of confusion, distress, and fear attendant upon the parental separation and related struggles around custody.

In addition to psychodynamic insight oriented therapy, mid-adolescents also respond well to cognitive therapy techniques. With achievement of formal operations, the adolescent becomes able to think about thoughts and to appreciate that there are multiple ways of thinking about a given situation. Cognitive therapy encourages adolescents to explore and adopt alternative, healthier ways of looking at various life experiences.

Psychotherapy can also assist the adolescent to utilize expanded cognitive capacities and insights to achieve increased separation from a dysfunctional family system by applying formal operations to the family system, understanding the dynamics, depersonalizing treatment received, and achieving extrication from enmeshment in the dysfunctional system. Many adolescents are able to achieve a healthier separation from a dysfunctional family system when they can view parental behavior as a product of the parents' own developmental experience.

Milieu

The inpatient treatment program for middle adolescents provides consistent supportive relationships and role models, an appropriate balance between external controls and encouragement for assumption of increased responsibilities, incorporation of prosocial values, and a decided peer group orientation.

As middle adolescents become more open to turning to adults for support and seek to discover a healthy balance between dependence and independence, the ready availability of consistent and caring adults represents a crucial component of the inpatient treatment program. These relationships provide a framework for treatment, a context within which the adolescent can feel controlled and cared for, respected, and safe to express, communicate, and learn to cope with feelings. Middle adolescence represents a developmental period marked by progressive growth of internalization. Middle adolescents who undergo psychiatric hospitalization due to a breakdown in self-controls require external reinforcement of control through consistent rules, expectations, and limit setting, as well as appropriate psychopharmacological interventions. Treatment program rules and the role modeling of staff members embody prosocial values. There is a treatment emphasis on progressive internalization based upon values, relationships, and self-interest. Even as the adolescents are provided with supplementary controls, they are being encouraged and supported to accept as much responsibility and autonomy as they can handle (which is often more than they think they can or are willing to assume).

The treatment program with older adolescents entails less structure and more self-direction than with younger adolescents. Older adolescents earn and budget their allowance, assume increased responsibility for monitoring their medications, and participate in patient government and activity planning. Reinforcers become less immediate and concrete and more symbolic, such as through a responsibility-level system. Activity therapy groups become more discussion-oriented and focus on the teaching and practice of independent living skills, values clarification, and stress management techniques. These groups also provide opportunities for processing of social interactions and development of interpersonal skills.

Middle adolescence is marked developmentally not only by progressive internalization, but also by consolidation in the establishment of identity. Treatment figures represent role models to be incorporated into the adolescent's developing sense of identity. Adolescents identify more with what adults do than with what they say. Treatment figures need to model prosocial values, healthy expression and management of feelings, flexible problem solving, and interpersonal communication, empathy, and respect.

Adolescent psychological disturbances clearly affect the development of identity (Erikson, 1968), and symptoms of psychopathology can become a central feature of the adolescent's sense of identity. While treatment is focused upon symptom alleviation, it is important to recognize that adolescents may experience symptomatic relief as a loss of identity. Treatment programs thus need to effect a balance between symptom relief and successful accomplishment of developmental tasks and incorporation of values and interests to support the growth of a new and healthier sense of identity.

A 16-year-old female adolescent was admitted to the hospital with suicidal ideation and multiple somatic complaints. She had faced multiple surgical interventions over a two-year period that included removal of a cancerous tumor. She was able to make use of psychotherapy to relate her somatic symptoms and suicidal thinking to the stress generated by her serious health issues. When placed on antidepressant medication, however, she noted that her body appeared to be "fighting the medication." Ensuing sessions focused on how her experience of depression had been integrated into her sense of identity and how she had come to seek secondary gains from her depression by eliciting caretaking. Subsequent work in psychotherapy then focused on developing skills for seeking support and building a healthier sense of identity.

As middle adolescents turn increasingly to peers for acceptance and support, the inpatient peer group tends to take on a life of its own. Appropriately managed, the patient peer group can come to assert a significant protreatment force (Lewis, 1970). The treatment program should clearly delineate between areas of staff and peer group responsibility and provide balanced opportunities for supportive contacts with peers and adults.

Education represents an important ingredient of the treatment program. As adolescents discover expanding cognitive abilities, they require intellectual stimulation and opportunities to experiment with and harness their creative energies. Sex education and male and female identity groups are designed to foster progress in the development of sexual identity while assisting adolescents to make healthy choices about sexuality.

Career choice begins to be an issue in middle adolescence. Vocational and educational assessment and counselling are available to assist adolescents in planning productively for their future.

Family involvement remains an essential ingredient of the inpatient treatment program. As adolescents approach adulthood, however, the treatment focus may shift to emancipation rather than reintegration into the family unit.

CONCLUSION

Enlightened and effective psychiatric treatment of adolescents must be offered in the context of a thorough understanding and appreciation of the developmental realities of adolescence. Each adolescent must be viewed as a total and developing individual. Treatment must incorporate a continuity of relationships with parents, extrafamilial adults, and peers.

Programming must respect the maturational level of adolescents and their developmental need for exercise of increasing autonomy, educational and physical activity, and creativity. The ultimate goal of treatment is to return the adolescent to a healthy, developmental course.

REFERENCES

Anthony, E.J. (1969). The reactions of adults to adolescents and their behavior. In A.H. Esman (Ed.), *The Psychology of Adolescence*. New York: International Universities Press.

Baittle, B. & Offer, D. (1971). On the nature of the male adolescent rebellion. *Adolescent Psychiatry*, Vol. 8, 184-199.

Berlin, I.N., Critchley, D.L., Rossman, P.G. (1984). Current Concepts in Milieu Treatment of Seriously Disturbed Children and Adolescents. *Psychotherapy*, Vol. 21, No. 1, pp. 118-131.

Blos, P. (1962). *On Adolescence*. Glencoe, Ill.: The Free Press.

Blos, P. (1967). The second individuation process of adolescence. *Psychoanalytic Study of the Child*, 22:162-186.

Blos, P. (1983). Intensive psychotherapy in relation to the various phases of the adolescent period. In A. Esman (Ed.), *The Psychiatric Treatment of Adolescents*. New York: International Universities Press.

Blotcky, M.J. & Gossett, J.G. (1980). Normal Female and Male Psychological Development: An Overview of Theory and Research. *Adolescent Psychiatry*, Vol. 8, pp. 184-199.

Blotcky, M.J. & Gossett, J.G. (1989). Psychiatric Inpatient Treatment of Adolescents. *The Psychiatric Hospital*, Vol. 20, No. 2, pp. 85-93.

Dulit, E. (1972). Adolescent thinking a' la Piaget: The Formal Stage. *Journal of Youth and Adolescence*, 1(4):281-301.

Elkind, D. (1974). *Children and Adolescents: Interpretive Essays on Jean Piaget*. New York: Oxford.

Erikson, E.H. (1963). *Childhood and Society*. New York: Norton.

Erikson, E.H. (1968). *Identity, Youth and Crisis*. New York: Norton.

Erlich, H.S. (1983). Growth opportunities in the hospital: Intensive inpatient treatment of adolescents. In A. Esman (Ed.), *The Psychiatric Treatment of Adolescents*. New York: International Universities Press.

Esman, A.H. (1985). A developmental approach to the psychotherapy of adolescents. *Adolescent Psychiatry*, 12(119-133).

Flavell, J. (1963). *The Development Psychology of Jean Piaget*. New York: Nostrand.

Freud, A. (1946). *The Ego and the Mechanisms of Defense*. New York: International Universities Press.

Gossett, J.T., Lewis, J.M. & Barnhart, F.D. (1983). *To Find a Way, The Outcome of Hospital Treatment of Disturbed Adolescents*. New York: Brunner/Mazel.

Halpin, R. & Rosenberg, G. (1990). A Cognitive Group Therapy Approach with Adolescents. Presentation at the Sheppard and Enoch Pratt Hospital.

Hartman, H. (1958). *Ego Psychology and the Problem of Adaptation*. New

York: International Universities Press.

Josselson, R. (1980). Ego development in adolescence. In J. Adelson (Ed.), *Handbook of Adolescent Psychology*. New York: Wiley.

Keating, D.P. (1980). Thinking Processes in Adolescence. In J. Adelson (Ed.), *Handbook of Adolescent Psychology*. New York: Wiley.

Kohut (1977). *The Restoration of the Self*. New York: International Universities Press.

Kottman, T.T., Strother, J. & Deniger, M. (1987). Activity Therapy: An Alternative Therapy for Adolescents. *Journal of Humanistic Educational and Development, 25*(4):180-186.

Lewis, J.M. (1970). Development of an inpatient adolescent service. *Adolescence*, 5:301-312.

Looney, J.G., Blotcky, M.J., Carson, D.I. & Gossett, J.T. (1980). A Family Systems Model for Inpatient Treatment of Adolescents. *Adolescent Psychiatry*, (8), pp. 499-511.

Mahler, M., Pine, F., & Bergman, A. (1975). *The Psychological Birth of the Human Infant*. New York: Basic.

Meeks, J. (1981). *The Fragile Alliance*. Malabar, Fla: Krieger Publishing.

Miller, D. (1983). *The Age Between: Adolescence and Therapy*, New York: Jason Aronson.

Neimark, E.D. (1975). Intellectual development during adolescence. In F.D. Horowitz (Ed.), *Review of Child Development Research*, (Vol. 4), Chicago: University of Chicago Press.

Noshpitz, J.D. (1983). Notes on the theory of residential treatment. In A. Esman (Ed.), *The Psychiatric Treatment of Adolescents*. New York: International Universities Press.

Offer, D. (1969). *The Psychological World of the Teenager*. New York: Basic Books.

Offer, D., Marcus, D., Offer, J.L. (1970). A longitudinal study of normal adolescent boys. *American Journal of Psychiatry, 126*(7):917-924.

Olds, J. (1982). The inpatient treatment of adolescents in a milieu including younger children. *Adolescent Psychiatry*, (10), 373-381.

Piaget, J. (1954). *The Construction of Reality in the Child*. New York: Basic Books.

Piaget, J. (1972). Intellectual evolution from adolescence to adulthood. *Human Development*, (15), 1-12.

Piaget, J. & Inhelder, B. (1954). *The Growth of Logical Thinking From Childhood to Adolescence*. New York: Basic Books.

Redl (1966). *When We Deal With Children*. New York: Free Press.

Rinsley, D.B. (1983). *Treatment of the Severely Disturbed Adolescent*. New York: Jason Aronson, Inc.

Sarnoff, C. (1976). *Latency*. New York: Aronson.

Schiffer, M. (1984). *Children's Group Therapy*. New York: MacMillan.

Weiner, I.B. (1980). Psychopathology in Adolescence. In J. Adelson (Ed.), *Handbook of Adolescent Psychology*. New York: Wiley.

Weiner, I. B. & Elkind, D. (1972). *Child Development: A Core Approach*. New York: Wiley.

Chapter 14

LIMIT SETTING WITH ACTING-OUT ADOLESCENTS

Harinder S. Ghuman
and Richard M. Sarles

"Got my word on that," said Makepeace Smith. "And you don't have to write it down. A man who keeps his word doesn't have to read and write. But a man who has to write down his promise, you got to watch him all morning. I know that for a fact. We got lawyers in hatrack these days."

"The curse of civilized man," said Taleswapper. "When a man can't get folks to believe his lies anymore, then he hires him a professional to lie in his place."

From Seventh Son *by Orson Scott Card*

Often, adolescent patients are admitted to inpatient hospital settings under the guise of receiving psychiatric treatment, but they are, in reality, trying to escape legal consequences of their actions. Often mental health professionals, knowingly or unknowingly, participate in such a patient's pathology. At any given time, there may be 20–30 percent of inpatients who are referred by juvenile courts or are actively involved in the legal process. Another 20–40 percent have been involved in antisocial activities in the past, which is sometimes known to authorities or parents but most often not. These activities include stealing, burglary, vandalism, selling drugs, violence, and even rape and murder. Some of these adolescents and their parents are genuinely interested and believe in psychiatric treatment. The mental health professional's dilemma is how to treat these youngsters without overprotecting them and/or participating in their psychopathology.

Included in this large group of patients are adolescents with diagnoses of conduct disorder, oppositional disorder, personality disorder, and other psychiatric diagnoses in which antisocial acting out is a part of their problem. Limit setting is probably the most important issue in managing such adolescents' behavior and in making significant changes in their maladaptive personality structures. The behaviors frequently bring these patients into conflict with others and society. During the inpatient stay, they often recreate situations in which they violate social norms, challenge authority, and act aggressively, and they are acutely aware of the hospital staff's response. Confronting such behaviors provides the hospital staff with an opportunity to send an explicit message that the adolescent must take responsibility for his/her actions; in doing so, they can help adolescents to think before they act.

It is imperative that the inpatient staff set clear expectations for these patients, with limits and consequences clearly defined if milieu norms and rules are violated. Limits can vary depending on the severity, frequency, and circumstances under which the limit testing behavior takes place. Limit setting can include loss of responsibility level and/or sign out, restriction of various activities, fines, and time out in the quiet room or in the patient's room. In some cases, it may mean temporary exclusion from the milieu and in extreme cases transfer to another hospital or return to the court for placement in the juvenile justice system.

Limit setting is crucial for successful inpatient adolescent treatment. In order for treatment or therapy to be effective, a patient's acting out has to be brought under control since acting out releases tension or painful affect, which is necessary for therapeutic work. Limit setting by staff also provides the patient with support and structure allowing patients to feel safe and secure and protected from their own impulses. Limits can also promote a sense of both individual and group responsibility. Lastly, limits can be used as a consequence for not taking responsibility or for not following social, institutional, and ethical rules. One of the main treatment team-related variables that result in successful outcome is how well the treatment team as a whole and team members individually are able to set limits on the patient's acting-out behavior.

Two overarching problems may occur with limit setting: (a) not setting appropriate limits at all; and (b) not setting consistent limits. Some of the common reasons for not setting limits are discussed below. There are, however, many more complex issues that interfere in limit setting, including internal issues of the individual or the treatment team as a whole, such as issues of trust, superego formation, development of control, and dealing with authority.

NORMALITY VS. PATHOLOGY AND LIMIT SETTING

Often, a new team member confuses what is normal age-related behavior and what is pathological behavior. According to Gralnick (1966,1969) adequate treatment is essential, as such patients are sick and not merely going through a developmental state. Rinsley & Inge (1961) described how adolescent patients resist treatment by acting like, or to be viewed as, a "typical adolescent." These adolescents can best be described as "Pseudo teenagers" and there is often a tendency and danger to give the youngster the benefit of doubt toward normality, resulting in underdiagnosis, false hope, and mismanagement. Such underdiagnoses would include adjustment disorder, identity disorder, and parent-child problems, for example, and the patient's acting-out behavior would be labeled as "typical teenage behavior" or "what you would expect from teenagers—they are into drugs, sex, and rock 'n roll."

Sometimes, an inexperienced staff member may look to normality or to his/her own teenage experiences as a point of reference. The problem created with such thinking is: (a) the staff member may be using denial or rationalization to deal with the patient's as well as with his or her difficulties; and (b) the staff member may be overlooking the intensity and frequency of acting-out behavior. These patients often barrage staff with question like, "Have you ever smoked grass?" or "Are you telling me you never did anything behind your parents' back?" Such questions often put staff members in a defensive position. They may start questioning their own identity and value system and if they are not sure or are conflicted about these self issues, they may get lost in these questions and not do what is required.

Most hospitalized adolescents, especially those on long-term units, suffer from chronic and serious psychiatric disorders. Eventually, to the surprise of an individual staff member or several team members, there is a realization of the seriousness of the patient's acting-out behavior, which may lead to staff feeling betrayed, and angry at themselves for playing into the patient's pathology. As a result, staff may set limits that may be too strict or severe.

CONFUSION REGARDING ROLE AND AUTHORITY

In a typical inpatient setting, it is the therapist who is vested with most authority to impose limits and it is the nursing staff who are responsible to set and enforce the limits. Nursing staff often look for the therapist's approval to set a limit on the acting-out behavior. There are times when staff brings an acting-out behavior to the therapist's attention and the therapist gives a very intelligent psychodynamic explanation of the behavior, since therapists are often fascinated with the dynamics of the behavior, and the issue is dropped without anyone's dealing with the acting-out behavior. This occurs when the therapist is using insight (therapist's insight not the patient's) as a substitute for limit setting. Inexperienced or passive staff may not question the therapist, and the therapist's nonchalant attitude may serve as an excuse for the nursing staff not to set the limit, thereby giving credence to a fact that all professionals (and parents) dealing with adolescents know—that limit setting is always one of the most difficult jobs.

There are times when nursing staff has to put a lot of energy into explaining the reason for limits to a particular therapist in addition to dealing with the patient's wrath for setting the limit. This can cause serious problems, especially if the therapist feels that his or her patients are treated unfairly and the patient recognizes that the therapist is not supporting the nursing staff. This may result in a reluctance on the part of the nursing staff to set limits with patients of that therapist. Usually, this culminates in: (a) the patient bringing the therapist and the nursing staff together by severe acting out; (b) the patient and the therapist initially being involved in a false grandiose sense of special relationship, thus losing the opportunity to work on the patient's problem; and (c) increased alienation between team members, resulting in premature discharge or a false sense of cure.

INPATIENT THERAPY AND LIMIT SETTING

Various authors (Kernberg, Gunderson & Stone, 1988) have stated the importance of clear limits and explicit treatment contracts regarding conditions of therapy, e.g., regular attendance, active participation, paid bills, etc., especially with outpatient borderline patients. Issues of limit setting become even more important with antisocial acting-out inpatients because a sense of boundaries is often lacking or defective in these patients to an even greater degree than in an "average borderline." In contrast to the borderline patient who frequently attempts to test or transgress boundaries, the antisocial acting-out patient has no regard for boundaries and often steals, vandalizes, rapes, or assaults with a sense of entitlement as if everything belonged to him.

All inpatient therapists (individual, group, family, and activity) and nursing staff need to approach the severely acting-out inpatient with a different therapeutic framework than one would use with an outpatient who is generally less disturbed. Passive, interpretative, and inactive approaches may not produce favorable results with an acting-out adolescent. There is no way that a therapist, especially an individual therapist, will be able to stay out of management issues regarding an acting-out patient. An experienced therapist may be able to use these management issues, including limit setting, as an important tool for individual psychotherapy, instead of viewing these issues as distractions. Even if the therapist is not actively involved in setting limits in the hall milieu, rules and limits need to be followed during individual therapy sessions. Often, these patients become involved in name calling, threatening aggressive behavior, stealing, and sometimes even exposing themselves during therapy sessions. While working with the acting-out adolescent who has poor impulse control and poor superego formation, and uses splitting as a defense, the therapist who does not set the same limits during therapy as set in the milieu is likely to confuse the patient and permit patients to experience the hospital environment to be as inconsistent as was their home.

Therapists are often hesitant to set limits due to concerns that it may adversely affect their therapeutic relationship with the patient, hold back the free flow of therapy, or encourage the patient to view limit setting as punishment. One therapist's dilemma regarding limit setting was best described by her saying, "I have been in the situation so many times of patients calling names or being abusive that I wasn't sure if I was going to be helpful if I didn't allow it. They needed to do this." There are several reasons given for setting limits during psychotherapy of borderline patients: (a) a failure to set limits allows reward with secondary gain; (b) to prevent turning the therapeutic relationship into an actual or real relationship; and (c) to bring negative feelings into therapy instead of letting them be acted out (Kernberg, Gunderson, & Stone, 1988). The same reasons apply to working with acting-out adolescents. In addition, limits are essential for building a trusting, safe, and mutually respectful relationship between the therapist and the patient. With limits, the therapist helps the patient to gain and internalize controls and helps lay the foundation for superego development.

CONFUSION REGARDING ISSUES OF CONFIDENTIALITY AND LIMIT SETTING

On occasion, a treatment team member may know from the patient of past or present acting-out behavior but is reluctant to share this information with other team members or to set limits, fearing that this will break the patient's trust. Nursing staff and therapists are aware that if a patient's behavior is a danger to self or others, then all team members must be informed. These behaviors may include stealing, sexual acting out, drug and alcohol use, and destruction of property. However, even with such dangerous behaviors, staff and therapists often explain the need to divulge the information in that it is against the law to keep such information secret. This type of explanation may play into the patient's psychopathology in that the patient may feel that the person does not personally care about the dangerous behavior or the patient himself, but is intervening only because of the law. Notwithstanding, the patient may benefit from seeing an adult obeying the law. One of the main objectives for the setting of limits on and consequences for the acting-out adolescent is to help him/her achieve a sense of responsibility for behavior even if it causes discomfort. The staff needs to show that they can deal with the patient's anger and still take personal responsibility for appropriate limit setting. Explanations for limit setting such as, "This is hospital policy" or "Staff or therapist did this, not me," or "It's team decision," are inadequate and misleading without a show of personal commitment to limit setting. If there is disagreement within the team regarding a limit, this needs to be thoroughly discussed and resolved before the limit is placed.

When one is dealing with the acting-out inpatient adolescent, the following guidelines can be helpful to address the question of limit setting and confidentiality:

1. Any behavior in which the patient indulges that is against milieu norms is not confidential.
2. When a patient does indulge in such behavior, it is imperative that the staff insist that the patient discuss this issue with the primary therapist in order to avoid patient-staff splitting and to provide the patient with the opportunity to examine the meaning of the behavior. Appropriate limits then need to be imposed, depending on the intensity and frequency of the behavior.
3. The patient should be encouraged to inform other team members and the peer group about this behavior. If the patient refuses, it is often useful to impose restrictions/loss of privileges. One needs to continually emphasize that it is the patient's problem and his/her responsibility to be open and honest.

FAILURE TO SET PRIORITIES

At times, the failure to set priorities in dealing with a patient's problem can interfere with proper limit setting. When a patient presents with multiple problems, staff often try to work on as many of the problems as possible. This approach may be successful in some cases; but often this can be an obstacle. For example:

> Sixteen-year-old Kate was admitted to the long-term adolescent unit because of a two-year history of runaway behavior, drug abuse, stealing, and vandalism. She had dropped out of school, had been sexually acting out, and was involved in prostitution during her runaways. Previous attempts at outpatient treatment and short-term inpatient treatment had been unsuccessful.
>
> Kate was adopted when she was six months of age, and information regarding her natural parents was limited. Development was described as normal except that she was a "clingy baby." She had above-average intelligence and achieved A's and B's in school until age 13. Kate was involved in various athletic activities, such as gymnastics and volleyball, and apparently did well in sports. Kate's father was discovered to have multiple sclerosis when Kate was approximately 10 years old, and he was confined to a wheelchair at the time Kate was admitted to the adolescent inpatient unit.
>
> Upon admission to the hospital, Kate initially made a good impression on the staff. She immediately expressed her wish to have off-hall privileges to attend the hospital school, which complemented her parents' wish for her to start school and function at the level she used to when she was 13 years old. The staff wanting to help Kate deal with her multiple problems and, sensing significant potential in her, decided to permit her off the unit so that she could attend school. Kate responded by eloping. Fortunately, within a few days, Kate was brought back by the police. After lengthy discussion by the team, it was decided to place Kate on hall restriction for an indefinite period to help limit her acting-out behavior and to help her form an attachment to the unit. The treatment team continued to assess her situation weekly and reevaluate the need for this limit. There was continuous pressure from Kate, her parents, the school staff, and various team members to permit Kate to be involved in various activities. But the team was able to focus on the issue of helping establish necessary relationships as a top priority before venturing into other problem areas. Kate required about 10 weeks of hall restriction, which provided the foundation for her to complete her treatment successfully. Three years following discharge, Kate had not been readmitted to any inpatient program, had completed high school, had a

part-time job, and was attending college. Her relationship with her parents had improved substantially.

In this case, without appropriate limits and focus on the major problems of forming relationships, the patient could have been predicted to elope and to continue her acting out behavior.

Following is an example of a treatment failure:

> Sam was 17 years old when admitted because of multiple problems, including several violent episodes at home and school, a history of stealing, vandalism, school failure, drug and alcohol abuse, and runaway behavior. He was identified as having a learning problem and hyperactivity at an early age. The patient had been in outpatient treatment intermittently and was treated with Methylphenidate and various major tranquilizers. He had had three hospitalizations totaling eight months in the three years prior to this admission.
>
> Sam's father, an alcoholic who physically abused Sam and his mother, left the family when Sam was four. Sam's mother had several male friends following her husband's deserting the family.
>
> During hospitalization, Sam threatened staff and peers and required seclusion on several occasions. He lied and stole from peers. He seemed to keep others away by poor hygiene. Different team members and school staff wanted to work with Sam, helping him with his various problems. Although Sam continued to show problems with aggression, major treatment focus was shifted away from this problem and the treatment team decided to involve Sam in school and an off-unit drug program. After this, Sam's aggression escalated, resulting in the serious injury of a staff member and his transfer to another facility. We believe that if the treatment team had continued to focus on the issue of aggression and provided necessary limits for Sam, the treatment outcome may have been different.

Often, there are pressures from external sources to modify or to make exceptions to the limit setting program prescribed by the staff. In addition to the problems mentioned above, sometimes the power of a limit can be undermined by making too many exceptions to the limit. These exceptions are made because of external pressures, such as, limited insurance coverage or pressure from third-party reviewers and distraught family members. The team may feel pressure to placate different members of the team. There are advantages to having different profes-sionals work with a patient, but it can also cause confusion as they may have different priorities depending upon their expertise. The treatment team needs to carefully assess what the priorities are during the different phases of treatment of an adolescent, and a consensus should be reached. If the team is unable to reach consensus, then the team leader has to decide, and everyone needs to support the decision.

LIMIT SETTING WITH THE ADOLESCENT GROUP

Until now, the focus of this chapter has been on the importance of limit setting with the individual patient. Limit setting with the adolescent group on an inpatient unit is also a very important consideration. Adolescence is a stage when influence of peers is at its maximum. Limits placed on the group are critical to bring about necessary changes in the individual adolescent, the adolescent group, and milieu conditions. Whenever there is suspiciousness and acting out either aggressive or self-destructive in nature, no one can feel safe in the milieu and benefit from treatment. Lewis et al. (1973) introduced and formalized the concept of "protreatment group process," which was characterized by making the group responsible for the behavior of each member and each member responsible to the group for his/her own behavior. Limits in the form of loss of privileges and restrictions were placed on the group. Lewis' group met four times a week and had the following rules:

1. When any patient physically hurts himself, hurts another, abuses drug, sets fire, or runs away, the entire unit was to lose all privileges except for going to school.
2. Group restriction continued until three conditions were fulfilled:
   a. Each member in the group had explored his own role in participating, either actively or passively, in the behavior that caused the group restriction;
   b. There had been an open expression of honest feeling for the patient whose behavior led to the restrictions;
   c. The group had attempted to help the patient or patients who caused the restriction to find out reasons for the behavior and ways of handling the feelings involved.

Limits on the group can help to build a cohesive group, increase peer accountability, and manage milieu effectively. A problem with this approach is that the new patient, families, and inexperienced staff may be resistant and unable to accept the reason for restriction on the whole group. This approach may not be appropriate for short-term treatment programs or when there is high staff turnover. Necessary modifications can be made to suit the program. These modifications include use of partial restrictions, shorter duration of restrictions, and one or two problem-specific restrictions. For example, it will be very difficult to put a whole unit on hall restriction if there are several patients being admitted and/or leaving.

The following is an example of setting limits with an adolescent group on a 12-bed long term unit:

> The nursing staff in consultation with the therapists decided to place all of the adolescents on hall restrictions after one of the adolescent females, Shelly, ran away during an off-grounds activity. The initial reaction of the adolescents was of anger and denial of any knowledge or participation in Shelly's plan to run away. The nursing staff held community meetings twice a day in addition to regular community meetings (1–2/week) and group therapies (3/week). As the hall restriction was continued, group members started to show concern about the possibility of Shelly getting into a bigger and more serious problem due to her impulsive nature. Three of the adolescents informed the staff how Shelly had tried to get them to run away with her. The group members examined their reasons for not informing the staff. One of them thought that Shelly was not serious about running away. Two other patients, after some initial defensiveness, expressed open hostility toward Shelly and relief that she had left. They were angry at some of Shelly's behavior on the unit, especially lying and stealing from them. The group restrictions were gradually lifted after the group members had talked about their responsibility towards Shelly's running away, their feelings toward Shelly and her runaway behavior, and what to do in similar circumstances should they arise in the future.

LIMIT SETTING WITH ACTING-OUT PARENTS

Many of the acting-out adolescents who come for inpatient treatment have parents who suffer from severe psychopathology and often are described as "personality disordered," "borderline," "narcissistic," or "antisocial," who often act out their conflicts, impulses, and painful feelings. Often, a major part of treatment of the adolescent is dealing with the parents who continue to act in a pathological manner with the adolescent even when the teenager is in the hospital. Limit setting on the parents' acting out can be more difficult than setting limits on the adolescent, since parents are not identified as patients and they have many more legal rights. Their legal rights can be suspended or terminated only in extreme situations and only after much time and energy invested by the hospital staff members. It is not uncommon and certainly understandable that the hospital's legal representative, administration, and clinical staff often try to avoid these confrontations.

One needs to understand the reasons for the parents' acting out and work on these issues in family therapy. There can be a number of reasons for parents' interference and acting-out behavior. These may include difficulty in trusting themselves and others in taking care of their adolescent, being too anxious, having difficulty in separating themselves from their adolescent, being overcontrolling, and/or having poor impulse control and superego deficits. So often, these parents provoke countertransference feelings among the team members, including anger, feelings of inadequacy, and the need to overcontrol. Team members also may lose proper perspective of the situation and what is required for good treatment when dealing with such parents. Therefore, it is an ongoing task for the hospital staff to constantly evaluate their countertransference feelings in relationship to limit setting for adolescent patients and their families.

There are times that family therapy is not enough and parents may require very specific limits to their interference and acting-out behavior. These limits may include shortening or stopping visits by parents, denial of sign-outs, limiting phone contacts, supervision of contacts, change of custody to a healthier parent or to Social Services, and certification of the adolescent. In some cases, if parents continue to act out despite the treatment team's best efforts and there is no legal course for the treatment team to take, then the parents may be required to arrange for transfer of the adolescent to another psychiatric facility. Hopefully, the adolescent and his/her parents will be able to learn from this process and support the treatment at the next facility.

The following are examples of limit setting with parents:

> Scott, a 16 year old, was admitted to the hospital for the second time due to increased aggressive behavior towards his parents, drug and alcohol abuse, school refusal, and not following house rules. The precipitating event for the hospitalization was a physical altercation Scott had with his father in which both received cuts and bruises. Scott's hospitalization, six months prior, was the result of a similar altercation and the father had

tried to run over his son with his car. Scott's father had a history of excessive drinking, was described as having a bad temper, and was physically abusive to Scott and Scott's mother. Yet he had never received any psychiatric treatment. Scott's mother had called the police several times at home after Scott's father's outbursts, but she never filed any charges.

On Scott's admission, his father was very angry, threatening, and argumentative to Scott and staff, and Scott himself was very provocative and overinvolved with his father. The treatment team had to set constant limits on Scott and his father by supervising and limiting their interactions, while the social worker tried to understand and clarify family dynamics to help the family deal more appropriately with their conflicts and persuade Scott's father to seek individual psychiatric treatment. Despite all efforts by the staff to limit Scott and his father, the father continued to escalate his threatening and aggressive behavior and threatened to inflict physical harm upon the staff, his wife, and himself.

The treatment team decided that in order to provide safety to Scott, his family, and the staff, it was necessary to prohibit Scott's father from access to the hospital grounds. Scott's father was informed about this decision as an absolute need to protect and ensure a safe treatment environment and was also notified that hospital security and the local police department had been informed about the father's threats. The treatment team made an unsuccessful attempt to have Scott's father hospitalized on an involuntary basis. However, Scott's father did respond to these limits and subsequently sought voluntary admission to a psychiatric facility. The limiting of acting-out behaviors allowed Scott the opportunity to examine and work on his own intrapsychic problems and his relationship with his father.

Robin, 14 years old, was transferred from an acute inpatient treatment facility to Sheppard Pratt Hospital for longer-term, intensive psychiatric treatment. She was admitted after an overdose of approximately 30 aspirin tablets. Robin had a two-year history of running away from home, skipping school, and sexually acting out, including having sex for drugs. The patient's mother had history of prostitution and drug and alcohol abuse and had died of a drug overdose a year prior to Robin's admission. The patient's father described himself as a recovered alcoholic and drug addict. However, during Robin's hospitalization the treatment team suspected that the father was involved in excessive drinking, and illegal activities, such as selling drugs, all of which he denied.

On the adolescent unit, Robin seemed very needy and in severe emotional pain, but most willing to work on her problems. The patient's father, although superficially supportive to Robin in her treatment, continually forced the treatment team to make exceptions for Robin. At the same time, he had great deal of difficulty understanding why Robin did not follow his directions at home. Despite family therapy, Robin's father continued with this behavior. As Robin became more engaged in her treatment, the treatment team decided that setting appropriate limits were crucial for Robin to be able to internalize controls on her previously out-of-control behavior. The team also decided not to give into her father's unreasonable demands, thus providing both Robin and her father the opportunity to internalize controls.

Robin's father requested a sign-out for Robin even though she had not fulfilled her responsibilities that week; his request was denied and he threatened to take Robin out of the hospital. The treatment team emphasized that the staff was willing to work with Robin and her father, but at the same time, the team would not be effective if he continued to undermine treatment. Robin told her father that she did not want to leave the hospital. After an initial standoff, he decided not to take Robin out of the hospital. Subsequently, Robin's father was more cooperative and worked on his relationship with Robin, allowing Robin to become more assertive and less acting out with him.

SUMMARY

Limit setting with acting-out adolescents is essential in their treatment so that a safe environment can be provided and necessary behavioral and internal changes made. There are a number of factors described in this chapter that can interfere in the staff's limit setting with adolescents. There is a danger that if proper limits are not applied, the patient's psychopathology may worsen. Limit setting with the adolescent group itself can be a very effective way of helping acting-out adolescents. Often, parents of acting-out adolescents are also in need of limit setting by the treatment team in order for the staff to work best with the patient.

REFERENCES

Card, Orson Scott (1987) *Seventh Son*. New York: Tor Books.
Gralnick, A. (1966). Psychoanalysis and the treatment of Adolescents in a Private Hospital. In J. Masserman (Ed.), *Science and Psychoanalysis*. (pp.

102-108) New York: Grune and Stratton.

Gralnick, A., Rabiner, E.L., Astillo, G.D. and Zawell, D. (1969). Treatment consideration in the Adolescent Patient, *Dis. Nerv. System*, *30*, 833-842.

Kernberg, O.F., Gunderson, J.G., Stone, M. (1988). Special Problems in Therapy of Borderlines-Conversations with the Experts. *Clinical Psychiatry News.*, *16*, 1.

Lewis, J.M. Gossett, J.T., King, J.W. and Carson, D.I. (1973). Development of a Pro-Treatment Group Process Among Hospitalized Adolescents. In Feinstein, S.C. and Giovacchini P.L. (Eds.), *Adolescent Psychiatry* (pp.351-362). Vol. 2. New York: Basic Books.

Rinsley, D.B. and Inge, G.P. III. (1961). Psychiatric Hospital Treatment of Adolescent: Verbal and Nonverbal Resistance to Treatment. *Bull. Menninger Clin.*, *25*, 249-293.

PART IV

Special Issues

Chapter 15

TEAMWORK WITHIN THE TREATMENT TEAM

Harinder S. Ghuman and Erika E. Wilmoth

Teamwork is an integral aspect of inpatient treatment. When the treatment team is not functioning at an optimal level, the most qualified staff and enthusiastic treatment plans will achieve only limited results. In this chapter, we will attempt to delineate the essentials for good teamwork, including role clarification, role of the leaders, issue of communication, and appropriate staff relationships.

ROLE OF A TEAM MEMBER

Lack of clarity regarding duties and responsibilities and the interface with team members of various disciplines is a major area of concern. Distribution of power and authority within the team and institution (hospital or residential setting) has a major effect on the role of team members and their ability to function within the team framework.

It is important for new staff joining the team to be clearly advised by the supervisor of his/her duties immediately. The new staff member should be given a written document outlining specific duties, tasks, and expectations, and what is unacceptable practice. It is useful to have a staff orientation booklet in addition to on-the-job training under supervision of a senior staff member. The following is an example of a written statement of job duties: "The staff nurse has assigned shift accountability for overall functioning of the milieu. Oversees the work of the paraprofessionals in person. Responsible for assessing, planning, organizing, administering, documenting, and evaluating patient care delivery. Staff nurse administers medication, performs prescribed treatments, provides patient teaching, and offers psychosocial support. Acts as a liaison between the head nurse and patients. Attends patient-related meetings as assigned. Meets regularly with the head nurse for the purpose of supervision, problem solving, and goal setting. The staff nurse is directly responsible to the head nurse" (Wilmoth 1987).

At times, there may be two sets of supervisors for a particular staff member, such as a staff nurse who may have a head nurse and a unit director as supervisors, or a social worker who may have the head of the social work department and the unit director as supervisors. Different agendas and expectations can cause confusion for the staff. For example, the unit director may want the staff member to spend time on the unit and deal with clinical issues, whereas the department head may assign duties to the staff member outside the unit (i.e., attending committee meetings, etc.). If the unit director and the department head are not in tune, unnecessary confusion, conflict, and friction for the new staff member may develop. The staff member may follow the direction of the supervisor, who has authority over his performance appraisal or may follow his own personal interest. This situation provokes the potential for splitting to occur and a staff member may take advantage of this opportunity to achieve other personal goals. Therefore, with two sets of supervisors, the need to have a clear view and understanding of what is being asked of the new staff member is imperative, as well as to know which supervisor has the ultimate right of decision-making for that employee.

Often, treatment team members' duties and areas of work overlap each other. The following are areas where confusion and role blurring can occur regarding duties and responsibilities of team members.

1. Confusion between the activity therapist and the nursing staff regarding who will coordinate, plan, and implement activities, and how much time each discipline will provide.
2. How much and what level of involvement nursing staff have with the patients' families, in contrast to social work. Although the nursing staff will generally communicate with families after standard workday hours, the nursing staff may expect the social worker to perform this task.
3. The extent to which the nursing staff participate in group therapies.
4. Conflicts between nursing staff and physicians regarding flagging orders, writing and renewing orders, and implementing orders. Although some of these conflicts may be due to other reasons, such as issues of dependency and control, it is useful to be clear about the expectations for each discipline.

5. Patient escorting. Does nursing staff have to escort patients all the time and everywhere? Can other disciplines assist with this duty?
6. Limit setting with patients. This important issue has been addressed in Chapter 14.
7. Conflicts regarding space and time. Often, there is limited space available on a unit, and competition for this space may develop. Therapists may want to see an adolescent on the unit due to the patient's unstable condition or for a matter of convenience. Yet, nursing staff may not have any designated area to take a break or work in a quieter, private environment. Therefore, adequate space in which to perform one's duties and negotiation for limited available space are critical for a well-functioning team.

Adolescents often attend school while in an inpatient setting, and all therapies and treatment activities generally have to be scheduled after school hours. This can cause tension and may create competition among various therapists about which therapist or what therapy is most important. The treatment team has to actively address these issues on an ongoing basis. There is always a need for flexibility, setting priorities, and giving respect and cooperation in order that problem solving and conflict resolution occur in a timely and effective manner.

TEAM LEADERSHIP, AUTHORITY, DEPENDENCY, AND CONTROL

On a psychiatric adolescent inpatient unit, there is usually one designated leader. The leader's authority or power depends upon three factors:

(1) How the *hospital authority structure* is defined: (a) if the unit leader is the primary supervisor, he/she hires, delegates duties, and appraises staff performances; (b) when staff members have their department head as their supervisor that person is responsible for the above functions, not the unit leader, although the unit leader may provide input. There are disadvantages to both of these reporting relationships. When the unit leader has sole responsibility and authority over staff, (a) the development of better working relationships may be hindered as the team leader may not feel the need to involve staff in decision making and thereby loses valuable input as well as motivation of staff. It can also hinder the development and refinement of leadership skills of various staff members if the leader invokes absolute authority. Disadvantages of the second kind of system, (b) can be that work may not be accomplished at a quicker pace and this can be an excellent media for splitting and acting out in case there is poor quality staff or the team is overstressed.

(2) The *leader's own personality* contributes to appropriate use of authority. A firm, consistent, flexible, fair, honest leader with interest in the staff and high quality care will be able to exercise authority effectively.

(3) Another component that contributes to effectiveness of the leader's authority is the level of *staff competency* working under the leader. Munich (1986) wrote that good fellowship can make a limited leader function at a higher level than predicted, while fellowship organized around collusive incompetence, chronic feeling of deprivation or intransigent psychopathy can make a good leader fail in spite of his best intentions and efforts.

There is often a team within the team and a team hierarchy exists that may be due to the large number of nursing staff who fall under the direction of the head nurse. The head nurse obviously provides a pivotal role. How issues of trust, power, and responsibilities are worked out between the unit director and the head nurse can be a major factor in determining the effectiveness of the treatment team. A collaborative management style and mutual respect for role responsibilities prove invaluable in both team building and goal setting and attainment.

In order to develop and maintain an effective working relationship between the unit director and head nurse, both must be motivated in forming a working alliance. A thorough understanding of and adherence to the established unit philosophy and a consistent mode of practice is essential. Mere agreement in decision-making is not the formula that promotes effective treatment planning and a smoothly functioning milieu. It is the blending of individual skills and expertise that enables each to perform duties separately, but in harmony with each other, thus effecting a positive and productive result.

The team leader must be aware of the treatment team's needs at all times and usually needs to deal concurrently with issues of dependency and control. It is useful for the team leader to keep in mind that whenever staff changes occur it may be of more importance to fulfill the dependency needs of staff than to become overly frustrated by maintaining high expectations of the team members at that time. These dependency needs become more evident during periods of stress, for example around holidays or losses. Adolescent patients and their parents are vulnerable to the same stresses and events. Staff may experience a higher level of stress and anxiety due to the cumulative effect of personal stresses, in addition to attending to the needs of their patients and parents. The treatment team leader may be addressing the needs of both groups simultaneously.

Control and how much authority the team leader needs to exert at any given time are important issues. When does the team leader direct the team or an individual staff to carry out an important task regardless of personal issues? If the treatment team is mature and working together smoothly, the team leader may be in a position to offer less direction and guidance. Exercising more control may be necessary when: (a) team members become involved in bringing personal issues to the treatment environment; (b) there is a clique formation within the team, interfering with the team or keeping it from working effectively; and (c) the team is looking toward the leader to provide necessary controls because of staff ambivalence, disharmony, or lack of experience.

THE ROLE OF THE UNIT DIRECTOR

Munich (1986) has written about the various aspects of the unit chief's responsibility, including boundary management, generation of resources, the mobilization of consensus, and consultation and evaluation. We have found it useful to define the role of the unit director as: (a) providing structure and framework; (b) providing direction, affirmation, and clarification; (c) acting as facilitator and mediator; and (d) role model.

Providing Structure and Framework

The unit director is responsible for setting up the structural framework in which the team may accomplish its task. This includes basic issues, such as adhering to times set for meetings, encouraging regular attendance, emphasizing the importance of few disruptions, and ensuring a safe and comfortable place for the treatment team to meet. On many adolescent units, the team meets one to three times a week. Team members are encouraged to focus their total attention directly on the teamwork; various activities, such as phone calls and writing notes, are accomplished either before or after the meeting. For lengthy meetings, it may be useful to institute a five-minute midpoint break for staff to take care of personal needs, answer pages, or attend to emergency phone calls.

"Total attention" in team meeting is vital, since this may be the only place and time all the treatment team components are present. The major focus is on the development and implementation of the treatment plan, assignment of duties, and the opportunity for resolution to questions related to the adolescent or family situation. The unit director needs to remain aware of how decisions are followed through by team members and address any inconsistency. The unit director must be ever vigilant to assure that the adolescents receive proper supervision and that their basic developmental and treatment needs are being met. Berlin (1991) wrote that clinical administrators need to be firm and fair in requiring others to carry out their obligations, and deal with problems directly, promptly, and nonpunitively.

Providing Direction, Reaffirmation, Clarification

The unit chief is responsible for the treatment team remaining on task. This may require the unit chief to direct the team's attention toward a given task or to filter out various disruptions that may be distracting. Often, team members may be doing what is essential, but need reaffirmation from other team members or the unit director. This reaffirmation is important for the individual team member's professional growth and development. Reaffirmation not only provides clarification and reassurance to staff that they are on the right track, but also serves as recognition and encouragement from the team leader.

Facilitator and Mediator

The unit director is in a unique position to resolve conflicts among team members. In order to be successful in this role, the unit director has to remain neutral and above all professional idiosyncrasies and prejudices. Often, psychiatrists fill the role of the unit director, which may prove quite beneficial as the psychiatrist is usually the most experienced and skilled in dealing with intricacies of interpersonal relationships. Conversely, the psychiatrist leader may create a blind spot in dealing with other psychiatrists or psychiatric trainees on the unit due to professional prejudices.

There are times that different professionals are locked into their individual opinions and positions and in those instances the unit director may have to intervene and make the final decision. Depending upon the outcome, one group may feel that the unit director is showing favoritism. To avoid misinterpretation and the potential for conflict, the unit director must clarify the specific reasons for the decision. The unit director also needs to ensure that all disciplines on the team are equally involved, acknowledging that the input of psychiatrists, nurses, activity therapists, social workers, and school personnel is essential and must be elicited so that a global view of the patient can be obtained. The unit director may have to direct the flow of conversation so as to allow each discipline ample opportunity to provide input in the team meeting.

Role Model

The unit director is responsible for providing a continued focus on the quality of care being administered. In today's world of financial constraints, the need to increase revenue and cut budgets places special demands on the unit director to maintain a clear mission of quality treatment. The team leader as an administrator may be in a unique position to demonstrate, by example, how something can be done by actually doing it. Munich (1986) described the unit director's role-modeling potential for both the resident and the general psychiatrist by demonstrating, for example, how one is able to shift back and forth from the clinical role to the managerial role of unit director.

TEAM DEFENSES

The team is a dynamic, multifaceted body composed of various individuals with different personalities and professional backgrounds. It is always in the process of developmental flux, which may be due to internal and/or external factors. Like any individual, the team uses various defense mechanisms to deal with struggles, conflicts, and threats. The healthier the team defense, the better the outcome. The following are some examples:

> The team discussed a 16-year-old male who had a long history of violent behavior and had been restricted to the unit due to repeated violent behaviors while on the unit. He had assaulted the unit staff and threatened his peers, and yet he requested off-hall privileges. The school staff expressed concern that the patient was missing too much school and might fail. The patient's therapist reported the patient was working in therapy on important issues and he would like to see if the patient could handle going to school. The nursing staff continued to observe and report numerous problems with the patient's behavior requiring repeated staff intervention. The patient's social worker stated that the patient's parents were getting restless with the restriction and might take the patient out of the hospital.
>
> After a lengthy discussion, the team members agreed to take the patient off hall restriction. To an onlooker, it may appear the team had reached a good decision through consensus. But if the situation were more clearly defined, one could readily see problems with this decision. The patient's behavior remained out of control. The nursing staff had expressed their concerns,

yet they agreed to the decision because of feeling frustrated working with this patient and not sensing sufficient support from the other disciplines. The social worker was concerned that the parents might follow through with their threat to remove the patient from the hospital, and the teacher was looking at the school situation and was exclusively preoccupied with the student's scholastic performance. The patient's therapist was focused solely on the patient's performance in individual sessions. By having this false consensus, the team had used denial and employed a common defense used by teams of "getting together for the wrong reasons." Team leaders need to remain constantly aware of this ever-present problem, because if consensus happens for the wrong reason, it will create numerous problems in the long run. In this example, the team leader should have decided to keep the patient on the unit instead of allowing him to go to school; considering his ongoing aggressive behavior on the unit.

Another area of concern relative to counterproductive teamwork is the use of excessive projection and splitting mechanisms employed by team members and the team leader. It can be, for example, "those administrators," "those parents," or "that social service department," that is against "us"—the team. Sometimes, these may be necessary defense mechanisms to use when dealing with team stresses or when the team needs to become more cohesive. However, if the team becomes totally dependent upon these mechanisms to feel good or cohesive, this approach may become counterproductive and negatively translated into work with the patient. Ideally and optimally, the treatment team will feel close and good depending upon the team members' genuine respect and warm feelings toward each other and on the basis of their joint ventures and accomplishments.

The team discussed a 16-year-old female who had a history of running away, sexual acting out, drug abuse, and involvement with a male peer who had a history of violence and drug abuse. She had been warned about breaking rules on the unit, such as borrowing from and lending personal articles to this boy. Although warned, she continued to be involved in this interaction. The patient's therapist asked the nursing staff to have the patient placed on restriction from this particular male and the patient was told by the nursing staff that her therapist had put her on restrictions. The patient did not have the reason explained, and staff's response to the patient's questioning was to direct the patient to the therapist because they were not responsible for setting this limit. This interaction provided a strong impetus toward splitting and proved to be of no value to either the patient's understanding and growth nor to the team's ability to provide a therapeutic milieu.

ISSUES OF COMMUNICATION

In order for team members to assist a patient in dealing with communication problems, they need to provide appropriate role models themselves by having good communication with each other. Usually on a unit, there are both verbal and written communication skills utilized, and priorities have to be set to decide what needs to be conveyed to whom and how fast. Communication relative to a patient's suicidal thoughts/ attempts, physical violence, death, acute physical illness, runaways, and drug abuse on the unit needs to be communicated immediately. To accomplish this, it is useful to have a "communication book" readily available to alert all staff of these issues or situations. The communication book should not be used for personal communication, or in situations when the whole team does not need to know specific information. Additionally, it is essential to have a separate summary of the patient's daily status. This written summary may alert others to seek detailed information in the chart when necessary. Keeping team meeting notes and nursing meeting notes can be useful for reference for staff who are not present in those meetings. It is essential that notes be written legibly in a clear, concise, simple language; "slangs" and "abbreviations" should be avoided, as confusion and misinterpretation may result.

The team and unit do not live in a vacuum. There are outside influences on the team and unit all the time. A team representative needs to have constant open communication with neighboring units and the school. For example, a clique was being formed in the school by a very aggressive, rebellious group of adolescents from various inpatient units as well as by some day students. The school did not have complete information regarding the situation. The unit treatment team had information regarding what the group was planning to do, and this information was transferred to the school staff through the school representative on the team. By communicating to the various disciplines in a clear, concise, accurate, and timely fashion, staff was able to avert the full destructive potential such clique formation can create. Rapid deescalation and maintenance of control to ensure a safe environment were made possible by the intense, cohesive teamwork of all disciplines involved in both the inpatient and school setting.

STAFF RELATIONSHIP

There is not much written regarding this important aspect of teamwork, although most mental health professionals would probably be able to give their own idea of what the "professional relationship" consists of. Staff relationships on adolescent inpatient psychiatric units are most important for a variety of reasons, among which are: (a) patient and staff are involved in close and intimate interactions with each other; (b) often one of the major problems for adolescent psychiatric patients is with interpersonal relationships; (c) adolescents are acutely aware of what transpires in the relationship of their caregivers who are serving as important adult role models; (d) relationships during adolescence are especially important, because at this developmental stage there is a renegotiation of earlier dependent relationships and interactions, setting the stage for more adult, intimate relationships; and (e) adolescents have a tendency to fantasize and as a result may misinterpret the interactions among staff.

There are two aspects of staff relationships—staff relationships among staff members and staff relationships with patients. A "professional relationship" for these two components dictates that staff-to-staff and staff-to-patient relationships be based solely upon interactions that are of benefit to the adolescent patient. Personal feelings and issues must be set aside, which does not mean that staff cannot talk with each other about weather, world events, and personal life. However, this should be done only during "free" time when patients do not require attention. Staff must also be mindful of what is being said in front of patients. Can unit staff become involved in intimate relationships with each other? Should they continue to work on the same unit? How should the information of the relationship be made known to the staff and patients? Theoretically, it is possible that two staff members may be involved in an intimate relationship, and it may not affect their work on the unit. There are, however, very practical considerations regarding this issue as it could result in gross interference in patient treatment. The following are three examples:

1. During a therapeutic camping trip, a female patient had sexual intercourse with a male patient. On investigation by the staff, it was discovered that two staff members of the opposite sex who had been

involved in an intimate relationship with each other for some time and who were supervising the trip had decided to sleep in one tent instead of being with the patient group.

2. There had been increased physical contact among patients on the unit, including touching and fondling. The treatment team was concerned that more intimate contact might also be occurring. Closer observation of the unit staff revealed that two or three staff members were attracted to each other, and both their verbal and nonverbal interactions were openly observed by patients. These behaviors included massaging each other's neck and receiving flowers, which provoked confusion and misinterpretation by the patients. Staff were role modeling behaviors appropriate in the development of intimate relationships, but totally unacceptable for the milieu.

3. Staff had been concerned about provocative behavior by several female patients on the unit with male peers. A young female staff member who had recently joined the team often wore revealing shorts, low-cut tops, and stylish leather clothes. This mode of dress continued for some time due to several staff feeling too uncomfortable to confront her and some staff covertly encouraging her in her inappropriate choice of dress by making confusing remarks based on their own anxiety or excitement.

Staff must be constantly vigilant with both verbal and nonverbal communication. "Clique formation" is a common barrier in formulating therapeutic relationships and alliances. There are always some staff members who share similar likes and dislikes and consequently tend to gravitate toward each other. Sometimes, such groupings can create a positive, constructive interaction helpful to the team. Conversely, cliques often exclude others, thereby setting one person/group against another person/group. Sometimes, these cliques involve professional disciplines such as one group of professional staff against the other; at other times, cliques may cross professional lines. It is interesting to observe that adolescents are often involved in clique formations on the unit. Closer observation of the adolescent clique formation can provide staff with increased knowledge and understanding of this phenomenon. These cliques usually allow patients to feel special or to deal with loneliness, insecurities, and anger. The team leader must exercise caution with the example he/she sets. Are some staff more favored than others? Is one professional favored over the other? It is likely that if one staff member is working harder or expresses viewpoints similar to those of the team leader, a natural gravitation by the leader toward that particular staff member may occur. The team leader should not be influenced by favoritism in thinking that a particular staff can do no wrong, while others who may have experienced problems in the past will continue to demonstrate difficulty regardless. Upon confirmation that a clique formation exists, the team leader and team members need to actively intervene and confront the situation so as to resolve the issue before it intensifies and becomes problematic.

It is common knowledge and accepted practice that staff should not be involved in a romantic, sexual, or violent fashion toward any patient. Areas of concern frequently arise with the more subtle interactions that occur between staff and patients. Problems occur when one staff member is trying to impress a particular patient. For whatever reasons, the patient has become special to him or her, making it difficult to remain neutral when dealing with this patient. At times, staff may not be in agreement with some aspects of treatment, and consequently may respond by treating the patient unfairly. Staff may be spending an inordinate amount of time with a particular patient who is socially more competitive while ignoring the needs of others. Staff may also become involved in the use of personal remedies to cure a patient rather than using those decided upon and prescribed by the team. For example, one staff member had a meeting with a patient in a dark room lighted only by a candle in order to meditate, another therapist let an adolescent patient sit on the therapist's lap, and another therapist conducted individual therapy in the middle of the busy cafeteria without any consideration for confidentiality.

All of the above examples can be extremely counterproductive and countertherapeutic. It is vital that one's personal preferences, beliefs, and self-need fulfillment be in total check prior to one's making decisions relative to patient care planning, development, or delivery. At times, staff may need encouragement and support to be open and direct toward a fellow team member when actions, motivation, or investment are in question. Often, staff demonstrate reluctance to confront a team member in hope that unpleasantness and conflict may be avoided. Initially, this avoidance provokes a style of nonverbal communication in direct response to individual team members' dissatisfaction. If the disharmony is allowed to continue, the team structure and stability may decompensate and be replaced by a very negativistic, self-defeating group.

SUMMARY

It is essential that treatment team members are "working together" in order to help disturbed adolescents. This "working together" can be accomplished by clearly defining roles and duties of each team member and having a clear understanding of the lines of authority. The team leader has to constantly monitor what the needs of both the adolescents and the team are, what distraction the team is facing, and how the team can accomplish the task at hand in a growth-promoting fashion. Relationships and communication among team members and with adolescents are an important variable in team functioning and treatment outcome.

REFERENCES

Berlin, I.N. (1991) Some Principles of Clinical Administration Derived From Therapeutic Insight. In R.L. Hendrin & I.N. Berlin (Eds.), *Psychiatric Inpatient Care of Children and Adolescents: A Multicultural Approach* (pp. 278–288). New York: John Wiley & Sons Inc.

Munich, R.L. (1986). The role of unit chief and integrated perspective. *Psychiatry, 49*, 325-36.

Wilmoth, E.E. (1987). Staff Orientation Booklet Older Adolescent Unit: The Sheppard and Enoch Pratt Hospital.

Chapter 16

ADMINISTRATION OF AN ADOLESCENT INPATIENT PSYCHIATRIC TREATMENT PROGRAM

Richard M. Sarles

The proper administration of an adolescent inpatient psychiatric treatment program is critical for the delivery of mental health services. The administration's primary function is to ensure that the setting, staff, and support services are conducive for the optimal safe and secure treatment of psychiatrically disturbed adolescents and their families.

There is much heterogeneity of inpatient adolescent units (see chapter on Inpatient Settings) ranging from an adolescent unit as part of a university medical school, to a unit as part of a general hospital, to a multi-unit program as part of a large psychiatric hospital. Each of these settings will require different levels of administrative support and the unit director or program director will participate in the administration and management of the overall system to varying degrees.

While the definitions of both manage and administer include the term "to direct," manage implies "to carry on business" and administer "to perform executive duties" and "dispense." For the purpose of this chapter, I will make a distinction between administration and management. Administration, I believe, takes a broader role in the total management of a program, ranging from strategic planning, to budget preparation and monitoring, to marketing, recruitment and retention, credentialing and privileging, hiring and firing, and the equitable and reasonable allocation of resources. The administrator must insure that the adolescent program is in concert with the general overall mission of the hospital and/or medical school. The administrator may or may not be a clinician, but I believe that the administrator of an adolescent inpatient psychiatric program should ideally be a clinician with administrative education and training. The administrator may perform some clinical care, but the primary role is to administrate. There are advantages and disadvantages to the clinician-administrator amalgamation which will be discussed later in this chapter.

Management, in contrast, has more to do with the everyday clinical operation of a unit or program and less to do with the more global issues, such as setting of the budget, marketing, and so forth. Management must be clinically based and has more to do with operational issues, whereas administration has more to do with planning and delegating.

In a simplistic mode, administration must ensure that the right things get done, whereas management must ensure that the things get done right.

LEADERSHIP

A quality essential to both administrators and managers is that of leadership. Managers must provide clinical leadership on the unit by direct example of delivering high quality psychiatric care, by ensuring the optimal functioning of the team with equal input from all disciplines, and by constantly teaching and supervising the staff. The unit manager must act as the interface between the clinical care delivery and general administration, advocating for scarce resources and at the same time helping the line level staff to understand the imperative that all businesses have to balance revenues with expenses.

The administrator must take a broader leadership role, with qualities of fairness with justness, flexibility with firmness, and cheerleader-like qualities while setting limits. The administrative leader must be a planner with a vision of the future balanced with the reality of the present needs of the organization as determined by the current phase of its institutional life. The administrative leader must be an excellent communicator and listener and an expert at working with others to help in problem solving and negotiating. The leader must *plan*, *delegate*, and *communicate*, and must have the knowledge, skills, and attitudes to balance conflicting needs and tensions in a health care system.

Leadership must create and set the image and culture of the program in concert with the overall organization. Values and expectations come from leadership and are articulated verbally and in writing while being demonstrated in practice. Leadership must always strive for excellence and should not tolerate mediocrity. A leader must be a combination of architect, orchestrator, and choreographer, bringing all parts of the organization together in a harmonious, smoothly functioning fashion.

Hard work must always be recognized and rewarded. The staff's devotion to the patients, program, and co-workers, and their teamwork should be constantly reinforced and applauded. Emphasizing values, symbols, and beliefs of an organization is a major role of leadership.

The administrator must also set priorities and know when to act and when not to. Talbott and Frosch (1980) believe that an administrator has "only so many chips to play" and knowing when to play and when to sit out is essential for successful administrative management. This approach does not imply administration by exception in which the leader selectively attends to only that which is unusual, different, or out of the ordinary, and is inattentive to routine everyday issues. Proper administrative leadership attends to operational issues, routine and problematic, and plans for future contingencies all at the same time.

Silver and Marcos (1989) described five distinct features in the development of a clinical administrator: individual personality traits; clinical psychiatric training and clinical competence; mentor relationships; administrative training; and on-the-job training and experience.

INDIVIDUAL PERSONALITY TRAITS

Perseverance

Social systems resist change and change slowly; bureaucratic systems are often the most impenetrable and most resistant to change. The administrator needs to help balance efficiency and effectiveness and to determine at what point cost cutting, restructuring, and reduction of resources negatively impact on clinical care. The administrator must be extremely sensitive to staff morale, but needs to have a tough skin in order to stay the course of solid business management while still maintaining morale and esprit de corps. The administrator needs to develop tolerance for hard knocks and disappointments, funding specialty areas for growth and change while making necessary cuts in other areas. Administrative priorities from higher positions on the table of organization always take precedence even after long-standing commitments for resources have been made. The administrator must be cautious not to personalize many difficult administrative decisions and must always be able to step back to separate the person making the decision from the position being taken.

Creativity

The administrator must constantly plan, always trying to enhance clinical programs while making them more cost effective. Administrators should always have a project on the "back burner" and a contingency "what if" list. The skill of how to take advantage of market shifts and trends is the sign of a good administrator as is the ability to maximize resources and revenues while maintaining quality clinical care. An example would be how the administration adjusts staffing to accommodate to seasonal trends by planning for ten-month staff contracts in order to reduce staff in the slower summer months.

Tolerance for Ambiguity

Very few issues are absolute in administration except perhaps for employee dereliction of duty, insubordination, and criminal behavior. The administrator must, therefore, be able to deal with both sides of an issue and tolerate the ambiguities of business administrative life. Although it has been said that most important decisions are made on the basis of insufficient data, administration must deal with the gray zone and weigh both sides of an issue, making the best tactical-strategic decision with the available data.

CLINICAL PSYCHIATRIC TRAINING AND CLINICAL COMPETENCE

In the past, clinicians interested in inpatient psychiatric work could anticipate a staff position in which patient care was the primary responsibility. The administrative functioning of an inpatient program was usually learned by direct observation with on-the-job training and little, if any, formal training in management theory and practice. Management skills of directing an adolescent inpatient unit were gained under the tutelage and supervision of a more senior person in a direct supervisory relationship. With the enormous expansion of adolescent inpatient hospital programs during the 1980's, particularly the for-profit national hospital corporations, the need for unit directors and managers increased dramatically, and many young professionals were recruited with the lure of large salaries and the promise of leadership. Unfortunately, this required a rapid rise from clinician to manager, which prevented young clinicians from achieving a firm clinical foundation and clinical competence. Instead, they handled administrative-managerial tasks for which they were totally ill prepared. In addition, the young clinician turned administrator rarely was given the all important mentoring relationship, which is so critical for professional development.

MENTOR RELATIONSHIPS

Crucial to professional growth and development is the opportunity to work and study with those who can pass down the wisdom and experience they have gained. Mentors help develop others, and mentors are concerned with the future of an organization. It is said that an organization that is not capable of perpetuating itself has failed and will decay and die. Mentoring aids in the institution's process of constantly renewing its human resources. Mentoring should promote creativity, develop independent thinking, allow risk taking, and encourage shared participation. A supervisory relationship is critical in this endeavor. In our cost-cutting environment, the old saying, "Time is money" takes on even greater significance, since mentoring-supervision takes time. As the profit margin of all mental health systems is reduced, especially in inpatient settings, the luxury of time to talk with patients in psychotherapy, time for team meetings, and time for grand rounds or in-service teaching is coming under tremendous pressure. The increasing demands of patient care with shortened lengths of stay, and the demands of constant utilization review and managed care monitoring are consuming larger and larger amounts of clinicians' time. Mentoring, however, must never be viewed as a luxury of time. Without mentoring, a unit, the staff, and the institution are doomed.

ADMINISTRATIVE TRAINING
AND ON-THE-JOB TRAINING

All general psychiatry training programs and child and adolescent fellowship training programs in the United States must offer clinical inpatient experiences. Although all trainees participate in ward management meetings and receive supervision from the unit director, the focus of training is primarily clinical. As is often the case, the unit director may also be gaining both clinical and administrative experience with supervision from a senior clinician-administrator. The trainee's experience and understanding of the actual managing of the unit are essentially gained through observation and seldom through formal didactic teachings or readings on management theory. An educational dilemma is created by this factor; on the one hand, clinical competence is the first and foremost goal of the trainee's experience, but there is no really convenient opportune time to really learn management and administrative principles. Along with an understanding of the already full curriculum in all training programs and the constantly increasing demands to develop new content areas, I believe that formal lectures on management principles, with ongoing supervision by the unit director and senior clinician-administrator, would be an invaluable experience. This combination of didactic and experiential learning would best prepare trainees for management positions in the future, whether they be in private practice, community mental health centers, or governmental programs and facilities. The American Association of Directors of Psychiatric Residency Training (AADPRT) has administrative psychiatry curriculum modules available.

Those clinicians who feel that they have acquired a firm clinical foundation and wish to follow a career path towards administration should pursue training in administrative psychiatry with the same rigor and commitment as they did in clinical psychiatric training. There are several options available to obtain training in administrative psychiatry: postgraduate fellowships in some academic departments, continuing medical education workshops of varying duration, and self-motivated education following the American Psychiatric Association Committee on Administrative Psychiatry recommended reading list. More intensive courses of study could include matriculation to obtain a degree of Master of Business Administration (M.B.A.) or Master of Health Administration. The American Psychiatric Association Committee on Administrative Psychiatric also gives a yearly written and oral examination to clinicians who wish to receive a certification of competence in administrative psychiatry.

THE CLINICIAN-ADMINISTRATOR

In the not-too-distant past, those clinicians who assumed administrative functions and positions were often viewed with suspicion and disdain by their clinical colleagues. Pejoratives, such as "paper pusher," "number cruncher," or "one of them," were often used to describe the clinician-administrator. The perception of the clinician as turncoat or traitor was not uncommon, and a we-they scenario often developed. Such a dichotomous view developed secondary to the misbelief that the task of clinical staff was exclusively to deliver quality care, while the task of administration was to conduct the business aspects of the program. Each side seemed sheltered from the reality of the other side, and each side seemed to believe the other side was uninterested or unconcerned about clinical issues or business issues respectively.

The clinician-administrator has the greatest opportunity to bridge this mistrust and misunderstanding gap. The clinician-administrator appreciates the struggles and hardships of clinical work, the taxing, draining nature of an adolescent inpatient unit, and the tremendous responsibility of medically and psychologically managing a seriously mentally ill, psychotic, or manic adolescent. The clinician-administrator understands the need for appropriate staffing with skilled professionals and the necessity for a safe, secure, yet pleasant inpatient setting and supporting environs. The clinician-administrator also knows and appreciates the demanding, taxing, draining nature of administrative work and the tremendous responsibility of maintaining the financial health and well-being of an adolescent program. The clinician-administrator also knows the requirements of various regulatory agencies, such as JCAHO and HCFA, is aware of risk management issues and patient rights policies, and is able to read, understand, and use the statements of operations and balance sheets.

The clinician-administrative provides the experience, skills, and knowledge for both clinician and administrative issues, gained from clinical training and experience as well as from administrative training and experience. The successful administration of an adolescent inpatient psychiatric treatment program demands such a clinician-administrator because careful attention to managing both clinical and administrative matters is essential to a well-run unit.

REFERENCES

Levinson, D.J., Klerman, G.L. (1967): The Clinician-Executive: Some Problematic Issues for Psychiatrists in Mental Health Organizations. *Psychiatry*, 30:3-15.

Silver, M.A., Marcos, L.R. (1989): The Making of the Psychiatrist-Executive. *American Journal of Psychiatry*, 146:29-34.

Silver, M.A., Akerson, D.M. (1990): Critical Factors in the Professional Development of the Psychiatrist-Administrator. *Hospital and Community Psychiatry*, 41:71-74.

Talbott, J.A., Frosch, W.A. (1980): The Three Monkey Solution to Administrative Problems. *Hospital and Community Psychiatry*, 31:9, 635-636.

Talbott, J.A., Kaplan, S.R. (1983): *Psychiatric Administration: A Comprehensive Text for the Clinician-Executive*. New York: Grune & Stratton.

Chapter 17

LEGAL ISSUES IN ADOLESCENT INPATIENT PSYCHIATRY

Daniel J. Moore

INTRODUCTION

A practitioner engaged in the psychiatric treatment of inpatient adolescents confronts several special legal issues. Although the most commonly confronted legal issues are not substantially different in kind or character from those implicated by the inpatient treatment of adults, the unique legal status of the minor always informs the legal analysis and frequently controls its conclusion.

Under state and federal constitutions, statutes, and common law, all persons are equally possessed of fundamental individual rights and theoretically enjoy equal access to established remedies for the enforcement of those rights. Nonetheless, not all classes of individuals enjoy the same rights or, concomitantly, the same remedies. Children and adolescents historically have not enjoyed in the United States the same rights that are well recognized for adults, and some of the rights afforded to minors are exercised by others on their behalf. Thus, citizens under the age of 18 are not afforded a right to vote, as the judgment of society as reflected in law holds that minors do not have the capacity to wisely exercise the franchise. The conduct of public affairs clearly impacts on the interests of children, yet the law presumes that the interests of children will be protected by the adult members of the community who hold the franchise. Similarly, in many states, unemancipated minors cannot enter into certain contracts for delineated goods or services, nor can they unilaterally terminate the parental rights of their parents or give consent to many types of medical or surgical intervention. The law deems the minor to lack capacity to freely exercise all of these rights; thus, the law recognizes a delegation in the exercise of these rights to parents or guardians.

A hospital or clinician providing inpatient psychiatric services to children and adolescents confronts, therefore, several fundamental legal questions that are particular, if not unique, to the legal status of this class of patients. In the first instance, the hospital or clinician must know who exercises personal rights on behalf of the patient, how those rights are exercised, and what must be the response of the therapeutic team to a perceived conflict in interest between the minor patient and his or her parents or guardians. If parents are legally empowered to act for the minor and admit the minor to inpatient services, is the minor's legal status voluntary or involuntary? Who is the intended beneficiary of the process of informed consent and who has the potential claim or cause of action when this process fails? If parents are empowered to exercise rights and choices on behalf of children, must both parents agree and exercise these rights jointly or, if only one parent is available, does the clinician or institution still need the assent of both parents prior to the provision of services? If two parents are involved in the process of making decisions on behalf of the minor patient, how does the clinician respond to an irreconcilable conflict between the parents or, in the event of an irreconcilable conflict between the child and parents or parent, what does the law require for the protection of the rights of all?

All of these questions and concerns and more arise frequently at the initiation of inpatient services for children and adolescents and throughout the provision of those services. Clinicians, therefore, must develop a relatively safe and practical process for the resolution of these issues lest the provision of necessary services be unduly frustrated by the fear of future claims for violations of patients' rights or for the negligent provision of care. If a clinician is fairly well versed in the legal principles and analyses that are operative in this area in his or her legal jurisdiction, the clinician can realistically reduce the risk of crippling lawsuits and, of equal importance, can reasonably make informed, clinical decisions based on the medical and psychiatric needs of the patients rather than on the vagaries and risks inherent in a very imperfect legal system.

In this chapter, the statutory and common law of Maryland will be used as a model or framework for the legal analysis of those issues that most commonly arise in the psychiatric inpatient treatment of adolescents. This use of Maryland law carries with it no endorsement that the law is either perfect or complete and, clearly, this body of law has no jurisdictional application beyond the borders of Maryland. Maryland's law does provide, however, a fairly reasonable and structured analysis that is similar in most significant respects to the law of other states; thus, it provides an understandable structure for the resolution of these issues.

THE VOLUNTARY OR INVOLUNTARY ADMISSION OF ADOLESCENTS

The admission of minors to state and private facilities raises a number of legal issues concerning notice, consent, the nature of the admission, and the competing interests of the parent and child. As minors are generally considered incapable of consenting to inpatient psychiatric treatment, the necessary consent is provided by parents or guardians who act in the minor's stead. Such an admission would be considered a voluntary admission, as appropriate consent from an appropriate individual with power to consent has been given.

This reality creates a circumstance rife with potential conflict. Clearly, the minor may not want inpatient treatment or either parent may not believe that such treatment is appropriate. Moreover, parents do not always act in the best interests of a child and, if hospitalization serves the interests of the parents yet is deleterious to the interests of the adolescent, how can the adolescent's rights be protected, and how can the interests of the institution be protected under circumstances of conflict that reasonably point to litigation?

Throughout the 1970's, courts of various jurisdictions attempted to strike a balance between the competing and often conflicting rights of minors and parents where an inpatient psychiatric admission was sought. These conflicts were finally resolved by the United States Supreme Court in *Parham v. J.R.*, 442 U.S. 584, 99 S.Ct. 2493 (1979). The Court recognized that the minor whose parent was seeking institutionalization had a constitutionally protected liberty interest in not being confined unnecessary for medical treatment, in being free from unnecessarily bodily restraints, and from being erroneously labeled as suffering from a mental disorder. The parents' presumed competing interest was the concern for the best interest of the child and their inherent authority as parents. Therefore, the Court recognized that the parent should retain a substantial role in the decision-making. The Court also balanced the consequences and risks of an erroneous admission and concluded that the voluntary admission of a minor to a mental health facility by a parent requires inquiry by a neutral fact-finder to determine if the requirements for admission are met.

This inquiry need not entail a hearing or require legal representation or necessitate a formal procedure. Rather, the constitutional dictates of due process can be simply met. The neutral fact-finder, such as a physician, psychologist, or social worker, must interview the minor and must have the authority to refuse the admission. Moreover, the Court held that the minor's continuing need for the commitment must be reviewed periodically through the same independent procedure. Thus, for the voluntary admission of a minor not statutorily empowered to voluntarily admit himself or herself, there must be a determination by a neutral fact-finder that the minor is eligible for admission under the criteria adopted by each state.

In Maryland, a minor 16 years of age or older has the same capacity as an adult to consent to admission to a mental health facility.[1] The individual 16 years of age or older and any adult who applies for admission cannot be admitted unless they are suffering from a mental disorder, the mental disorder is susceptible to treatment or care, the individual understands the nature of the request for admission, the individual is able to give continuous assent to the admission, and the individual is able to ask for release.[2] If these criteria are met, then the individual may be admitted to the facility.

Maryland has specifically addressed the voluntary admission of minors less than 16 years of age as well (Md. Health Gen. Code Ann. § 10-610 [1982]). In that circumstance, the parent or guardian may apply for admission to nonstate facilities or to the child or adolescent unit of a state facility. The individual less than 16 years of age can be admitted only if the individual suffers from a mental disorder, if that disorder is susceptible to care or treatment, if the applicant understands the nature of the request for admission, and if assent is given by the admitting physician of the facility.[3] If the minor is being admitted to a child or adolescent unit of a state facility, then assent must be given by a physician and a psychologist, or by two physicians. Moreover, the admission to the child and adolescent unit of a state facility cannot exceed 20 days.

Maryland's statutory scheme is typical of those adopted in response to *Parham v. J.R.* States have adopted various ages at which minors may consent to their admission or mental health treatment. If the minors do not have the statutory capacity to consent to their treatment, then that treatment may be requested by a parent or a guardian. If the parent or guardian requests treatment, then a physician, psychologist, or social worker will be required to determine that the statutory criteria for admission are met.

Similarly, statutory schemes for involuntary commitment to mental health facilities are designed with recognition of the constitutional rights of individuals, including due process and liberty protections. Involuntary commitment requires that certain criteria for admission be met, that the existence of those criteria be certified by neutral parties, and that the individual be given notice and a hearing on the propriety of the admission and continued custody of the individual.[4] These involuntary commitment procedures are as applicable to children and adolescents as they are to adults. One of the required criteria is that an individual be dangerous to himself or herself or others. If a child or adolescent presents such a danger, then involuntary commitment may be sought.[5]

An additional criterion is that the individual be unable or unwilling to voluntarily seek inpatient treatment.[6] If a minor is younger than 16, then he or she is unable to consent to voluntarily seek inpatient treatment. If the parent or guardian of such a minor does not consent to treatment, then requirement of unwillingness is also met, and the minor can be involuntarily admitted. Similarly, if the minor is 16 or older, his or her consent can be given or refused; thus, the minor is treated as an adult and the adult involuntary procedure is applicable. In all of these circumstances, the health care provider is considered a neutral third party who gathers information and determines whether criteria for admission are met. Those criteria may vary based on the type of admission, and it is important that facility personnel understand the state's statutes concerning admission and consent for treatment.

After admission of the patient to an inpatient facility, the potential for conflicts between the minor patient and parents or guardians remains. Conflict issues most typically surface concerning questions of confidentiality and access to psychiatric records, informed consent to specific treatment modalities, and the reporting of suspected child abuse or neglect. The issues of consent to treatment and the reporting of abuse or neglect will be treated separately later in this chapter.

As to the confidentiality and access to psychiatric records, the law presumes that a minor who has capacity to consent to medical treatment also has the capacity to control access to the records pertaining to that treatment. In Maryland, that general proposition of law is subject to one statutory exception, namely, a minor 16 years of age or older can block access to his or her psychiatric records to all persons except his or her parents or guardians. Parents and guardians have the right to such records unless the clinician, in the exercise of his or her judgment, believes that access to the records would be deleterious to the interests of the patient.[7]

One area in which the specific conflicts of interests have been recognized is divorce and custody litigation. In many cases, parents who are in the process of divorce and are determining visitation and custody issues will seek the mental health records of their children to be used in evidence in any court proceedings. Under these circumstances, the interests of the minor in confidentiality may conflict with the parents' interests and objectives in the divorce litigation. For these reasons, Maryland requires that before records can be produced, an attorney must be appointed for the minor to make the determination as to whether the mental health records will be disclosed and under what circumstances they will be disclosed (*Nagle v. Hooks*, 296 Md. 123, 460 A.2d 49 [1983]). This is despite the fact that in Maryland parents are given the right to consent to the release of their children's mental health records.[8] Medical records custodians and health care providers should be aware of similar provisions in their state and should ascertain the purpose of a parent's acquisition-of a minor's records.

NEGLECT AND ABUSE

Anglo-American jurisprudence has historically been hostile to the imposition of generalized duties mandating that individuals act for the benefit of others. Parties to a transaction can allocate rights and duties by way of contract and if that contract is breached and damages flow from the breach, the principles of contract law provide a remedy for an aggrieved party. Similarly, in accordance with the law of negligence, a party injured by the lack of due care of another may recover in damages.

Absent the allocation of duty by private yet publicly enforceable agreements and the generalized duty to refrain from injuring another, few affirmative duties to help, protect, or secure the person or property of others have historically been imposed by the American legal system.

As an exception to this general animating spirit of law, certain classes of individuals deemed to be under a disability are frequently protected by statute or common law, and duties may well be imposed on others to facilitate the protection of those who are deemed less able at protecting their own interests. Minors and individuals of diminished capacity fall within such groups. As a consequence, most states have expanded the scope of protection afforded to persons under a disability by imposing on select third parties an obligation to further the protection of minors or affirmatively assist in the prevention of harm to them.

Beginning in the mid-1960's, all 50 states enacted some form of statutory reporting of child abuse.[9] Most of these statutes contain similar provisions regarding who must report, to whom the reports must be made, and the circumstances that require reporting. Moreover, those statutes generally provide to the reporting person or institution two key protections: a waiver of the privilege and a grant of immunity from civil suits for good faith reporting. These provisions and protections are critical lest compliance with reporting regulations or statutes place the reporter in jeopardy for potential claims of breach of privacy, defamation, false arrest, or intentional infliction of emotional distress. As strict compliance with the terms and conditions of the statutes or regulations ordinarily is a condition precedent to the protection afforded by the law, the regulations of each state must be carefully examined and followed.

In Maryland, the starting point regarding a health care provider's obligation to report physical, sexual, or mental abuse is set forth in Md. Fam. Law Code Ann. § 5-704 (1990). Under that statute, it is mandatory for a health care provider acting in his or her professional capacity who has reason to believe that a minor is subject to abuse or neglect to make an oral report to the Department of Social Services or an appropriate local law enforcement agency.

In determining a health care provider's responsibilities under this statute, a number of factors must be met. First, the abused person must be a minor as defined by Maryland law, that is any individual under the age of 18.[10] The obligation to report is imposed on a health practitioner, educator, or human service worker. Human service workers include teachers, counselors, social workers, case workers and any person authorized to practice healing in accord with state law.[11]

The statute also defines the type of abuse that must be reported. Abuse includes physical injury and sexual abuse. Reportable physical injury and sexual abuse are defined both in terms of the prescribed conduct and in terms of the identity of the actor. Physical injury is defined as physical injury by a parent or other person having permanent or temporary care or custody or responsibility for the supervision of the minor, or by any household or family member under circumstances that indicate that the minor's health or welfare is significantly harmed, or at risk of being significantly harmed.[12] Sexual abuse is defined as any act involving sexual molestation or exploitation of a minor by a parent or other person who has permanent or temporary care, custody, or responsibility for supervision, or by any household or family member. Sexual abuse includes conduct defined by Maryland's Criminal Law Code: incest, rape, sexual offense in any degree, sodomy, and unnatural or perverted sexual practices.[13]

In determining whether the physical or sexual abuse is committed by a person within the household, the statute defines the household as where the minor resides, where the abuse or neglect allegedly occurred, or where the suspect believed to have abused the minor resides. Similarly, a household member is defined as one who lives with or is a regular presence in a home of a minor at the time of the alleged abuse or neglect. For example, this might include extended family members who are living with the parents and children, live-in boyfriends or girlfriends, or siblings.

Finally, the statute defines neglect as leaving the minor unattended, or failing to give proper care and attention to the minor by its parents, guardian, or custodian under circumstances that indicate that the minor's health or welfare is significantly harmed or placed at risk or significant harm.[14]

Under the Maryland statutory scheme, reportable abuse or neglect is limited to acts or omissions of individuals who stand in some custodial role to the minor. Acts and omissions by relative strangers do not fall within the ambit of reportable offenses. The Maryland statute has as its principal goal the facilitation of intervention on behalf of a minor to provide an opportunity for the minor's protection and healing. Abuse by relative strangers is not subject to mandatory reporting, and such conduct remains a matter for the criminal process. In this regard, a clinician ought not to ignore the strict language of the applicable reporting statute and ought not to err on the side of caution. If a clinician were to report any and all cases of abuse regardless of whether the abuse technically fell under the reporting provisions of the statute or not, the clinician may well put himself at risk by voiding the protections and immunities provided under the statutory scheme. As strict compliance with the provisions of a given reporting statute protects both the minor and the reporter, shortcuts in terms of the statutory language ought not to be taken.

Once all the statutory definitions have been met, the health care providers must determine what reports should be made, when the reports must be made, and to whom the reports must go.

With respect to abuse as defined above, the health care provider must immediately make an oral report by telephone or direct communication to the Department of Social Services where the minor lives or where the abuse occurs, or to an appropriate law enforcement agency.[15] The statute defines law enforcement agencies as state, city or municipal police departments, sheriffs' offices, states' attorneys, or the attorney general's office. In instances of neglect, the health care provider is obligated to report only to the Department of Social Services. In either case, however, if the reporter is acting as a staff member of a hospital or related institution, the staff member must also immediately notify and give all information to the director of the institution, or to the director's designee.

Once the oral report has been provided to all appropriate parties, the health care provider is then obligated to provide a written report not later than 48 hours after the individual formed his or her belief of abuse or neglect. In cases of abuse, the written reports must go to the Department of Social Services and the appropriate law enforcement agency. In cases of neglect, the written report need be sent only to the Department of Social Services.

The contents of the report must include the following: the name, age, and address of the minor; the name and address of the parent or person responsible for the care of the minor; the whereabouts of the minor; the nature and extent of the abuse or neglect, including any evidence or information available to the reporter concerning possible previous instances of abuse or neglect; and all other information helpful to determine the cause of the suspected abuse or neglect, and the identity of the person responsible for the abuse or neglect.

In some instances, the communication by the health care provider to the Department of Social Services and law enforcement officers implicates the psychiatrist/patient privilege. However, the reporting statute specifically, explicitly, and clearly indicates that it overrides the psychiatrist/patient privilege.[16] In addition to the override of the privilege, the statutes also explicitly and expressly provide for immunity to all persons reporting suspected abuse or neglect pursuant to the statutes.[17]

Once the Department of Social Services and the appropriate law enforcement agency receives the reports, they will investigate the information contained therein. Pursuant to statutes, the Department of Social Services "shall be provided upon request" the medical records of the abused child.[18]

Reporting abuse may implicate some difficult questions regarding disclosure to the parents of the abused child. In cases where the minor is abused by a third person, there may be some inclination to tell the parents or to seek their permission to make the report to the appropriate individuals. However, as the statutes are mandatory in nature, no consent issues are implicated and, therefore, parental consent is not required.

Given the mandatory language of the reporting statutes, no consent from any person, the minor, his or her parents, or guardians, or anyone else is required as a precondition to reporting. However, prudent practice may well dictate the sharing of certain information. If appropriate, the abused child or adolescent ought to be told of the report that is being made and ought to be further advised that he or she can exercise no veto over the reporting of the information. In fact, it may frequently be therapeutically valuable to have the affected adolescents report the abuse themselves. Such a report does not obviate the duty imposed on the health care provider, but does allow the reporting process to become a part of the therapeutic process. Similar considerations may well obtain with the parents or guardian of the affected minor.

The obligation to report reportable abuse and neglect applies regardless of whether the minor is a patient, resident, or otherwise associated with the hospital or other health care facility. Similarly, the statute does not distinguish in any meaningful way among various sources of information. If the information is gleaned through examinations or interviews with any person and is reasonably believed and is otherwise reportable, the information must be reported.

Maryland law does distinguish, however, between a clinician's obligation to report abuse that occurred independent of the adolescent's status as an inpatient and abuse or neglect that occurs while the adolescent is a resident in an inpatient facility (Md. Health Gen. Code Ann. § 10-705 [1990]). Under this section, abuse is defined differently than in the general reporting provisions. Pursuant to § 10-705, abuse includes any physical injury or any sexual abuse, sexual act, sexual contact, or vaginal intercourse. The reporting obligations are also different. Here, any "person" who believes that an individual in a facility has been abused shall promptly report to the appropriate law enforcement agency and the administrative head of the facility. By imposing the reporting obligations on any "person," the reporting obligation goes beyond counselors, social workers, or persons authorized to practice healing under the Health Occupation Code. The persons to whom the report is given are also different. The statute requires the report to go to an appropriate law enforcement agency and the administrative head of the facility. The administrative head is then responsible to ensure that a report has gone to the appropriate law enforcement agency. The appropriate agencies are the same as defined above—local police and state's attorneys' offices.

The substance of the report under Health General § 10-705 is less defined than under the prior reporting sections. The report can be oral or written and must simply contain as much information as the reporter can provide regarding the abuse of the resident.

The immunities discussed in the prior section also apply here as well. Any reporter is immune from liability for making the report, participating in the investigation of the report, and in any judicial proceedings that follow thereafter. It is significant, however, to note that no immunity is provided to any abuse or potential abuser who makes a report or participates in the investigation or judicial proceedings.[19]

The final statutory provisions dealing with reporting requirements are included in the "patient's bill of rights."[20] Once again, the abuse and reporting requirements are fairly similar. Abuse is prohibited by the patient's bill of rights and is defined as nontherapeutic infliction of physical pain or injury, or a persistent course of conduct intended to produce, or resulting in, mental or emotional distress.

The reporting requirements are imposed on any person believing that a resident of a hospital has been abused. That person shall promptly report the alleged abuse to an appropriate law enforcement agency, the Secretary of Health and Mental Hygiene, or the Office on Aging. In determining what constitutes a prompt report, it is important to note that the statute provides that the failure to make a report in three days of learning of the abuse renders the person liable for a civil penalty of not more than $1,000. None of the prior reporting statutes carry any penalty for failing to report.

The report once again may be written or oral and shall contain as much information as the reporter is able to provide. The recipient of the report, whether the Secretary or law enforcement agency, shall notify the other entity not receiving the report. The recipient must also notify the administrator of the institution where the abuse allegedly occurred, unless the administrator is the alleged abuser.

Once again, the reporters are immune from liability for making the report or participating in investigations or judicial proceedings. The immunities section also includes immunity for the institution from participating in transferring, suspending, or terminating the employment of any individual who is believed to have abused or aided in abusing a resident.

INFORMED CONSENT

All patients or their designee have the legal right to be fully informed of the need for various treatment modalities, the nature of the treatment, and what adverse consequences could follow from the treatment in order to allow the patient to make an informed consent to treatment. As minors are not generally deemed to have the capacity to exercise informed consent, persons under the age of 18 exercise the process of informed consent by a legally established delegation of that process to a parent or guardian. The parent or guardian is fully advised of the need for treatment and its consequences, and that individual has the power to accede to or reject treatment on behalf of the minor. In response to the conflicts concerning treatment between minors and parents, most states have established by statute exceptions to the general rule. Those exceptions in Maryland are fairly typical, as they empower minors to take a more active role in consenting to certain treatments and concomitantly diminish the role, authority, and importance of a parent or a guardian's decision-making ability.

In accord with Md. Health Gen. Code Ann. § 20-103 (1982), any person 16 years or older is capable of consenting to treatment for mental or emotional disorders. Implicitly, any individuals who are 16 or older also have the right to refuse treatment for mental or emotional disorders. The consent of a parent or guardian is not necessary, nor is that consent controlling for any minor 16 or older. The statute does provide, however, that disclosure of the treatment may be provided by the clinician to the parents or guardian if the clinician believes that such a disclosure is warranted in his or her clinical judgment.[21] As a practical matter, such a disclosure, if not injurious to the patient's treatment, ought to be made in order to better ally the parents or guardians with the treatment process.

Additionally, any minor who is married or who is the parent of a child is deemed under Maryland law to have the capacity to consent to medical treatment and need not delegate that right or power to any other person.[22] Similarly, if the minor is in need of emergency treatment, capacity to consent is again presumed regardless of age. In other specified instances, treatment and advice may be provided to a minor without the parents' consent. Those specified instances include treatment for or advice regarding drugs, alcohol, venereal disease, pregnancy, conception, rape, and sexual offenses.[23] As treatment in all of those instances can present conflicts between parents and adolescents (conflicts that may jeopardize the rights and health of adolescents), treatment can be provided without parental consent. In those instances, parents or guardians can be informed of treatment, however, if the clinician believes in the exercise of his or her clinical judgment that disclosure would benefit the patient. Similarly under Maryland law, if a parent or guardian has consented to the treatment of a son or daughter for alcohol or drug abuse, that consent cannot be voided by the minor, as the minor under those circumstances has no legal right to refuse treatment.[24]

The process of informed consent is a good therapeutic tool, and it exposes the clinician to few legal risks. The documentation of informed consent is essential and easy. Most acute care and long-term hospitals present to a patient in the admission process a generalized form of near universal consent that the patient then executes. Although such forms are prudent and necessary, they frequently are insufficient. Informed consent is a process. Consequently, a patient's chart ought to contain specific entries documenting informed consent at the initiation of any treatment modality or at the time of any significant change in treatment. The chart should reflect the reasons for the treatment, an indication that all reasonably probable effects of that treatment were discussed with the patient, and the fact that the patient consented to the treatment. No specific form is required; it is merely necessary that the record entry be clear and complete. Additionally, specific forms may be required to document informed consent for the initiation of particular treatment modalities that are more controversial or more invasive; consequently, hospital administrators need to be fairly conversant with the statutory mandates that have been enacted in their jurisdiction.

If treatment is initiated without an informed consent, the health care provider can be answerable in damages for violation of the patient's rights. Moreover if the patient who has not given informed consent to treatment is in any way harmed or injured by the treatment, damages are recoverable in a malpractice action regardless of whether the treatment in question complied with the applicable standard of care. In those general circumstances in which a minor is presumed to lack capacity to consent and the consent is secured through a parent or guardian, a failure to secure the appropriate informed consent can generate a claim prosecuted on behalf of the minor. As a parent or guardian is acting for the minor, any claim or potential cause of action inures to the benefit of the minor, not the parent or guardian.

AVOIDING MALPRACTICE AND WORKING WITH THE LEGAL SYSTEM

Many clinicians view the legal process with disdain and apprehension and the courthouse as an arcane and adversarial arena that produces nothing more than delay and an opportunity for gamesmanship. Such a view in and of itself cripples a clinician's ability or the ability of a psychiatric institution to deal effectively with the legal process.

Statutorily and judge-made law and procedure are often a product of the need to balance competing interests in a procedural framework that embodies a notion of fundamental fairness. Moreover, the orientation or perspective of the law frequently competes with the orientation of the clinician. Physicians concern themselves with the health of patients, lawyers with the rights of individuals. In the litigation context, physicians focus on the patient and what was known about the patient's condition and what was done in response to that knowledge. In litigation, lawyers focus on the patient's medical records, on what was written about that patient, and on what was not known about the patient's condition or on what was not done. In the first instance, therefore, clinicians must recognize this difference in perspective in order to effectively work within the legal system.

In devising institutional policies and procedures that are animated in principal part by statutory provisions or the common law, administrators and clinicians ought not to sacrifice their judgment or their commitment to sound clinical decisions. Where the law directly affects the admissions, treatment, transfer, or discharge of patients, administrators must decide what is in the best interests of their patients and their institutions and *then* consult with their attorneys.

Administrators or clinicians should ask the attorneys how they can best accomplish their goals, what risks are created by the accomplishment of their goals, and how those risks can best be minimized. If attorneys are merely asked what an institution can or cannot do, they may in fact tell the hospital and may inappropriately set policies and practices that are deleterious to the best interests of the patients. Similarly, the medical community must appreciate a simple fact known to most practicing attorneys; namely, most conduct falls within the interstices of definitive law, and thus, easy and certain answers rarely exist.

The crafting of careful and explicit procedures in conjunction with informed legal analysis can reduce institutional legal risk, but to reduce that individual legal risk that may arise in dealing with a particular patient, more needs to be done. In this regard, no function is more important than the total education of every member of the staff of the treating institution.

Litigation is necessarily adversarial. Claims for violation of individual rights or for malpractice require, in the first instance, a complaining party. Patients and their families who believe that they have been provided complete information and involved in every step of a decision-making process concerning treatment are less likely to assert a claim than those who feel excluded from any portion of the therapeutic process. A good, caring, and communicative bedside manner is the best insurance any clinician can ever obtain. If the patient and key family members are involved in the decision-making process and the treatment process, they develop a stake in the success of the outcome and are more likely to perceive themselves as essential members of a caring team. Teammates ordinarily do not sue one another.

Just as increasing the size of the circle of care can lessen the risk of litigation, so, too, can increasing the circle of consultation reduce the risks confronted in litigation. Consultation should be freely sought and freely given, and all consultations, formal or informal, ought to be recorded. In court, it is easier for a litigant to attack the judgment of one clinician than it is to attack the informed judgment of several clinicians. In order to recover in a malpractice action, a plaintiff must establish by a preponderance of evidence that the clinician's conduct breached the applicable standard of care. In all jurisdictions, the standard of care references the reasonable and ordinary response that most clinicians would make to most patients under similar circumstances. Consequently, the greater the number of professionals who participate in treatment decisions, the greater the likelihood that a judge or jury will find that the treatment comported with the standard of care.

Nearly all interactions with the patients need to be recorded. In the courtroom, the patient's medical records can save or destroy a clinician. In the first instance, the records must be complete; in the second instance, they must detail the decision-making process. Negative findings or conclusions as well as positive findings must be noted. In litigation, the plaintiff will not merely attack the propriety of what was done but will attempt to impeach the process by which it was done. Expert witnesses retained by the plaintiff will testify as to those factors that should have been considered before treatment was initiated or discontinued. From this slender evidentiary thread, the plaintiff's attorney will argue that had the clinician known what they did not know or had the clinician considered what he or she did not consider, then the outcome would have been different. If the medical records detail the decision-making process, this facially appealing argument is negated.

Moreover, lawsuits are rarely initiated immediately after a bad outcome. More often than not, a period of time, including years, may go by before a claim formally surfaces by way of a court filing. The eventual trial may still be another year or two distant. As memories fade over time, the medical records will be used by all parties as the embodiment of the now distantly remembered reality. Clinicians frequently cannot recall with absolute assurance every aspect of the patient's care or of the decision-making process that mandated that care. Consequently, the medical records must be complete and ought to be written as effective and defensible summaries for subsequent legal proceedings. Similarly, as legal claims follow bad outcomes, institutions ought to establish regular procedures for the review and investigation of bad outcomes. Additional and supplemental information that may be of use ought to be recorded; if recorded, it should be noted in such a way that its discovery and subsequent admission into evidence at trial will not injure the interests of the institution or clinicians.

In the formulation of policy, in the education of staff, and in the defense of legal claims, hospitals should work closely with their attorneys and constantly seek from counsel better ideas and strategies to reduce risk while providing the highest level of psychiatric care. Similarly, if the hospital counsel is better educated to the needs, practical realities, and concerns of the hospital practice, then counsel will be better able to protect the hospital's interest.

[1]   Md. Health Gen. Code Ann. § 10–609(a) (1982).
[2]   Md. Health Gen. Code Ann. § 10–609(c) (1982).
[3]   Md. Health Gen. Code Ann § 10–610(c) (1982).
[4]   *See e.g.*, Md. Health Gen. Code Ann. § 10–613, *et seq.*
[5]   *See e.g.*, Md. Health Gen. Code Ann. § 10–617(a)(3) (1982).
[6]   *See e.g.*, Md. Health Gen. Code Ann. § 10–617(a)(4).
[7]   Md. Health Gen. Code Ann. § 20–104 (1982).
[8]   Md. Health Gen. Code Ann. § 4–302(a)(4)(ii) (1982).
[9]   Davis, Rights of Juveniles § 5A.3(b) (2d ed. 1992).
[10] Family Law § 5–701(d). Md. Health Gen. Code Ann. § 5–701(d).
[11] Family Law § 5–704(a); § 5–701(f), (h); Md. Fam. Law Code Ann. §§ 5–704(a); 5–701(f), (h).
[12] Md. Fam. Law Code Ann. § 5–701(b)(i) (1992).
[13] Md. Fam. Law Code Ann. § 5–701(b)(ii) (1992).
[14] Md. Fam. Law Code Ann. § 5–701(n) (1992).
[15] Md. Fam. Law Code Ann. § 5–704 (1992).
[16] Md. Fam. Law Code Ann. § 5–704(a) (1992).
[17] Md. Fam. Law Code Ann. § 5–708 (1992); *Freed v. Worchester Co. Dept. of Social Services*, 69 Md.App. 447, 518 A.2d 159 (1986). In an earlier case, *Catteron v. Coale*, 84 Md.App. 337, 579 A.2d 781 (1990), *cert. denied*, 321 Md. 638, 584 A.2d 67 (1991), the Court held that allegations that reporting done in bad faith or maliciously, overcame the statutory immunity. The Court's rationale was based in part upon the prior statutory language that explicitly required the reporting to be done in "good faith." Subsequent to the *Catteron* decision, the Maryland Legislature amended the statutes to delete the "good faith" language from the reporting statutes. As the Legislature is deemed to have acted in response to judicial decisions when amending statutes, a fair reading of this course of events indicates that the good faith requirement to immunity has been abolished, and that any and all reporting is privileged.
[18] Md. Fam. Law Code Ann. § 5–711 (1992).
[19] Md. Cts. & Jud. Proc. Code Ann. § 5–370 (1991).
[20] Md. Health Gen. Code Ann. § 19–347 (1982).
[21] Md. Health Gen. Code Ann. § 20–104(b) (1982).
[22] Md. Health Gen. Code Ann. § 20–102(a) and (b) (1982).
[23] Md. Health Gen. Code Ann. § 20–102(c) (1982).
[24] Md. Health Gen. Code Ann. § 20–102(c)(1) (1982).

Chapter 18

RESEARCH ISSUES IN ADOLESCENT INPATIENT PSYCHIATRY

Wells Goodrich

INTRODUCTION

Studies (Milazzo-Sayre, 1986; Almqvist 1986) of the hospitalization of severely disturbed adolescents estimate that between three and six percent of adolescents are psychiatrically hospitalized. The actual number of adolescents placed in various types of hospitals and treatment settings fluctuates over time due to political and funding patterns (Woolston, 1991). The best estimates are that at least 50,000 adolescents are placed in residential treatment each year in the United States and perhaps a larger number in inpatient psychiatric hospital settings (Lewis & Summerville, 1991; Cates, 1991). An analysis by Edwards (1991) of 10,898 youths being treated in 1987 by 162 institutions reported the duration of treatment averaged 16 months, with a median of 14 months.

In a survey of hospital admission data of 800 adolescents from 12 private psychiatric hospitals in 1985 and 1987, Miller (1988) revealed that the disturbed behavior that led to hospitalization consisted of school failure (85 percent of cases), self-destructive and assaultive behavior (50 percent), drug or alcohol abuse (50 percent) and difficulties with the law (40 percent). Over one-third presented symptoms of sexual acting out or running away from home, and one-fifth demonstrated psychotic symptoms. Fifty-five percent were male, and the patients ranged in age from five years to 18 years, with a median age of 15 years. Prior to admission, families reported an average four-year duration for serious symptomatic behavior and a prior outpatient-plus-inpatient treatment duration of two years. Only one-third of these adolescents were living with both their biological parents; 20 to 30 percent were adoptees, in contrast with the expected frequency in the general population of approximately 5 percent adoptees.

Research on such treatment is at an early exploratory stage. This chapter will review research studies relevant to the complex enterprise of inpatient psychiatric hospitalization. Methodological issues will then be discussed, followed by a suggested model (Goodrich, 1987) for hospital or residential treatment that has been applied at Chestnut Lodge Hospital over the past decade.

REVIEW OF THE LITERATURE

The literature on inpatient hospitalization of adolescents can be considered either unmanageably voluminous or incredibly scant depending on one's perspective. Adolescent inpatients have served as subjects for hundreds of studies investigating personality traits, diagnoses, genetics, family patterns, and so on. But if we look at the research about processes and outcome of inpatient treatment, the field suddenly narrows to a few compromised exploratory studies. Why is this?

In order to be useful to the clinician, the research investigator must answer the following questions: 1) Diagnostically, how can one describe adolescents on admission to the hospital? 2) How severely disturbed are these groups of adolescents? 3) How do these adolescents differ among themselves in significant aspects of their developmental histories? 4) How do the above data serve to predict response to treatment interventions carried out during hospitalization? 5) How do clinicians make judgments about discharge planning and about the necessity for extended inpatient or outpatient follow-up treatment? 6) How do these cohorts of adolescents appear after having received hospital treatment when studied at one-, three-, and five-year follow-up assessments?

Appropriate methods for use in research designs aimed at answering the above questions have only recently been developed. Most hospitals have enough difficulty financing the complex treatment itself and have not considered research studies to be an essential enough part of the hospital treatment program to fund this expensive enterprise.

Only recently has the field of child and adolescent psychiatry begun to realize the wide significance of dual, triple, or even quadruple diagnosis (Biederman et al., 1992). Kaminer (1991) studied the co-morbidity of substance abuse with mood disorders, conduct disorder, anxiety disorders, adjustment disorders, and personality disorders. He concluded that substance-abusing adolescents suffer in addition from a 25 to 50 percent frequency of conduct disorders, a 25 to 60 percent frequency of mood disorders, and a 12 to 17 percent frequency of mood plus conduct disorders. From his review of the literature, he estimates that perhaps as many as 70 percent of hospitalized adolescents may also suffer from substance abuse.

In a similar vein, Salyer Holmstrom & Noshpitz (1991), commented upon the frequency of learning disabilities among patients with severe psychopathologies, particularly borderline personality disorders. Biederman et al. (1991) have documented the co-morbidity of Attention Deficit Hyperactivity Disorders with Conduct, Depressive, Anxiety, and other disorders. Thus, it becomes apparent that in order to do justice to the question of diagnosis at the time of hospital admission, all investigations will have to report patterns of diagnostic combinations.

One significant area for research is to investigate how admission characteristics of adolescents may vary depending upon the hospital setting. Inamdhar et al. (1982), at the public Bellevue Hospital in New York City, investigated the association between intensely destructive behavior to self and others with the diagnosis of psychosis. They found that 85 percent of their psychotic patients showed either intense hostile destructiveness to others or self-destructive behavior, or both. Delga et al. (1989), in a rare replication study, repeated this design in a private hospital setting and found that psychotic adolescents admitted to this private hospital did not show significant frequency of self-destructiveness or destructiveness to others. Since more affluent families have easier access to inpatient treatment prior to the emergence of extreme forms of maladaptive behavior, violence and suicidality as expressions of psychotic pathology may be more frequently observed in public hospitals than in private hospitals.

To what extent can admission history data be used to predict the patient's behavioral response to treatment interventions within the hospital? Using a reliable rating scale to capture admission self-destructiveness and hostile aggressive behavior, Fritsch et al. (1992) demonstrated that preadmission high levels of external aggression predicted high levels of hostility and unmanageability after one month on the inpatient unit. Similarly, preadmission histories showing high levels of self-destructive behavior predicted self-destructive behavior while hospitalized.

The question of how clinicians evaluate the patient's need for longer length of hospitalization has been addressed in studies by Barber et al. (1992) and Ghuman et al. (1989). Barber studied experienced clinicians' criteria for longer length of hospitalization and showed that longer hospitalization was recommended when the patient suffered from multiple diagnoses, including personality disorders plus substance abuse. Additional factors were chronicity and severity of illness, the absence of family stability, and poor response to medication. In a study of hospital records contrasting the characteristics of short-term versus long-term patients, Ghuman et al. discovered 11 significant characteristics of long-term patients which included chronicity, younger age of onset, substance abuse, severe family pathology, and previous hospital elopement.

The best outcome data have been provided by Gossett et al. (1983) whose persistence led to their locating 85 percent of 176 hospitalized adolescent patients who were studied an average of five years postdischarge. At follow-up, 80 to 90 percent of least severely ill adolescents ("neurotics") were functioning adequately, 50 to 60 percent of moderately ill adolescents ("personality disorders") were functioning adequately, and only 25 to 30 percent of chronic psychotic adolescents were functioning adequately. Poor outcome was predicted by severity and chronicity of psychopathology upon admission, as well as by severity of family pathology and dysfunction. Good outcome was predicted by intelligence quotient, by completing the recommended treatment program, and by the patient having continued outpatient psychotherapy following hospital discharge. Gossett et al.'s study serves as a model for research on the long-term results of inpatient hospitalization. Replication studies and research improving upon their design are needed.

More recently, Pfeiffer and Strzelecki (1990) discussed Blotcky et al.'s (1984) narrative review of outcome studies for adolescent hospitalization and applied statistical procedures intended to integrate the results of these studies as well as adding more recent reports. The results in review involve 34 studies of both children and adolescents in residential psychiatric treatment. Similar to previous authors, Pfeiffer and Strzelecki (1990) concluded that neurological dysfunction (organicity), diagnosis of psychotic disorder or undersocialized aggressive conduct disorder, and symptoms felt to be bizarre or antisocial were most important in predicting poor outcome. Family functioning and family involvement in treatment, and treatment variables such as planned discharge, completion of a treatment program, and involvement in aftercare services were all related to improved outcome. Cornsweet (1990), Gable and Shindledecker (1992) agree with these conclusions in their reviews.

In the most extensive review to date of problems in outcome research on residential treatment and inpatient hospitalization, Curry (1991) comments that although these studies have made significant contributions to our knowledge, "because of the lack of a comparison group, within-program and between-subject designs are inherently incapable of addressing the question of the effectiveness of a specific program or treatment." Yet, he believes that most adolescent patients appear to improve and only a few appear to get worse. "Subject variables including the severity of illness and the type of disorder . . . appear to set limits on what can be achieved with such treatment." The adjustment of the patient within the program does not predict adjustment at follow-up period, but the degree of support and continuity of significant relationships following hospitalization does seem to predict better adjustment at follow-up. Other implications can be derived from research findings to date, such as: 1) hospitalized adolescents need extensive aftercare treatment; and 2) continued therapy with the family for extensive periods of time is critical to long-term outcome. Curry concludes that further studies require more attention by investigators to the conceptualization of treatment programs and processes as well as to more frequent follow-up observations.

METHODOLOGICAL AND DESIGN ISSUES

Research on psychiatric inpatient hospitalization requires reliable observations on the short-term and long-term impact upon the patients of hospital interventions. Such research involves observations applied repeatedly from admission to discharge and follow-up. A repeated-measures design can establish whether positive or negative changes have occurred in these patients. In preparing a research design, investigators need to consider routine application of reliable methods to all patients to assess: 1) demographic data; 2) diagnosis; 3) severity of illness; 4) inventory of earlier developmental stresses, deficits and personality strengths; and 5) inventory of symptoms that become targets for clinical concern and intervention. During hospitalization, staff can obtain observations repeatedly over time on the patients' adaptations within the milieu. If resources are available, it is also valuable to set up reliable indices of patients' performances within each of the specific programs, e.g. responses to school, to group or individual therapy, and to medication. The theoretical convictions of the clinicians guiding the program can be evaluated by the recording of the specific changes in the patients that are anticipated in response to programs and interventions believed to be mutative.

Patients who improve rapidly in the hospital can be seen as demonstrating the effectiveness of the program, as well as demonstrating their own preadmission strengths. Patients who fail to improve can be seen as demonstrating the limits of the effectiveness of the hospital program as well as their own preadmission deficits. Since most follow-up studies have demonstrated a closer relationship between admission and follow-up data than between data gathered at hospital discharge and at follow up (Lewis et al., 1980), it is important not to use data gathered at the time of discharge to make predictions about the patient's future in the community. This is not to underestimate the significance of improvement observed within the hospital (Robinson et al., 1990). These investigators studied depression and severity of illness in 22 hospitalized children and adolescents and found a high frequency of improvement demonstrated at the time of discharge. Similar data using the DSM-III-R GAF Scale on over 60 patients showed an average improvement in its GAF Scale from a mean of 40 at admission to 60 at discharge (Goodrich & Fullerton, 1986). In general, a patient's condition at discharge is positively influenced by hospital containment; however, the true index of improvement is autonomous functioning after a considerable postdischarge period.

A basic research design for studying adolescent inpatient treatment must include reliable and valid instruments for characterizing the patient in regard to numbers 1 to 5 below, for assessing change across time in the hospital, as in number 6 below, and for evaluating the patient after return to the community, number 7:

1. *Demographic and Family Data*: Age, sex, socioeconomic status, adoption, family genetic history of psychiatric disorders. The current literature demonstrates significant differences in diagnoses, as well as in treatment effects, related to these variables.

2. *Diagnosis*: Two validated reliable structured interviews with rating scales for each interview question are suitable for obtaining an Axis I diagnoses from DSM III-R. These are the Diagnostic Interview Schedule for Children and Adolescents (DICA) (Reich et al., 1982) and the Schedule for Affective Disorders and Schizophrenia for School Age Children (6-18 years) K-SADS-P (Orvaschel & Puig-Antich, 1987; Ambrosini et al., 1989). Either method covers most of the Axis I diagnoses and can be carried out by interviewing the patient or a close relative. Time required is 40 to 60 minutes.

   For Axis II, DSM-III-R, the Millon et al. (1989) questionnaire or the Loranger et al. (1987) interview may be considered. The Millon is less thorough but more convenient, taking only 15 minutes for the patient to complete; the more detailed Loranger interview takes two hours for clinician and patient to complete.

3. *Severity of Illness*: The Global Assessment of Functioning Scale

(abbreviated either GAS or GAF) from DSM-III-R (1987), is a valuable tool for demonstrating improvement or failure to improve when it is administered repeatedly. Robinson et al. (1990) and Fritsch and Goodrich (1990) have demonstrated the efficiency of the GAS with the Nurses' Behavioral Rating Scales (see number 6) to demonstrate improvement between admission and discharge. The GAS can also be used in follow-up studies.

4. *Developmental and Family History*: Milestones and specific trauma and stresses should be documented for each developmental stage of the patient. Such inquiry can balance information about the family environment with concrete description of the patient's pattern of behavior and responses at each stage. Death and other severe stresses, such as geographical moves or parental conflict or divorce and changes in family composition, need to be recorded. These may correlate with treatment-relevant responses. For example, Yates et al. (1989) on a sample of 114 inpatient adolescents, demonstrated among patients most severely ill on admission a significant increase in grandparent death during the first two years of life, accompanied by maternal depression.

Pfeiffer and Strzelecki (1990), in a review of outcome studies, noted the close relationship between level of family functioning and outcome. Van Hasselt et al. (1992) established the very high rate of physical and other family abuse in earlier childhood when adolescents are hospitalized for substance abuse plus various psychiatric disorders. Lewis (1989) provided instruments for assessing family psychopathology and Edman et al. (1990) for family cohesion and adaptability.

5. *Symptom Rating Scales*: Achenbach and Edelbrock (1983) have developed the "*Child Behavior Checklist*" (CBCL), which is a useful and reliable instrument that accurately surveys the range of child behavioral difficulties. It can be filled out within 15 minutes by school teachers and parents as well as by other observers. Repeated measures can demonstrate progress or lack thereof.

6. *Nurses Behavioral Rating Scale*: Since nurses are more intimately involved with the adolescents than other staff, it is important to establish their observations of the patients. Fritsch and Goodrich (1990) have combined scales covering relevant domains of inpatient behavior including antisocial behavior, depression, and psychotic behavior. This instrument has shown a significant relationship with preadmission data (Delga et al., 1989) and postadmission psychological test data (Fritsch et al., 1990).

7. *Follow-Up Methods*: Gossett et al. (1983) used a structured interview with the patient or close relative, tape recording the data when possible (confidentiality is guaranteed and informed consent signed). Blotcky (1988) has also developed a questionnaire for follow-up purpose.

If all of the above methods were to be combined, this design would provide an expensive and ambitious undertaking requiring significant funding. Nevertheless, a simple design including selected methods for establishing admission psychopathology and using a repeated measures design with CBCL and GAS, along with the brief nurses' scale, will generate much new knowledge relatively inexpensively. Even a brief telephone tape-recorded follow-up interview or postdischarge questionnaire is far more useful than no data at all about the patient's condition one or more years following discharge.

EVALUATION OF TREATMENT PROCESSES

Despite the present preoccupation with accumulating reliable behavioral observations on disturbed adolescents without regard to the adolescent's internal experiential states and personality changes (Dalton & Forman, 1992), mental health providers must come to understand the "how" and "why" of success or failure in treatment. Woolston (1989) has provided a pragmatic model to guide treatment planning during short-term hospitalization which advocates prioritizing a focus on readily modifiable aspects of patient responses and environmental stresses in an attempt to return the patient rapidly to the community. Blotcky and Gossett (1989) has reviewed four common conceptual frames of reference included in most long-term hospital programs. They refer to these as the: 1) Developmental Model emphasizing "corrective emotional experience" and learning improved, age-appropriate adaptation; 2) Delinquency Model, including concepts of resocialization through "lifespace interviews"; 3) Family Systems Model, focusing on improved separation-individuation processes; and 4) Psychoanalytic Model, focusing on insight and new identifications. They also comment on the widespread use of the concepts of resistance and phases of working through defenses and conflicts. Unwin (1968) suggested five stages of change: (a) resistance and engagement; (b) testing the milieu; (c) learning to inhibit maladaptive behavior; (d) consolidating the therapeutic relationship; and (e) development of health or neurosis. Masterson and Costello (1980) preferred the constructs: (a) testing; (b) working through; and

(c) separation, whereas Rinsley (1980) suggested: (a) resistance; (b) definitive phase; and (c) resolution.

For research purposes, the Chestnut Lodge research group has proposed a simplified version of current psychodynamic, interpersonal, and developmentally based concepts (see Figure 18.1). This model assumes that the patient's ability to develop new and more rational self-and-other percepts will require a prolonged period of careful self-scrutiny and self-questioning about past patterns of interpersonal relationships. To contain the psychopathologically based patterns of disturbed behavior sufficiently to permit such an internal focus of interest and a restructuring of personality requires the adolescent to develop and maintain a working alliance with treatment team members over a prolonged period of time. The close connection between dependent attachment ("positive transference") and the therapeutic alliance has been commented on by Freud (1912) with respect to adults in psychoanalysis and reported by Luborsky et al.'s (1983) research on outpatient psychotherapy with adults. Improved scientific understanding of positive changes during hospital-based treatment, therefore, will arise after investigators have learned more about the conditions that support adolescent attachment, alliance, self-observation, insight, and change in self-and-other perceptions.

A systematic survey of values and concepts used by clinical staff to guide their interventions with severely disturbed children and adolescents in residential treatment revealed a similar treatment process model. This model grew out of an investigation of 240 behavioral reports of child interventions obtained from all disciplines with direct inpatient responsibilities (Goodrich and Boomer, 1958). This study, carried out on Fritz Redl's (1991) unit at the National Institute of Mental Health, revealed that staff interventions were designed to support patients with anxiety or depression; to prevent, limit, or contain disruptive behavior; to promote self-observation and self-evaluation; to encourage positive relatedness and motivation; and to promote insight and more adaptive self-concepts.

Clinical experience indicates that adolescent patients tend to show different changes depending upon the phase of treatment (see Figure 18.1): early, middle, or late (Goodrich, 1987). During the first phase, the assessment and containment phase, efforts are made by the treatment team to develop a treatment alliance with the patient and the family. This working collaboration grows out of a trusting attachment. This alliance supports the patient and family in their acceptance of the staff's assessments, limit setting, and interpretations. Over the early weeks in the hospital, less disturbed patients often show amelioration of symptomatic behavior resulting from this engagement and from the structure, support,

Phases	Patient Processes	Staff Interventions	Disturbed Concepts of Self and Others
1)	<u>Attachments</u> <u>Therapeutic Alliances &</u> <u>Transferences</u>	<u>Limit Setting</u> <u>Support</u> with anxiety-laden conflicts Intensive Observation and Assessment	
2)	<u>Improved Communication</u> <u>& Observation</u> <u>New Identifications &</u> <u>New Insights</u>	<u>Clarification/Confrontation</u> about repetitive transference conflicts/ defenses <u>Resocialization</u> (Promoting new coping adaptive behavior)	
3)	<u>Testing</u> new self-concepts & <u>Separating</u> from the hospital	<u>Interpreting</u> unconscious meaning of symptomatic behavior <u>Supporting New Adaptive Capacities</u>	More Realistic Concepts of SELF and OTHERS

Figure 18.1. Work of Treatment

and containment of the inpatient unit. Staff support with issues of conflict and anxiety, opening up communication, and identifying sources of difficulties, as well as staff members beginning to suggest solutions, may lead to greater self-control, a diminishing of disturbed behaviors, and the reemergence of hope in the patient.

During the second phase of treatment, whether the adolescent is an inpatient or outpatient, the treatment processes continue but with an emphasis on improving communication barriers within the family, teaching both patient and family better self-observation, and modifying long-standing conflicts. Resolving the patient's distorted self-perceptions as well as his or her inaccurate perceptions of family members and others is centrally relevant to this middle phase. The treatment team pays special attention to the emergence of repetitive transference processes which are projected into the treatment relationship.

These need clear labeling and tactful interpretation, otherwise the alliance may be lost and the patient's progress toward honest self-evaluation blocked. The phase is a prolonged one; when successful, it promotes the emergence of a new sense of self in the adolescent—more positive and resourceful with accompanying concrete future life plans.

The third phase of the treatment process emerges when the patient demonstrates greater insight, as well as a stable period of greater self-control, diminished anxiety, and improved relationships with the family and the community. The patient begins to take greater responsibility for his or her work and school, as well as care in selecting friends. The treatment team encourages the patient in these developments and collaborates in a plan for hospital discharge. During this phase of diminished supervision, the patient may regress and show a return to initial symptoms. At such a time, the treatment team will, with collaboration from the family, temporarily reinstitute greater support and control over the patient.

Recent data gathered at Chestnut Lodge Hospital are consistent with this model of process. Over the past decade, Goodrich, Fritsch, and Fullerton have developed a maturity of attachment scale for use in rating the quality of adolescent attachment experiences as regards mature-integrated attachment versus immature-disorganized attachment. This scale can be reliably rated from a semistructured interview with the patient. The interview focuses on reports of actual experiences of attachment, support, possessiveness, separation anxiety, and dependency. In a sample of 77 patients, Fritsch, Goodrich and deMarneffe (1992) studied correlates of this *maturity of attachment* measure with 16 demographic, behavioral, psychopathological, and other treatment variables. Attachment scores were significantly correlated with the adolescents' therapeutic *alliance* (collaboration with the work of the treatment program), internal *locus of control* (a sense of self-direction in the adolescent rather than the adolescent experiencing his or her behavior as being controlled by outside forces), symptomatic *improvement* over the first three months' hospitalization, and older *age* at admission. These findings are consistent with the earlier study (Fritsch & Goodrich, 1990), which observed adolescents after three months and after 15 months in the hospital and found that less severely ill patients, i.e., those with higher Global Assessment Scale scores, made more mature attachments earlier in treatment.

These data also showed that maturity of attachment observed during the third month of hospitalization was more likely to occur in depressed adolescents than in narcissistic or psychotic adolescents. Note the similarity of this finding to the findings from reviews of follow-up studies by Gossett, Blotcky, Pfeiffer, and others that psychotic patients and personality-disordered adolescents have poorer outcomes. A recent study used hospital runaway behavior as an indicator of impulsive and treatment-resistant behavior in hospitalized adolescents. Here, the data showed that runaway behavior is highest among adolescents who initially form friendships with peers only and avoid positive relationships with staff (Goodrich & Fullerton, 1984).

What begins to emerge from these studies is that the overall severity of illness tends to undermine both the positive attachment and the working alliance with these patients. Severity of psychiatric illness may also interfere with improved communication, self-observation, the development of insight, and more adaptive percepts of self and other.

DIRECTIONS IN RESEARCH

Nearly all existing studies of inpatient treatment can be criticized as containing the effects of specific hospital environments or admission policies, or the effects of specific cohorts within a larger, heterogeneous hospital population. The answer to such criticism of inadequate sampling lies in carefully designed interhospital collaborative studies. Planning of such interhospital collaborative efforts must be informed by preparatory research on the course and outcome of specific Axis I and Axis II diagnoses. Patterns of psychopathology in severely disturbed adolescents that involve common clusters of diagnoses require careful study. For example, one could compare treatment process and outcome data on the complex of conduct-disordered, narcissistic personalities with and without depression, since such contrasting patterns are widely represented in most hospitals.

There is a need for studies of specific treatment programs and interventions that comprise most hospitals' treatment approach. The field requires more information about the changes that identifiable groups of adolescents show within the special school setting, within family therapy, within the nursing milieu, and in response to medication (see Table 18.1). It appears that many patients improve first within the school situation, often reversing an average of two years' loss in achievement level within six to 12 months. Patients vary in whether their growth and development is more enhanced in family therapy as compared with individual or group therapy. Research investigations are needed to clarify the significance of each of these programs within the overall hospital efforts at fostering improvement.

Clinicians shy away from clinical research for many reasons. However, research is quite feasible in most clinical settings and might focus on the effectiveness of specific interventions. Confidentiality can be assured and informed consent for research obtained conveniently at the time of hospital admission. If the program is particularly invested in family therapy, the patient's response to family therapy interventions could be the focus. If the program is a behavioral reward program, responses to that can be systematically recorded. Short-term and long-term changes in severity of illness and in social adaptation can be systematically rated

Table 18.1: Model for Hospital Treatment

PERSONALITY DYSFUNCTION	TREATMENT INTERVENTION
1. COGNITIVE SKILLS	SCHOOL
2. AFFECT MODULATION }	
3. IMPULSE EXPRESSION }	MILIEU
4. SELF-OTHER PERCEPTS }	
5. CONFLICTS/DEFENSES }	PSYCHOTHERAPY
6. PSYCHOPHYSIOLOGY	MEDICATION
7. FAMILY PATHOLOGY	FAMILY THERAPY

using a Global Assessment Scale, Child Behavior Checklist, nurses' rating, and brief structured interviews. If these observations are controlled for diagnosis and severity of illness on admission, information will emerge about the effectiveness of these treatments. Periodic inpatient reassessment will provide mean change scores for specific types of patients. While the condition at discharge has been demonstrated to be largely an effect of hospital containment and support, the patient's condition following discharge from hospital reflects the patient's ability to function freely and autonomously in the community. Follow-up data test the patient's true gains from hospitalization and evaluate the longer-term effectiveness of inpatient adolescent hospitalization.

REFERENCES

Achenbach, T.M. and Edelbrock, R.C. (1983). *Manual for the Child Behavior Checklist and revised Profile*, Univ. of Vermont Dept. of Psychiatry.

Almqvist, F. (1986). Psychiatric hospital treatment of young people. *Acta Psychiatrica Scand.*, 73, 289-294.

Ambrosini, P.J., et al. (1989). Videotape Reliability of the Third Revised Edition of the K-SADS. *J. of Amer. Acad. Child Adolescent Psychiatry, 28*, 723-728.

Barber, C.C., Allen, J.G. and Coyne, L. (1992). Optimal length of stay in child and adolescent psychiatric hospitalization. *American Journal of Orthopsychiatry, 62* (3), 458-463.

Biederman, J., Newcorn, J., and Sprich, S. (1991). Co-morbidity of attention deficit hyperactivity disorder with conduct, depressive, anxiety, and other disorders. *American Journal of Psychiatry, 148,* 564-577.

Biederman, J. et al. (1992). Research forum on "Psychiatric Co-morbidity." Annual Meeting Program, American Academy of Child and Adolescent Psychiatry, Washington, D.C.

Blotcky, M.J. (1988). Personal communication.

Blotcky, M.J., Dimperio, T.L. and Gossett, J.T. (1984). Follow-up of children treated in psychiatric hospitals: A review of studies. *Amer. J. Psychiatry, 141,* 1499-1507.

Blotcky, M.J. and Gossett, J.T. (1989). Psychiatric inpatient treatment for adolescents. *Psychiatric Hospital, 20,* 85-93.

Cates, J.A. (1991). Residential treatment in the 1980s, part II: Characteristics of treatment centers. *Residential Treatment for Children and Youth, 9,* 75-84.

Cornsweet, C. (1990). A review of research on hospital treatment of children and adolescents. *Bull. Menninger Clinic, 54,* 64-67.

Curry, J.F. (1991). Outcome research on residential treatment: Implications and suggested directions. *Amer. J. Orthopsychiatry, 61,* 348-357.

Dalton, R., & Forman, M.A. (1992). *Psychiatric hospitalization of school-aged children.* (pp. 61-70). American Psychiatric Press.

Delga, I., Heinssen, R.K., Fritsch, R.C., Goodrich, W., Yates, B.T. (1989). Psychosis aggression and self destructive behavior in hospitalized adolescents. *American Journal of Psychiatry, 146,* (4), 521-525.

Diagnostic and Statistical Manual of Mental Disorders (1987). Third Edition, American Psychiatric Association, Washington, D.C.

Edman, S.O., et al. (1990). Convergent and discriminant validity of FACES-III: Family adaptability and cohesion. *Family Process, 29,* 95-104.

Edwards, J. (1991). Use and administration of family therapy in residential treatment for older adolescents. *Residential Treatment for Children and Youth, 9,* 55-73.

Freud, S. (1912). The dynamics of transference. *Standard Edition, 12,* 97-108. London: Hogarth Press, 1953.

Fritsch, R.C., Goodrich, W. (1990). Adolescent inpatient attachment as treatment process. In S.C. Feinstein (Ed.), *Adolescent Psychiatry, 17,* pp. 246-263.

Fritsch, R.C., Goodrich, W., deMarneffe, C. (1992). Concurrent validity of an adolescent attachment scale. *International Annals of Adolescent Psychiatry, 2,* 298-316.

Fritsch, R.C., Heinssen, R.K., Delga, I., Goodrich, W., Yates, B.T. (1992). Predicting adolescent hospital adjustment by adolescent hospital inpatients. *Hospital and Community Psychiatry, 43,* 49-53.

Fritsch, R.C., Holmstrom, R.W., Goodrich, W., Rieger, R.E. (1990). Personality and demographic differences among different types of adjustment to an adolescent milieu. In S.C. Feinstein (Ed.), *Adol. Psychiatry, 17,* pp. 202-225.

Gable, S. and Shindledecker, R. (1992). Adolescent psychiatric inpatients: Characteristics, outcome and comparison between discharged patients from a specialized adolescent unit and nonspecialized units. *J. Youth and Adolescence, 21*, 391-407.

Ghuman, H.S., Jayaprakash, S., Saidel, D.H., Whitmarsh, G. (1989). Variables predictive of the need for placement in a long-term structured setting for adolescents. *Psychiatric Hosp., 20*, 31-34.

"Global Assessment of Functioning Scale" (1987). *Diagnostic and Statistical Manual of Mental Disorders (DSM-III-R)*. American Psychiatric Association, Washington, D.C., p.12.

Goodrich, W., & Boomer, D.S. (1958). Some concepts about therapeutic interventions with hyperaggressive children. *Social Casework, 39*, 207-213, 286-291; also in P. Fellin, (1969) (Ed.), *Exemplars of social research*, (pp.285-304). Illinois: Peacock Press.

Goodrich, W. and Fullerton, C. (1984). Which adolescent borderlines in residential treatment will run away? *Residential Group Care and Treatment, 2* (3), 3-14

Goodrich, W. and Fullerton, C. (1986). Unpublished study.

Goodrich, W. (1987). Long-term psychoanalytic hospital treatment of adolescents. *Psychiatric Clinics of North America, 10* (2), 273-287.

Gossett, J.T., Lewis, J.M., and Barnhart, F.D. (1983). *To Find a Way*. New York: Brunner/Mazel.

Inamdar, S.C., Lewis, D.D., Siomopolous, G, et al. (1982). Violent and suicidal behavior in psychotic adolescents. *Amer. J. Psychiatry, 139*, 932-935.

Kaminer, Y. (1991). The magnitude of concurrent psychiatric disorders in hospitalized substance abusing adolescents. *Child Psychiatry and Human Development, 22*, 89-96.

Lewis, J.M. (1989). *The Birth of the Family—An Empirical Inquiry*. New York: Brunner/Mazel.

Lewis, M., et al. (1980). The undoing of residential treatment: A follow-up study of 51 adolescents. *J. Amer. Acad. Child Psychiatry, 19*, 160-171.

Lewis, M. and Summerville, J.W. (1991). Residential Treatment, Chapter 78, *Child and Adolescent Psychiatry, A Comprehensive Textbook* (Ed. M. Lewis), Williams & Wilkins, 895-902.

Loranger, A.S., Sussman, V. and Oldman, J., et al. (1987). The personality disorder examination: A preliminary report. *J. Personality Disorders, 1*, 1-13.

Lefcourt, H.M. (1982). *Locus of Control: Current Trends in Theory and Research, 2nd edition*. Hillsdale, New Jersey.

Luborsky, L., et al. (1983). Two helping alliance methods for predicting outcomes of psychotherapy. *J. Nerv. Mental Disease, 171*, 480-491.

Masterson, J.F. and Costello, J.L. (1980). *From Borderline Adolescent to Functioning Adult: The Test of Time*. New York: Brunner/Mazel.

Milazzo-Sayre, L.J. (1986). Use of inpatient psychiatric services by children and youth under age 18. *Mental Health Statistical Note, 15*, Rockville, MD; U.S. Dept. Health and Human Services Publicat. No. (ADM) 86-451, April 1986.

Miller, P. and PACTE (Hospital Coalition for Psychiatric Adolescent and

Child Treatment and Education) (1988). Paper on admission profile; presented at annual meeting of National Association of Private Psychiatric Hospitals, Phoenix, AZ.

Millon, T., et al. (1989). New diagnostic efficiency statistics: Comparative sensitivity and predictive/prevalence ratio. *J. of Personality Disorders, 3,* 163-173.

Orvaschel, H. and Puig-Antich, J. (1987). Fourth Version of K-SADS-E. Western Psychiatric Institute, Pittsburgh, PA 15213.

Pfeiffer, S.I. and Strzelecki, S.C. (1990). Inpatient psychiatric treatment of children and adolescents: A review of outcome studies. *J. Amer Acad. Child Adol. Psychiatry, 29,* 847-853.

Redl, F. (1991). Crisis intervention in residential treatment: The clinical innovations of Fritz Redl (Morse, W.C., Ed.). *Residential Treatment for Children and Youth, 8,* (4).

Reich, W., Herjanic, B, et al. (1982). Development of a structured psychiatric interview for children: Agreement on diagnosis comparing child and parent interviews. *J. Abnormal Child Psychology, 10,* 325-336.

Rinsley, D.B. (1980). *Treatment of the Severely Disturbed Adolescent.* New York: Jason Aronson.

Robinson, R.M., et al. (1990). Inpatient psychiatric treatment for depressed children and adolescents: Preliminary evaluations. *Psychiatric Hospital, 21,* 107-112.

Salyer, K.N. Holmstrom, R.W. and Noshpitz, J.D. (1991). Learning disabilities as a childhood manifestation of severe psychopathology. *American Journal of Orthopsychiatry, 61,* 230-240.

Unwin, J.R. (1968). Stages in therapy of hospitalized acting out adolescents. *Canadian Psychiatric Association Journal, 13,* 115-119.

Van Hasselt, V.B., et al. (1992). Maltreatment in psychiatrically hospitalized dually diagnosed adolescent substance abusers. *J. Amer Acad. Child & Adol. Psychiatry, 31,* 868-874.

Woolston, J.L. (1989). Transactional risk model for short and intermediate term psychiatric inpatient treatment of children. *J. Amer. Acad. Child Adol. Psychiatry, 28,* 38-41.

Woolston, J.L. (1991). Psychiatric Inpatient Services for Children. Chapter 77, *Child and Adolescent Psychiatry, A Comprehensive Textbook* (Ed. M. Lewis), Williams & Wilkins, pp. 890-894.

Yates, B.T., Fullerton, C.S., Goodrich, W., Heinssen, R.K., Friedman, R.S., Butler, V.L., Hoover, S.W. (1989). Grandparent deaths and severe maternal reaction in the etiology of adolescent psychopathology. *Journal of Nervous and Mental Diseases, 177* (11), 675-680.

Chapter 19

FUNDING, THIRD-PARTY PAYERS, AND MANAGED CARE

Steven S. Sharfstein

Our health care system is in the state of crisis. Double-digit inflation, combined with many millions of Americans with no access to health insurance, are symptoms of a system in a state of collapse. Perhaps the most egregious example of our ailing health care system is the lack of opportunity for treatment for children and adolescents with mental and substance abuse disorders.

This class of disorders simultaneously combines the problem of growth of costs and allegations of profiteering with unmet need and lack of access. This chapter will review the dimensions of the costs and access problem, describe the "managed care" solution, and point to an approach that may lead us in a new direction.

COSTS OUT OF CONTROL

Many articles in the media have highlighted the high costs of questionable hospitalization of adolescents. Today, we are witnessing a strong backlash from the payers against the growth of extended hospitalization of adolescents. Nineteen percent of all discharges from psychiatric hospitals in 1986 were for children and adolescents. This increased to 22 percent in 1988 and 25 percent in 1989. During this three-year time period, the number of psychiatric beds in private hospitals increased by 40 percent, with the increase due mostly to the growth of adolescent beds in for-profit chains. Between 1984 and 1988, there was an increase of 160 hospitals, with an average yearly 13 percent growth in hospitalization and an 11 percent growth in admissions.

A recent study (Frank, Salkeaver & Sharfstein, 1991) utilizing data on 1.3 million employees and their dependents from the years 1986 and 1989 examined more closely the relation of cost increase, payer reaction, and trends in access. Although the data were not entirely reflective of the U.S. population since they focus on the self-insured, it provides information on costs and use for a large and well insured segment of the population.

Substance abuse and psychiatric treatment were covered by health insurance plans during the study period. Benefits did not change significantly between 1986 and 1988. At the beginning of 1989 however, benefits did change significantly for a portion of the population. That year, insurance benefit limits were imposed on mental health and substance abuse care. Over half of the enrolled populations had their benefits curtailed during that time period.

During 1986 and 1988, the charges for psychiatric and substance abuse treatment rose at substantially higher rates than for all health care, 20.1 percent for psychiatric and 32.4 percent for substance abuse, compared to an overall health cost increase of 13 percent. Inpatient care for both psychiatric and substance abuse problems increased more rapidly than charges for all inpatient care. Most of this increase in payments, almost three-quarters for psychiatric between 1986 and 1988, was due to an increase in utilization by children and adolescents. Days for inpatient psychiatric care for children and adolescents grew by three to five days per 100 enrollees. The growth in inpatient care to children and adolescents accounted for all the growth in the use and costs for psychiatric care.

In 1989, however, the picture changed dramatically. Limits on benefits led to sharp declines in inpatient use by children and adolescents. The introduction of such limits was the first step in major curtailments for health insurance coverage for mental disorders since the expansions of the 1970's and 1980's.

UNMET NEED AND LACK OF ACCESS

In 1982, the Children's Defense Fund estimated that three million children or five percent of all children were severely mentally ill and in need of care. Serious mental illness was defined as having a duration of over one year and known to two or more agencies. In 1986, the Office of Technology Assessment estimated that 12 percent or nearly eight million of the nation's children and adolescents under the age of 18 were in need of mental health services. In 1989, the National Academy of Sciences, Institute of Medicine estimated that 22 percent, or 14 million children and adolescents, were in need of mental health services. They further estimated that two million were in need of immediate care, but only one-quarter to one half million were actually in treatment. This extent of need exposes a deficiency in our health care system that is of critical and unethical proportion.

So, we have a twin problem of high costs for some patients, but gross underutilization in other areas of our society. One solution to address the problem of high cost that has expanded dramatically in the last five years is managed care.

MANAGED CARE

The term "managed care" denotes a wide range of review and service delivery systems designed to control costs. Third-party payers, both governmental and nongovernmental, are shifting the economic risks from themselves to the patients or providers through such approaches (Usdin, 1991).

Utilization management is defined by the Institute of Medicine as "a set of techniques used by or on behalf of purchasers of health benefits to manage health care costs by influencing patient care decision-making through case-by-case assessment of the appropriateness of care prior to its provision." The essence of this effort is to limit payment for care by a case-by-case assessment prior to the provision of that care (Tischler, 1990).

This approach includes preadmission certification before hospitalization is authorized and second opinions before expensive care is undertaken. In addition, intensive discharge planning is necessary to facilitate early discharge and minimize costly inpatient stays if the patient is admitted.

Referral to hospital or office-base practitioners often requires screening by gatekeepers for mental health care. The gatekeeper's main goal is to contain costs by finding the most economic treatment provider and treatment plan. Increasingly, managed care entities contract with professionals who work for discounted rates and abide by strong managed care controls. Patients whose health benefit providers have contracted with managed care systems have economic incentives to receive their mental health care from these providers, because if they consult providers outside the system, they must pay more through higher deductibles and co-payments.

Other forms of managed care include health maintenance organizations (HMOs) and preferred provider organizations (PPOs).

HMOs provide health care services to a group of enrollees in return for predetermined payment which is calculated on a per-head (person) or capitated basis. The payment amount is unaffected by the volume or price of services subsequently received. This prospective payment approach distinguishes HMOs from other health care delivery systems. Because enrollees pay a fixed amount to the HMO independent of their actual use of services, the HMO assumes the financial risk for providing care. Stringent utilization review is prominent in all HMOs in an effort to contain costs.

Most HMOs restrict mental health benefits to a greater extent than traditional private insurance. Such benefits typically consist of a limit of 30 inpatient days and 20 outpatient visits per year, and if it appears that care is going to be required beyond these limits, referral is made immediately to community service agencies. Thus, mental health care utilization rates in HMOs for adults as well as children and adolescents are a good deal lower than in traditional fee-for-service insurance.

PPOs are a provider response to the pressures for cost containment. In PPOs the providers join together to negotiate with payers for discounted fees in return for a guaranteed volume of patients with an agreement to abide by strong utilization review guidelines. Patients are usually not required to receive care from a preferred provider, but if they consult such a provider, their cost sharing is a good deal less than if they select an outside provider. PPOs are sponsored mostly by physician group practices as well as by independent entrepreneurs, insurance companies, and, increasingly, other nonphysician mental health professionals.

Both HMOs and PPOs have experienced significant growth in the late 1980's as Americans have searched for a variety of ways to contain their medical costs.

One form of managed care that may be of use to children and adolescents and change their opportunities is "high cost case management." High cost case management concentrates on the few individuals in any insured group who are likely to generate very high expenditures. This patient population might exhaust the insurance benefits rather rapidly, with their care then being shifted to the public sector. A case manager under the system determines whether extra assistance in planning, arranging, or coordinating a specialized treatment plan would permit less costly care that may be longer term and more appropriate. In selected instances, extra-contractual benefits may be granted to cover services not technically covered by a patient's insurance policy. This approach for severely ill children and adolescents can be quite important for those patients who need alternatives to hospital care, such as residential services, day treatment, and outpatient visits. This approach may be one way to address the current dilemma of high costs and lack of access.

Children and adolescents are particularly vulnerable to utilization management and managed care. Utilization management refers to the concept of a case-by-case allocation of resources and is often involved in outside review of care and denial of treatment based on medical necessity and appropriateness criteria. The trend to shortened length of stay is reinforced by frequent case reviews, often conducted over an 800 line with criteria that are not made explicit. Managed care, on the other hand, refers to the combination of utilization management with a select provider network. These networks are expected to deliver a full range of services and a continuum of care for children and adolescents.

In the process of utilization management, there are critical issues related to the treatment plan. The treatment plan included in the medical record should distill the many assessments and evaluations into a coherent statement of the patient's diagnosis, deficits, and assets, and then establish a series of treatment objectives. It outlines the treatment program and the specifics with regard to methods and clinicians responsible for specific segments of the treatment. Time frames should be included for reaching specific treatment objectives and discharge criteria described even within the first 24 hours of admission. As the medical record is submitted to the utilization management entity for approval, it is important that the clinician dealing with the managed care organization understand the appeals process. This process should be made clear in writing; if the clinician disagrees with the concurrent review by the utilization manager, then it is important that he make a cogent appeal.

The recently published book, *Utilization Management: A Handbook for Psychiatrists*, by the Committee on Managed Care of the American Psychiatric Association (APA, 1992) goes into great detail about the obligations and responsibilities of psychiatrists who work with outside reviewers.

It is important to fully engage the family in this process of utilization review and management. They need to be aware from the first day of hospitalization about the medical benefits and the contract to review care, and they should have a copy of the criteria the clinician possesses or request a copy of the criteria from the managed care organization. Families should be full collaborators with the clinician in helping with the treatment plan as they are obviously a critical part of the discharge plan, as well. In cases of arbitrary and capricious denial, they are almost always the most effective and articulate appealers not only to the utilization management company but also directly to their employer. It is best, however, to try to negotiate a compromise among the treating clinician, the family, and the utilization management group and arrange for extra-contractual benefits, sometimes called flex-benefits, so that additional outpatient, day treatment, and residential care become available for the child or adolescent. This is a delicate process, since a too-aggressive, antiutilization management or managed care perspective can easily lead to a "demarketing" of the provider from the network of approved treatment. On the other hand, if patients are being harmed by denials of care, clinicians as well as families should surface these issues through the appeals process as well as directly to the employer who is in charge of paying the benefits in order to secure necessary care (Quaytman & Sharfstein, 1990; Sharfstein, 1991; Hood and Sharfstein, 1992).

SYSTEM REFORM—POINTING IN THE DIRECTION OF AN IMPROVED TREATMENT SYSTEM FOR CHILDREN AND ADOLESCENTS

The current system of care largely consists of three options—hospitalization, residential treatment and outpatient care (Figure 19.1). This is so because most private insurance reimburses on the basis of hospital stays, to some extent residential care, and to a lesser extent outpatient treatment. These artificial financial barriers convert into the only available settings for treatment and care of adolescents and children, seriously disturbed children and adolescents who are either hospitalized, treated in costly extended inpatient or residential care, or inadequately handled through spotty outpatient services. Often, they are totally abandoned and neglected in the social welfare and juvenile justice systems, and in state mental health programs. Therefore, it is imperative that we conceptualize a broader array of appropriate services and reprogram resources that have been devoted to the expensive few for resources devoted to many of those in need of a much more diversified continuum of care.

An improved system for children and adolescents is indicated in Figure 19.2. This system not only includes acute short-term hospitalization, but residential treatment in group homes, specialized foster care, day treatment on a full- and half-day basis, therapeutic school and vocational placements, evening treatment, and expanded outpatient care. Innovative approaches, such as in-home crisis stabilization, are necessary so that expensive hospital stays may be avoided. The full funding of this range of treatment for children and adolescents requires the use of high-cost case management of private insurance and a collaboration of the public and private sectors through single streams of funding. The entire system needs to be refinanced in a way consonant to the needs of a majority of children with severe emotional problems.

CONCLUDING COMMENTS

Twenty years ago, I was a director of a community mental health service in a small, comprehensive, neighborhood health center in a working-class neighborhood in Boston. I worked closely with an idealistic pediatrician who had received a grant from the state government to conduct a comprehensive physical and psychological screening of the children in three elementary schools located in our neighborhood. There were almost 900 children in all, and this screening required an extensive mobilization of families, teachers, and others. From the beginning, I had misgivings about the project, since any program of case funding might lead to high expectations from the parents and teachers for care and treatment way beyond the resources of our small health program. The results of the study fulfilled my worst nightmare. It was determined from the study that 600 of the 900 children suffered from "emotional problems." When the pediatrician colleague tried to reassure me by focusing on the 50 of the 600 who were in need of immediate diagnosis and treatment for severe emotional disturbance, I indicated that at this point in the growth of the program, we were able to take only two additional referrals. This gap between expectation and reality struck me as the fundamental issue for clinicians, policymakers, concerned parents, and advocates for children and youth.

The Present Mental Health Service Is on the Horns of a Dilemma

Expanding services without cost constraints under health insurance has proven to be a costly and inefficient solution. Restricting these benefits under restricted public funding leads to the public health disasters and clinical tragedies that we are experiencing today. Managed care has many pitfalls, particularly when care is denied and no alternatives are found for a disturbed child or adolescent. Only through a more thoroughgoing financing reform, perhaps through the passage of universal health insurance, can we grope our way out of this morass.

Universal health insurance would provide a floor for all Americans to access psychiatric care, both inpatient and outpatient. In principle, the coverage should be "nondiscriminatory," especially as it relates to the cost containment provisions within such legislation. Cost sharing for physical and mental illness should be equal. Unfortunately, most plans have "inside limits" for psychiatric care—the best being the current Kennedy-Mitchell bill which provides for 45 inpatient days, a two-for-

---

HOSPITALIZATION
RESIDENTIAL TREATMENT
OUTPATIENT

Figure 19.1. Current "system" for children and adolescents

HOSPITALIZATION
RESIDENTIAL TREATMENT
    * **GROUP HOUSE**
    * **SPECIALIZED FOSTER CARE**
DAY TREATMENT
    * **FULL and HALF DAY**
    * **THERAPEUTIC SCHOOL**
    * **THERAPEUTIC VOCATIONAL PLACE-**
      MENT
EVENING TREATMENT
OUTPATIENT
IN-HOME CRISIS STABILIZATION

Figure 19.2. Improved system for children and adolescents

one split of day treatment for inpatient and 20 outpatient visits. For the "medical management" of mental disorders, however, coverages are paid for on the same basis as all conditions. Managed care would be part of whatever universal health plan that is passed, but administrative redundancy and high overhead costs would be reduced through a single-payer system.

For children and adolescents, the major issue will be coverage for those parts of the continuum of care not readily reimbursed through such a universal plan. A variety of school services, home care, and other specialized cognitive services would have to be financed through some alternative system. Social welfare services, particularly for children and adolescents who do not have families, is another critical area that must be attended to if those with psychiatric problems are going to make use of good mental health benefits.

Psychiatric care for children and adolescents has come of age. More effective diagnosis and treatment should justify better levels of funding. Accountability for the level of care is essential and managed care is a part of that accountability.

REFERENCES

American Psychiatric Association, Committee on Managed Care: *Utilization Management: A Handbook for Psychiatrists.* Washington, D.C., 1992. American Psychiatric Association

Frank, R., Salkever, D., Sharfstein, S.S. (1991). A new look at rising mental health insurance costs. *Health Affairs*, Summer, 116–123.

Hood, L., Sharfstein. S.S. (1992). Managed care for patients who are treatment resistant. *Hospital and Community Psychiatry, 43:8, 774–775.*

Quaytman, M., Sharfstein, S.S. (1990). Managed patient care. *Hospital and Community Psychiatry,* 41:12, 1296–1298.

Sharfstein, S.S. (1991). Assessing the outcome of managing costs: An exploratory approach. Psychiatric Hospitalization: *Advances in Outcome Research* 19, 311–320.

Tischler, G. (1990). Utilization management of mental health services by private third parties. *American Journal of Psychiatry, 147,* 967–973.

Usdin, G. (Ed.) (1991). Managed care: Impact on psychiatry. *Medical Information Systems, Inc., 11,*1-10.

AUTHOR INDEX

Achenbach, T., 283
Ackerman, N., 55
Adam, R., 74
Adler, J., 56
Aldershof, A., 115
Allen, C., 133
Allen, R., 108, 133
Almqvist, F., 277
Alt, H., 29
Ambrosini, P., 282
Anderson, L., 118
Anthony, E., 12, 38, 218

Bailey, H., 199
Baittle, B., 207
Baker, L., 168
Ballenger, J., 121
Barber, C., 279
Bardill, D., 57
Barker, P., 6
Barnhart, F., 204
Barr, E., 108
Baruch, S., 195
Bateson, G., 90
Beaumont, P., 169
Beglin, S., 167
Beitel, A., 57
Bender, L., 104, 193, 194
Bendtro, L., 189
Benfer, B., 77
Bergman, A., 216
Berkovitz, I., 53
Berlin, I., 203, 246
Berman, E., 194
Berman, I., 56
Bertagnoli, M., 194

Bettelheim, B., 12
Biederman, J., 109, 278, 279
Birch, N., 117
Birmaher, B., 124
Black, D., 194
Black, M., 134
Black, N., 195
Blaustein, F., 53
Blos, P., 205, 216, 217
Blotcky, M., 280, 287
Boenheim, C., 55
Bolding, D., 75
Boomer, D., 285
Borchardt, C., 194
Borison, R., 122
Bowen, M., 93, 96
Bowers, M., 119, 120
Boyer, J., 135
Bradley, W., 104
Brindad, E., 74
Brooks, A., 71, 72
Brown, G., 106
Brown, S., 181
Burton, B., 120
Button, E., 166
Buxbaum, E., 52

Campbell, J., 194
Campbell, M., 110, 115, 116, 118
Canino, I., 115
Cantwell, D., 107
Capozzoli, J., 115, 190
Carlsen, P., 133
Carlson, G., 107
Caroff, S., 119
Carr, V., 194

Casey, N., 76
Casper, R., 166, 169
Cates, J., 277
Clardy, E., 193, 194
Clark, P., 133
Clement, P., 166
Clinton, J., 120
Cockcroft, D., 115
Cohen, D., 122
Cohen, I., 115
Cole, J., 113
Collins, N., 76, 85, 87
Connors, M., 166
Cooper, P., 167
Cornsweet, C., 280
Costello, A., 110
Costello, J., 283
Cotton, N., 189, 190
Coyle, J., 104–125, 115, 190
Crimson, M., 123
Crisp, A., 166, 168
Critchley, D., 203
Cromwell, F., 134
Curry, J., 280

Dalton, R., 75
Dare, C., 168
Daruna, J., 75
Dauphin, M., 194
Davis, D., 169
Davis, J., 166
Davis, R., 119
Davison, K., 194
Delga, I., 279, 283
Delong, G., 115
deMarneffe, C., 287
Deniger, M., 213
Dermer, S., 121
Deutsch, S., 110
deZwann, M., 167
Dimpero, R., 72
Donlon, P., 120
Dooher, L., 117
Dostal, T., 115
Dowling, J., 117

Dubin, W., 120
Dulit, E., 206
Duncombe, L., 135

Ebert, M., 167
Eckert, E., 166, 167, 169
Edelbrock, R., 283
Edwards, J., 277
Eisler, I., 168
Elkind, D., 206, 214, 216
Ellis, M., 53
Ellsworth, R., 76
Erikson, E., 205, 216, 220
Erlich, H., 213
Errera, P., 38

Fahl, M., 135
Fairburn, C., 167
Faretra, G., 117, 118
Fava, M., 113
Feguine, R., 112
Feld, J., 120
Fichter, M., 167
Fidler, G., 135
Flavell, J., 206, 216
Folkart, L., 13
Forbes, O., 117
Frank, R., 294
Freidman, J., 119
Freud, A., 167, 203
Freud, S., 285
Fritsch, R., 279, 283, 287
Frosch, W., 256
Fullerton, C., 282, 287

Gabbard, G., 28, 32
Gable, S., 280
Gair, D., 189
Gallineck, A., 194
Gardner, D., 123
Garfinkel, P., 167, 168
Garner, D., 167, 171
Garrison, W., 189
Gault, M., 115
Gazda, G., 132

Geller, B., 112
Geraty, R., 6
Ghuman, H., 3–15, 18–33, 52–68, 189–200, 224–236, 241–253, 279
Gillis, A., 194
Gittelman-Klein, D., 111
Glaun, D., 169
Glod, C., 113
Goldberg, H., 123
Goldberg, S., 166, 169
Goldbloom, D., 167
Goodrich, W., 277–289, 282, 283, 285, 287
Gorman, J., 124
Gossett, J., 204, 280, 283, 287
Gralnick, A., 226
Grant, E., 132–147
Green, W., 110, 116
Greenberg, L., 107, 110
Greenhill, L., 107, 108, 109, 115
Greenstone, J., 53
Grold, L., 53
Gross, J., 168
Gualtieri, C., 110, 118
Gunderson, J., 12, 76, 227, 228
Gunn, S., 141, 144
Gutheil, T., 189

Halikis, J., 182
Halmi, A., 169
Halmi, K., 166
Halpin, R., 214
Hamill, P., 108
Hamilton, M., 112
Hanton, R., 74
Hardison, J., 135
Harper, G., 6, 13
Harrison, P., 181
Hartman, A., 93
Hartman, H., 205
Hassanyeh, F., 194
Hatsukami, D., 167
Hawkins, R., 166
Heuyer, G., 194
Hickey, R., 76

Hift, E., 194
Hift, S., 194
Hill, J., 110
Hodes, M., 168
Hoffman, N., 181
Hogarth, C., 73, 75, 81, 87
Hollis, F., 93
Holmes, D., 38, 42
Holmstrom, R., 279
Hood, L., 298
Hopkin, J., 120
Hopkins, L., 90–103
Hsu, G., 166, 167, 168
Hudson, J., 168
Hunt, R., 122
Hyer, L., 76

Inamdhar, S., 279
Inge, G., 226
Inhelder, B., 206, 216

Jaffe, S., 107, 181–188
Jaskulski, J., 132–147
Jefferson, J., 115, 116, 117
Johnson, C., 166, 168
Jonas, J., 168
Jones, J., 72
Joshi, P., 104–125, 189–200
Josselson, R., 205, 216

Kafantaris, V., 121
Kalucy, R., 166
Kaminer, Y., 278
Kanner, A., 111
Kashani, J., 112
Kassoff, A., 56
Kastenholz, K., 123
Katma, A., 85
Kearny, G., 132–147
Keating, D., 216
Keck, P., 119
Keilhofner, G., 133
Keller, M., 112
Kernberg, O., 227, 228
Kester, B., 6

Kilgalen, R., 195
King, J., 29
King, R., 114
Klein, D., 111
Klein, R., 108
Klerman, J., 193
Koplewica, H., 111
Kottman, T., 213
Kramer, A., 112
Kranzler, H., 123
Kremer, E., 135
Kuperman, S., 124
Kupietz, S., 108
Kutcher, S., 123

Laessle, R., 167
Laird, J., 93
Lansing, S., 133
Law, W., 112
Lebovici, S., 194
Leckman, J., 122
Lena, B., 115
Levine, I., 38
Lewis, J., 5, 78, 204, 221, 232, 283
Lewis, M., 277, 282
Liebowitz, M., 112
Lipton, E., 199
Llorens, L., 132, 135
Looney, J., 218
Loranger, A., 282
Luborsky, L., 285
Lucas, A., 111
Lunde, D., 92
Lupafkin, W., 112
Lynch, M., 13

McElroy, S., 119
McHale, P., 121
McKeith, I., 122
MacKenzie, S., 123
Mahler, M., 216
Main, F., 13
Mandelbaum, A., 21
Mansheim, P., 194
Marcos, L., 256

Marcus, D., 205
Masterson, J., 283
Matsutsuyu, J., 134
Mattson, M., 189
Meyer, A., 132
Mikkelsen, E., 110, 115
Milazzo-Sayre, L., 277
Miller, D., 205
Miller, P., 277
Millon, T., 282
Millstein, K., 190
Minderaa, R., 122
Minuchin, S., 93, 168
Mitchell, J., 167
Moore, D., 261–276
Mordock, J., 53
Mosey, A., 132, 135
Mumford, M., 132
Munich, R., 244, 245, 247
Mutani, R., 119

Nakhla, F., 13
Nasar, S., 189
Neimark, E., 216
Nelson, D., 135
New, P., 74
Newton, R., 123
Nicol, A., 122
Noshpitz, J., 12, 211, 279
Nurcombe, B., 13, 74
Nylander, I., 168

Offer, D., 205, 207
Offer, J., 205
Olds, J., 213
Olmstead, M., 171
O'Malley, F., 38, 42
O'Morrow, G., 141
Orvaschel, H., 282
Oursted, C., 13

Palmer, R., 166
Pasley, F., 111
Paul, S., 123
Pearson, G., 72

Pentz, T., 203–222
Peplau, H., 75
Perel, J., 112
Perry, R., 116
Peterson, C., 141, 144
Petti, T., 6, 22, 112
Pfeiffer, S., 280, 283, 287
Phillips, P., 189
Piaget, J., 206, 216
Pine, F., 216
Pinel, P., 189
Pirke, K., 167
Plutchik, R., 189
Polivy, J., 171
Pool, D., 118
Pope, H., 119, 168
Popper, C., 120
Post, R., 121
Potter, H., 6, 121
Potter, W., 122
Powles, W., 54
Preskorn, S., 111
Puig-Antich, J., 109, 111, 112, 282
Pyle, R., 167

Quaytman, M., 298

Rabiner, C., 111
Rabinovich, H., 109
Rapoport, J., 110, 115
Rauss-Mason, C., 168
Realmuto, G., 118
Redl, F., 189, 211, 212, 285
Reich, W., 282
Reid, J., 112
Reidl, F., 12
Reilly, M., 132
Remschmidt, H., 121
Resnick, M., 120
Riblet, L., 123
Richard, M., 199
Rinsley, D., 5, 12, 42, 53, 203, 204, 226, 285
Robinson, R., 282, 283
Rogeness, G., 124

Rolfe, R., 76
Rose, R., 193
Rosen, A., 168
Rosenbaum, J., 113
Rosenberg, G., 214
Rosman, B., 168
Ross, D., 196, 199
Rossman, P., 203
Roth, D., 165–178
Roth, V., 132–147
Rubenfeld, S., 56
Rubin, E., 132
Rubin, R., 78
Rudorfer, M., 122
Rumpf, E., 193, 194
Ryan, N., 109, 112

Sacks, M., 189
Safer, D., 108
Saidel, D., 37–51
Salkeaver, D., 294
Salyer, K., 279
Saraf, K., 109
Sarles, R., 3–15, 64, 224–236, 254–260
Sarnoff, C., 213
Schiffer, M., 213
Schroder, P., 77
Schroeder, J., 109
Schulman, I., 55
Sechi, G., 119, 120
Seidel, R., 168
Serrano, A., 117
Shaffer, D., 110
Sharfstein, S., 293–301
Sheinin, J., 167
Shekim, W., 112
Shellow, R., 56
Shindledecker, R., 280
Sillanpaa, M., 122
Silver, L., 6, 9
Silver, M., 256
Simeon, J., 114
Singer, H., 118
Singh, H., 196, 199
Skolnick, P., 123

Slavson, S., 56
Small, A., 115, 118
Smith, B., 56
Soloff, P., 189
Specker, S., 167
Spiel,W., 194
Steinberg, D., 13
Steinhausen, H., 168
Steinschneider, A., 199
Stephans, J., 110
Stewart, M., 124, 194
Stone, M., 227, 228
Strober, M., 115, 167
Strother, J., 213
Strzelecki, S., 280, 283
Sugar, M., 53, 55
Summerville, J., 277
Sverd, J., 108
Swift, W., 167
Sylvester, E., 12
Szmuckler, G., 166

Taghizadeh, F., 165–178
Talbott, J., 256
Tanda, F., 119
Taylor, D., 123
Teicher, M., 113
Thorpe, J., 56
Tischler, G., 295
Tollefson, G., 119
Touyz, S., 169
Towle, C., 93
Treischman, A., 189
Tunks, E., 121
Tupin, J., 120
Turner, S., 189

Unwin, J., 283
Usdin, G., 295

Van Hasselt, V., 283
Vitiello, B., 115, 120
Wagner, R., 119

Waizer, J., 118
Walkup, J., 104–125
Waltos, D., 71–88
Ward, J., 56
Wardle, C., 6
Warneke, L., 194
Webster, J., 13
Weinberg, W., 111
Weiner, I., 207, 214
Weiner, J., 107
Weintrob, A., 6
Weiss, S., 167
Weissman, B., 123
Westman, J., 54
Whitehouse, A., 166
Whittaker, J., 189
Wilcox, J., 194
Williams, A., 122
Williams, D., 124
Williams, E., 165–178
Wilmoth, E., 52–68, 189–200, 241–253
Wilson, P., 37, 39
Wineman, D., 189
Winnicott, D., 12
Winsberg, B., 108
Wittchen, H., 167
Wolff, H., 53
Wolpert, E., 194
Wonderlich, S., 167
Woods, J., 75
Woods, M., 93
Woolston, J., 277, 283

Yager, J., 167
Yalom, I., 56
Yates, B., 283
Yatham, L., 121
Youngerman, J., 115
Yudofsky, S., 124

Zeitlin, S., 190
Zvosky, P., 115

SUBJECT INDEX

Abuse: alcohol, 4, 8, 24, 181–188, 277; child, 100, 265; dietary, 165; diuretic, 166; drug, 4, 8, 14, 24, 29, 78, 80, 94, 109, 113, 167, 181–188, 217, 277, 278, 279, 294; emotional, 186, 267; laxative, 166; and neglect, 100, 186, 265, 266–271; physical, 186, 190, 267, 270, 283; reporting, 100, 266–271; sexual, 4, 171, 186, 267, 270

Acting out, 22, 46–47, 52, 207, 217, 224–236, 277; as defense, 62; discharge related, 30; in therapy sessions, 57

Activities: adaptations to, 133–134; cognitive, 81; competing, 158–159; in early adolescence, 212–214; motor, 135; multiple, 77; occupational, 52; outpatient, 29; physical, 81, 143, 213; prevocational, 133; purposeful, 132–133; risk-taking, 8; social, 81

Activities of daily living, 23, 77–78, 133, 136

Admission: and diagnosis; diagnostic conference, 24–25; and discharge planning, 74; emergency, 74; involuntary, 20–21, 263–266; process, 20–22; rates, xiii, 4; voluntary, 101, 263–266

Adolescence: as developmental stage, 205; early, 208–214; implications for treatment, 207–215; middle, 215–221; physical changes, 206; substages, 205–221

Adult Children of Alcoholics, 94, 185

Aggression, 4, 80, 113, 117, 118, 120, 121, 279; controlling, 12; management of, 78, 115, 121; and medication, 105; passive, 59

Agoraphobia, 111

Agranulocytosis, 122

Akathesia, 118

Alanon, 94, 185

Alateen, 94

Alcohol abuse, 4, 8, 24, 181–188, 277

Alcoholics Anonymous, 94, 183, 184, 187

Ambivalence, 61–66

Amenorrhea, 166

Amoxapine, 109

Amphetamines, 106

Anafranil, 114–115

Anger, 49; as defense, 62; expressing, 39; management of, 81, 143, 213

Anorexia nervosa. See Eating disorders

Anticonvulsants, 105, 113, 121–122; side effects, 121

Antidepressants, 105, 122–123, 175–176; clomipramine, 114–115; dosage, 110, 111; fluoxetine, 113–114; heterocyclic, 109; indications, 110–112; monoamine oxidase inhibitors, 112–113; serotonin selective re-uptake inhibitors, 113; side effects, 109–110, 113, 115; tricyclic, 109–112

Anxiety, 8, 30, 105, 167, 183, 204, 208, 278, 285; conflictual, 72; discharging, 46–47; interpersonal, 168; necessity for treatment, 46, 225; separation, 111; and therapy, 60

Approaches: behavioral, 11; eclectic, 10–11; family-oriented, 13; intermediate, 10, 54; long-term, 10, 28, 54; medical, 11; problem-oriented, 9, 13–14; psychodynamic, 12–13; short-term, 10, 54; time-oriented, 9, 10; treatment-oriented, 9, 10–11

Art therapy, 136, 137–141

Asendin, 109

Assertiveness training, 136

Assessment. See Evaluation

Authority, 72, 137, 226–227, 241; institutional, 56; opposition to, 49; parental, 95

Autism, 115, 118

Autonomy, 175, 205, 216, 218; age-appropriate, 74

Aventyl, 109

Behavior: adaptive, 82; aggressive, 4, 12, 120, 124, 279; alternative, 75, 82; appetite, 166; assaultive, 190, 191, 277; causes of, 60; contracts, 57; dangerous, 6–7, 18, 25, 38; destructive, 52, 53, 190; disorders, 104; disorganized, 7; disruptive, 285; expectations for, 47, 78; group control of, 59–60; high-risk, 183; impulsive, 7; indications for treatment, 6–8; intensification of, 68; maladaptive, 204, 284; modification, 11, 82–85, 92, 135; normal age-related, 226; norms for managing, 75; obsessive/compulsive, 7; oppositional, 190; presenting, 8; rationalizations for, 44; responsibility for, 229, 232; school, 23; self-assessment of, 82; self-destructive, 114, 200, 217, 277, 279; self-injurious, 191, 193, 195–200; self-mutilating, 115, 199; sexual, 7, 171; social, 135; socially responsible, 78; stereotypic, 118; theories, 92

Benzedrine, 104, 106

Boundaries, 95, 227; maintaining, 68, 73

Brain: damage, 23, 104; injury, 14

Bulimia nervosa. See Eating disorders

Bupropion, 122–123

Butyrophenone, 120

Carbamazepine, 121

Case management, 90, 92, 101; high-cost, 296

Catapress, 122

Chlorpromazine, 117

Chlorprothixene, 117

Chronicity, 15, 280

Cognition: deficits in, 23, 29; evaluation of, 22–23; limited, 206, 208, 215; skill development, 75

Communication: action, 209; book, 249; with family, 92; improving, 25; interpersonal, 220; nonverbal, 55, 213; in psychotherapy, 37, 39; between shifts, 157; skills, 81; treatment team, 249–250; understanding, 50; verbal, 209, 218

Community meetings, 66–68

Co-morbidity, 109

Confidentiality, 57–58, 66, 78, 80, 100, 228–229, 265, 266

Conflict, 284; dependency, 210, 217; identity, 73; internal, 39, 43, 50, 208; interpersonal, 56; oedipal, 55; resolution, 66, 215; unconscious, 39

Confrontation, 47, 53, 63, 183

Consent: for ECT, 194–195; informed, 109, 118, 262, 265, 271–273; for medication, 106

Contracts: behavioral, 11, 57, 83; family, 28; treatment, 227

Coping mechanisms, 74, 75, 175, 190, 216

Cost-containment, 4, 5, 10, 293–294

Countertransference, 39, 49–51, 72–73, 210, 234

Cylert, 106

Decalage, 216

Defenses, 22, 23, 43, 61–66, 183, 208, 216, 228, 284; acting out as, 62; anger as, 62; intellectualization as, 62; strengthening of, 208

Delirium, 119

Delusions, 106

Denial, 22, 50, 208, 226

Depression, 4, 18, 105, 111, 112, 121, 123, 167, 176, 193, 194, 204, 207, 217, 285; intensity of, 23; psychotic, 106; refractory, 113

Desipramine, 109, 110, 111

Desyrel, 109

Development: adolescent, 92, 205; cognitive, 11, 206, 208; deficits in, 32, 203–204; disorder(s), 105, 117, 118; ego, 38, 205; gross motor, 143; of identity, 220; normal, 72, 82; psychosexual, 23; psychosocial, 11; superego, 39; theories, 92; and treatment, 203–222

Dexedrine, 106

Diagnosis: and inpatient admission, 8–9; multiple, 278; procedures, 22–25

Diagnosis Related Grouping, 4, 5

Diaphoresis, 119

Discharge, 13, 28–31; early, 295; family reaction to, 29–31; patient reaction to, 29–31; planning, 74, 81, 92, 101–103, 176, 295; unplanned, 30–31

Disinhibition, 114

Disorder(s): adjustment, 226, 278; affective, 115, 119, 171; anxiety, 105, 123, 167, 278; attention deficit, 91, 105, 106, 107, 109, 110, 111, 117, 279; behavior, 104; bipolar, 115, 117, 121; conduct, 12, 225, 278, 279, 280; development, 105, 117, 118; dysthymic, 167; eating, 14, 24, 165–178; genetic effect, 92; identity, 12, 226; manic-depressive, 4; mood, 115, 193, 278, 279; obsessive-compulsive, 7, 24, 105, 113, 114, 115, 176; oppositional, 12, 225; pan-

ic, 111; personality, 12, 225, 233, 278, 279, 280; seizure, 24; separation anxiety, 111

Documentation, 144; of informed consent, 272–273; in litigation, 275; medico-legal, 13; necessity for treatment, 3; regulatory, 13

Dosage: antidepressants, 110, 111; lithium, 116; neuroleptics, 117–118; stimulants, 108, 109

DRG. See Diagnosis Related Grouping

Droperidol, 117, 120, 121, 192

Drug abuse, 4, 8, 14, 24, 29, 78, 80, 94, 109, 113, 167, 181–188, 217, 277, 278, 279, 294

Drug holidays, 108

DSM-III, 4, 11, 94, 166, 282, 283

Due process, 264

Dysarthria, 121

Dysphoria, 109, 207, 217

Eating disorders, 14, 24; clinical features, 166–167; co-morbidity factors, 167, 169; mortality rate, 167; physical complications, 167; prevalence rate, 167; treatment program, 169–178

Education, xiv, 81; accessing services, 99–100; departmentalized classrooms, 152; evaluation, 23–24; funding, 157, 160–162; home instruction, 152–153; leisure, 143; mainstreaming, 153–154, 156; models, 151–154; nutrition, 85; planning, 145; postdischarge, 99–102, 156–157; programs, 154–157; self-contained classrooms, 151–152; services, 85; sex, 85, 215, 221; special, 23, 99–100, 149–162; support services, 156

Education of the Handicapped Act of 1975, 99, 101, 160

Ego: building, 208; deficits, 212; development, 38; function, 39; observation, 218; skills, 205, 216; strength, 208, 215; tasks, 205; weak, 204

Electroconvulsive therapy, 25, 193–195

Empathy, 207, 215, 216, 220

Enuresis, 110, 115, 116

Environment: consistency in, 157; growth-promoting, 12; home, 91; least restrictive, 5; modification, 94–98; overstimulus of, 190; pathogenic, xiv; safe, 12, 75; social, 90; supportive, 12–13

Evaluation: cognition, 22–23; daily functioning, 23; emotional status, 22–23; of family, 23; neurological, 21, 24; nursing, 73–75; outpatient, 146; physical, 21, 24–25; process, 18–25; program, 77; psychiatric, 8–9; psychoeducational, 134; psychological, 22–23; recreational, 143; self, 74, 143; streamlining, 74; task-oriented, 134; of treatment, 284–288; vocational, 144

Exhibitionism, 7

Externalization, 22, 43, 208

Family: acting out parents, 233–236; communication with, 92, 94; consent for treatment, 272; disclosure of abuse, 269; dysfunctional, xiv, 92, 168, 219; evaluation of, 23, 94, 95; functioning, 280, 283; history, 21; involvement in treatment, 28, 280; and limit setting, 234; as pathological agent, 13; pathology, 185, 283; reaction to discharge, 29–31; response to admission, 21, 94; therapy, 12, 90, 92, 95, 175, 185, 234; use of behavior modification, 92

Fluphenazine, 117, 118

Fluvoxamine, 114

Foster care, 100; therapeutic, 101

Funding, 293–301; cost-containment, 4, 5, 10; Diagnosis Related Grouping, 4; educational, 150, 157, 160–162; federal, xiii; insurance, 15, 20, 33, 171, 294; for post-discharge services, 101; state, xiii, 15, 102; third-party, xiii, 4, 19, 295

Goals: behavioral, 75; daily, 75; long-term, 75, 144; setting, 13, 73, 81; short-term, 75, 144, 212

Group homes, 28; therapeutic, 101

Guilt, 22, 25, 31, 49

Hallucinations, 106

Haloperidol, 117, 118, 120

Health Maintenance Organizations, 5, 295–296

Health services, 100–101

Hepatotoxicity, 108

History: developmental, 73; family, 21; sexual, 73

HMOs. See Health Maintenance Organizations

Homicide, 181

Hospitals: admission rates, xiii, 4; competition among, 5; for-profit, 4–5, 15; not-for-profit, 15; "profiteering," 5; public, 15, 279

Hydrotherapy, 12, 25, 195–200; indications, 196–197

Hyperactivity, 91, 106, 110, 114, 115, 117, 118; rebound, 110

Hyperthermia, 119, 120

Hypothyroidism, 116

Identity, 215; conflict, 73; consolidation of, 205; development, 220; disorders, 12, 226; gender, 221; loss of, 28; self, 135; sense of, 216, 220; sexual, 205

Imipramine, 109, 110

Impulsivity, 7, 121, 204, 211, 212, 234

Inapsine, 120

Independent Practitioners Associations, 5

Indications: absolute, 8, 53; antidepressants, 110–112; hydrotherapy, 196–197; for inpatient treatment, 3–15; relative, 8, 53

Individual Education Plans, 151, 159

Individuals with Disabilities Education Act of 1990, 149

Information release, 20

Insurance, 3–4, 15, 20, 33, 101, 171,

294, 299, 300. See also Funding

Interaction: nonverbal, 27; peer, 80, 183; social, 143, 220; staff, 183; staff-patient, 27, 212; systems of, 75; verbal, 27

Internalization, 219

Intervention: acute, 38; behavioral, 11, 25, 156; pharmacological, 18; preventative, 74; proactive, 74; psychotherapeutic, 25–28; verbal, 212

IPAs. See Independent Practitioners Associations

Isolation, 11

Juvenile services, 100, 224

Learning disability, 24, 279

Legal issues, 261–276; admissions, 263–266; confidentiality, 265, 266; due process, 264; litigation, 265, 273, 274, 275; malpractice, 273–276; rights, 261–262, 264

Legal system, 224, 277

Length of stay, 5, 32, 54, 74, 95, 102, 157, 297; managed care denials of, 30

Leucopenia, 122

Leveling, 42, 45

Limits: and priorities, 229–232; setting, 12, 25, 46, 56, 63, 67, 73, 190, 210, 214, 220, 224–236; testing, 53, 78

Lithium, 105, 113, 115–117; side effects, 116

Lithobid, 115, 116

Litigation, 265, 273, 274, 275

Loxapine, 117

Magnesium pemoline, 106, 107

Managed care, 5, 10, 18, 30, 101, 295–298, 299, 300

Meaning, 50–51

Medicare, 4

Medication, 30–31. See also Pharmacotherapy; lowering reliance on, 87

Mental retardation, 109, 117

Methylphenidate, 106, 107

Milieu, program: containment in, 76; functions, 12–13, 76; multiple activities in, 78; order and organization, 77–78; stability of staff assignments in, 85–87; structured elements, 76–87; structure of, 76; support in, 76; unstructured elements, 75–76

Naranon, 94, 185

Narcissism, xiv, 233; attention-seeking in, 59; paranoid, 59

Narcotics Anonymous, 94, 183, 184

Nardil, 112

Neuroleptic malignant syndrome, 119–120

Neuroleptics, 117–121; butyrophenones, 117; dosage, 117–118; phenothiazine, 104, 117; side effects, 118, 120, 121; thioxanthenes, 117

Neuroleptization, rapid, 120–121

Nihilism, 50

Norpramine, 109

Nortriptyline, 109

Nursing services, 71–88; responsibilities for safety, 40

Nurturing, 73

Occupational therapy: activity analysis and adaptation, 133; assessment, 134–135; interdisciplinary interaction, 136–137; programming, 135–136; purposeful activity in, 132–133

Organicity, 23, 24, 280

Pamelor, 109

Parents. See Family

Parnate, 112

Passive aggression, 59

Peer(s), 206; acceptance, 135, 168, 221; accountability, 232; influence of, 52, 232; interaction, 80, 183; pressure, 64, 78; relationships, 12, 118, 214, 215

Perseveration, 105

Personality: borderline, 14, 171, 279; changes, 12; disorders, 12, 225, 233, 278, 279, 280; maladaptive, 168;

multiple, 14, 24; organization, 50; testing, 146

Pharmacotherapy, 25, 104–125; anticonvulsants, 121–122; antidepressants, 109–115, 175–176; beta blockers, 124; bupropion, 122–123; buspirone, 123; clonidine, 122; clozaril, 123–124; contraindications, 105; indications, 105; neuroleptics, 117–121; noncompliance, 116; stimulants, 106–109; toxicity in, 116, 122, 123

Phenelzine, 112

Phenothiazines, 117

Phobias, 172

Placement: alternative, 28; post-discharge, 31

Planning: discharge, 176, 295; education, 145

Polyuria, 116

PPOs. See Preferred Providers Organizations

Preadmission, 19–20

Preferred Provider Organizations, 5, 295–296

Privacy, 41, 78, 80

Privileges, 78

Problem-solving, 66, 81, 135, 211, 212, 214, 215, 220

Projection, 22, 27, 137, 210

Prolixin, 118

Promiscuity, 7, 217

Propanalol, 124

Prostitution, 7

Protective services, 100

Prozac, 113

Psychotherapy: acting out phase, 64; co-ed, 55; contraindications, 52–54; in early adolescence, 208–211; exclusion from, 53; gender factors, 55; goals, 54; group, 25, 52–68, 214–215; group rules and limits, 56–57; group sizes, 56; indications, 52–54; individual, 25, 37–51, 92, 174; location of groups, 56–57; in middle adoles-

cence, 217–219; overactivity in, 58–59; patient age as factor, 55; patient reluctance to participate, 57–58; resolution phase, 64; silence factor, 58–59, 208; structural issues, 40–42; treatment-alliance phase, 26–27; trust in, 57–58; working through phase, 27–28, 64

Psychotropics, 105

Public Law 94–142, 99, 101, 160

Public Law 101–476, 152

Quiet rooms, 11, 190, 191, 192, 193

Rationalization, 44, 226

Reality: adaptation to, 45; clarification, 208; as defense, 44; distorted, 45; in treatment, 44–45; vs. feelings, 59–61

Recreation, 52, 136. See also Therapeutic recreation

Referrals, 91

Regression, 28, 30, 73, 213

Reinforcement, 75, 83

Relapse, 28

Relationship(s): age-appropriate, 37, 45; avoidance of, 32; cause-and-effect, 193; development of, 12, 29–30; family, 13; interpersonal, 53, 175; mentor, 258; object, 23, 37, 39, 45, 47, 49, 92, 204, 212, 214; peer, 118, 214, 215; staff-patient, 72, 250–250; staff-staff, 250–250; therapeutic, 27, 71; therapist-patient, 37–51; unstable, 204

Repression, 208

Research issues, 277–289; methodology, 281–284; treatment outcomes, 279–281

Residential care, 28, 31, 101

Resistance, 12, 15, 42–44, 61–66, 145, 146, 217, 284, 285; mechanism, 42; sources of, 42

Restraint, 12, 25, 53, 189; chemical, 106; dietary, 166; physical, 120, 121, 192

Restrictions, 46

Rhabdomyolysis, 119, 120

Rights: to education, 99, 101–102; individual, 261, 264; of minors, 261–262; patients', 20, 262, 271; to privacy, 41; to withhold, 44

Ritalin, 106, 109

Role: models, 219, 220, 247, 249; play, 136, 213, 215

Runaways, 4, 7, 8, 30, 277, 287

Schizophrenia, 105, 106, 119, 123, 124, 193, 194

Seclusion, 12, 25, 189–193

Self: assessment, 74; awareness, 212; control, 190, 220; development of, 23; esteem, 143, 168, 175, 212, 213, 215; expression, 143; identity, 135; maintenance, 133, 134, 143; mutilation, 105, 115; observation, 207; regulation, 205; revelation, 53; seclusion, 190

Separation, 21, 30, 31, 42, 205, 216, 219, 285

Separation/individuation, 137, 167, 175, 215

Sertraline, 114

Setting: problem-oriented, 9, 13–14; therapy, 54–57; time-oriented, 9, 10; treatment-oriented, 9, 10–11; types, 3–15

Side effects: anticonvulsants, 121; antidepressants, 109–110, 113, 115; lithium, 116; neuroleptics, 118, 120, 121; stimulants, 107, 108

Skills: adaptive, 134; affect management, 168, 212, 213, 215; assertiveness, 136; building, 75, 81; cognitive, 75, 134, 206; communication, 81; coping, 175; daily living. See Activities of daily living; deficits in, 168, 171; ego, 204, 205, 213, 216; emotional, 134; independent living, 220; interactional, 75; job-seeking, 145; leisure, 171; maintenance of, 133; motor, 134; perceptual, 134; prevocational, 145; psychological, 75;

readiness, 134; social, 75, 134, 135, 143, 204, 212, 214; thinking, 206; verbal, 11

Social: activities, 81; behavior, 135; environment, 90; functioning, 74; interaction, 143, 220; skills, 75, 134, 135, 143, 204, 212, 214; withdrawal, 118

Socialization, 133, 136

Social Security, 4

Social work services, 90–103; in admission process, 21; practice, 94–98

Speech therapy, 136, 156

Splitting, 228

Staff: interaction, 183; morale, 87; nursing, 40; patient complaints about, 45; to patient ratio, 87; training, 14, 81, 211; turnover, 233

Stimulants, 106–109; and appetite suppression, 107, 109; side effects, 107

Stress management, 136, 143, 220

Sublimation, 204, 213

Suicide, 4, 7, 23, 113, 169, 181, 191, 193, 279

Superego: deficits in, 32, 234; development, 39; formation, 228

Tardive dyskinesia, 117, 118

Tegretol, 121

Testing: achievement, 146; Adolescent Role Assessment, 134; aptitude, 145, 146; Bender Gestalt, 23; Benton Revised Visual Retention Test, 23; Connors' Teacher Rating Scale, 107; Eating Disorders Inventory, 171; educational, 154; Global Assessment Scale, 282, 287, 289; Hamilton Anxiety Scale, 123; interest, 146; Luria-Nebraska Neuropsychological Test, 23; Nurses' Behavioral Rating Scale, 283; personality, 146; Rorschach, 23; TAT, 23; vocational, 146–147; WAIS, 23; Wide Range Achievement Test, 23; WISC, 23; Woodcock Johnson Psychoeducation Battery, 23

Therapeutic recreation, 141–144
Therapy, 81; activity-based, 25, 135, 212, 213, 219, 220; art, 136, 137–141; cognitive, 219; directive approach, 208; electroconvulsive, 25, 193–195; expressive, 137; family, 12, 25, 90, 92, 95, 175, 185, 234; group, 12, 25; individual, 12, 25, 174; insight-oriented, 208, 217–218, 219; intermediate, 54; long-term, 54; occupational, 132–137; outpatient, 100, 101, 280; play, 209, 213; psychoanalytically oriented, 12; recreation, 136, 141–144; settings, 54–57; short-term, 54; speech, 136, 156; structure, 54–57
Thinking: abstract, 206–207, 215, 216; concrete, 207; disorganized, 7; formal operational, 206–207, 216, 217, 218; skills, 206
Thioridazine, 117
Thiothixene, 117
Thrombocytopenia, 122
Time-out, 78, 193
Tofranil, 109
Tourette's syndrome, 105, 117, 118
Training: administrative, 258–259; assertiveness, 136; on-the-job, 258–259; psychiatric, 257; staff, 14, 81, 211
Transference, 37, 44, 47–49, 72, 210, 214, 218
Tranylcypromine, 112

Trazadone, 109
Treatment, 25–33; biopsychosocial, 105; consent for, 272; developmental, 203–222; eating disorder, 169–178; economic factors, 32–33; evaluation of, 284–288; failure, 22; groups, 135–136; implications for middle adolescence, 217–221; indications for, 3–15; lack of access to, 294–295; limit setting in, 224–236; milieu, 211–212, 219–221; multidisciplinary, 73; outpatient, 28, 29, 38; program administration, 254–260; reality in, 44–45; refusal of, 272; termination of, 22; and unplanned discharges, 30
Treatment plans, 75, 77
Treatment team, 19, 95; communication on, 249–250; defenses, 247–249; demoralization on, 32; leadership, 243–245; member roles, 241–243; therapist's role on, 38
Trifluoperazine, 117
Trust, 61, 204; development of, 26–27, 40; in therapy, 57–58
Twelve Step Programs, 94, 181–188
Utilization review, 33, 295, 296, 297

Vocational services, 144–147

Withdrawal, 7; dyskinesia, 118